We're Not Sick, We're Being Sold

How Industry Hijacked Our Plates, Rewrote Nutrition, and Made Us Sicker in the Name of Health

David Lawton Etheridge

Side B Publishing

Copyright © 2025 by David Lawton Etheridge

All rights reserved.

No portion of this book may be reproduced in any form without written permission from the publisher or author, except as permitted by U.S. copyright law.

Disclaimer

The information contained in this book is for educational and informational purposes only. It is not intended as medical advice and should not be used to diagnose, treat, cure, or prevent any disease or health condition.

The author is not a licensed healthcare provider. The content presented represents the author's research, analysis, and personal experience, not professional medical guidance. Individual health needs vary, and what works for one person may not work for another.

Before making any changes to your diet, exercise routine, medications, or medical treatments, consult with qualified healthcare professionals. Never stop taking prescribed medications or ignore medical advice based on information in this book.

The author and publisher disclaim any liability for adverse effects or consequences resulting from the use of the information contained herein. Readers assume full responsibility for their health decisions.

If you are experiencing a medical emergency, seek immediate professional medical care.

For Misty

Who listened with endless patience as I ranted about cholesterol myths and seed oils, never once rolling her eyes when I read aloud from yet another study. Who didn't just tolerate my obsession with health—she embraced it, standing beside me as we threw out everything in our pantry and learned to cook real food together.

When I was lost in criticism and frustration, you asked the question that changed everything: "What are you going to do about it?" Without that gentle challenge, this would have been just another complaint. With it, it became hope.

Thank you for seeing possibility where I saw only problems, for choosing this adventure with me, and for saying yes to a lifetime of figuring it out together. I can't wait to marry my best friend and spend forever discovering what healthy and happy really look like.

This book exists because you believed it should. Our future exists because you believed we should.

Contents

1. Introduction — 1
2. Part 1: Food Lies We Swallowed — 9
3. The Sugar Myth — 25
4. The Fat Myth — 40
5. The Seed Oil Myth — 59
6. The Calorie Myth — 75
7. The Low-Fat Myth — 93
8. The Plant-Based Myth — 110
9. The Red Meat Myth — 125
10. The Breakfast Myth — 144
11. Part 1 Summary — 159
12. Part 2: Medical Dogma and Systemic Failures — 168
13. The Statin Myth — 173
14. The Cholesterol Myth — 181
15. The Salt Myth — 190
16. The Antidepressant Myth — 200
17. The Hormone Replacement Therapy Myth — 212
18. The Peanut Allergy Myth — 224
19. The Supplement Myth — 233

20.	The Intermittent Fasting Myth	246
21.	GLP-1s	259
22.	Part II Summary: Medical Dogma and Systemic Failures	270
23.	Interlude: Follow The Money	282
24.	Part 3: The Way Forward	292
25.	Building Your Health Team	297
26.	Biomarkers That Actually Matter	309
27.	Transitioning to Real Food	323
28.	Navigating Resistance	344
29.	Emergency Protocols	359
30.	Raising Healthy Children	375
31.	Part 3 Summary: Your Implementation Roadmap	395
32.	Appendix	407
	About the author	419
	Action Guide	420

Chapter One

Introduction

We're Not Sick, We're Being Sold

My coronary calcium scan had just come back with a score of 450—meaning 92% of people my age had less arterial plaque than I did. I'd been on a statin for twenty years. Twenty years of following doctor's orders, taking my pills, avoiding the foods I was told would kill me. And here I was, sitting across from my cardiologist, being told I needed a *stronger* statin.

No curiosity about why two decades of cholesterol-lowering medication had failed to prevent the exact problem it was supposed to solve. Just a more powerful drug to chase the same failed strategy.

That's when I stopped asking *what's wrong with me* and started asking: **What if I'm not sick? What if I've just been sold a lie?**

Let me be clear: I'm not a doctor. I don't have letters after my name or a white coat in my closet. What I do have is a story—and I've lived every word of it. I've spent a lifetime on the receiving end of a system that told me I was broken and then tried to sell me pills as the cure.

But as I dug deeper into why the medical advice I'd faithfully followed for decades had failed so completely, I discovered something that changed everything: **I wasn't alone. And this wasn't an accident.**

The Lie That Broke a Nation

This book isn't another diet manifesto or wellness guide. It's an investigation into the greatest medical and nutritional fraud of our time—how an entire population was systematically taught to fear the foods that sustain health while embracing the products that destroy it.

For over half a century, we've been sold a story so elegant in its simplicity that it became unquestionable truth: fat makes you fat, cholesterol clogs arteries, red meat causes cancer, salt raises blood pressure, and you need to eat six small meals a day to keep your metabolism humming. We were told that our ancestors, who built civilizations without chronic disease epidemics, simply didn't understand nutrition like our modern experts do.

Meanwhile, as we dutifully followed this advice, something unprecedented happened. Despite spending more on healthcare than any nation in history, Americans became the sickest population on Earth. Obesity rates tripled. Diabetes became epidemic. Children developed diseases that were once exclusive to adults. Heart disease remained our leading killer despite decades of low-fat diets and cholesterol-lowering drugs.

This wasn't bad luck. It was the predictable result of replacing traditional foods with industrial products, prioritizing pharmaceutical profits over prevention, and mistaking marketing for medicine.

When the Script Flipped

I didn't always see it. Like most people, I trusted the experts. I started blood pressure meds in my early 30s—first one, then two, then three. Every increase came with a shrug and a line like, "You've maxed out the last dose." I asked, "Shouldn't it be getting better?" No real answer.

Then came cholesterol. My numbers weren't terrible, but I was prescribed a statin anyway. I didn't question it. The doctor knows best, right?

Fast forward to that calcium scan. Twenty years on a statin, and my arteries were worse than ever. That wasn't a fluke—it was a failure. A failure I paid for with time, trust, and side effects.

Then, almost as an afterthought, my cardiologist mentioned I was pre-diabetic. No conversation. No warning. Just a quiet label tucked in my chart.

INTRODUCTION

That's when I called bullshit. I started digging.

The first book that cracked things open for me was Dr. Robert Lufkin's *Lies I Taught in Medical School*. He revealed how medical education had been corrupted by industry influence. But his explanation of mTOR—a cellular master switch that controls growth, aging, and disease—blew my mind. Suddenly, my fatigue, weight gain, and mounting prescriptions weren't signs of personal failure. They were signs of a system that didn't understand—or didn't care about—metabolic health.

Next came *Blind Spots* by Dr. Marty Makary. He pulled back the curtain on how well-meaning doctors get trapped in a web of bad research, liability fears, and outdated guidelines. The truth hit hard: this system doesn't reward prevention. It rewards management.

Then I reread *Salt, Sugar, Fat* by Michael Moss. That book exposed the food industry's manipulative playbook. These companies don't just use sugar, salt, and fat for flavor—they weaponize them to hijack our biology and engineer addiction.

These weren't fringe authors or conspiracy theorists. They were respected physicians and journalists documenting a system-wide failure hiding in plain sight.

I remembered a moment years earlier when I'd asked a physician assistant for help losing weight. She said, "We don't manage weight loss. You have to go to a weight loss clinic for that."

I blinked. "So you treat the *problems* caused by obesity—but not the obesity itself?"

She gave me a sympathetic shrug. That shrug still haunts me. This system isn't set up to heal people. It's designed to manage them.

In April 2024, I hit my breaking point. I was driving back from Nashville with my soon-to-be fiancée after a great weekend—good music, food, friends—but I felt awful. Tired. Heavy. Off.

Somewhere between Nashville and Atlanta, I looked at her and said, "I'm done feeling this way." She agreed. We made a pact. Not a resolution. A decision. Right now.

Next morning: 310 pounds. That was my number.

We started cutting processed foods, cooking more, trying the Mediterranean diet. It didn't stick—too much planning. So I went back to low-carb. I'd lost weight on it before, and it worked again.

By January 2025, I'd lost 30 pounds. Not bad, but I knew this story. I'd been here before. Twice in the last 20 years, I'd managed to lose over 80 pounds, only to watch it creep back. I knew that cutting carbs would help me lose weight, but I didn't really understand *why*. And not understanding the why is exactly why I couldn't keep it off.

Without the science, carbs and sugar remained tempting treats I was "depriving" myself of. Eventually, you start justifying cheat days. You convince yourself an occasional dessert won't hurt. The cravings return because your body is literally designed to crave what's been driving your insulin response wild for decades.

After reading Dr. Lufkin's book, everything changed. He didn't just tell me to cut carbs—he explained exactly what they do to my body. How they spike insulin. How insulin blocks fat burning and promotes fat storage. How sugar hijacks my brain's reward system, creating genuine addiction patterns. How processed carbs trigger inflammation that damages my arteries—the same inflammation that no amount of statins could prevent.

Suddenly, I wasn't "giving up" bread and pasta. I was *protecting myself* from them. When I understood that every time I ate sugar, I was essentially telling my body to store fat and stay hungry, the desire for it just... disappeared. You don't miss poison once you recognize it as poison.

This is the power of understanding the mechanisms behind the myths. When you know that the "heart-healthy" whole grains are spiking your blood sugar higher than table sugar, you stop seeing them as health food. When you understand that your constant hunger isn't a lack of willpower but a hormonal response to insulin resistance, you stop blaming yourself and start addressing the cause.

I bumped my fasting from 12:12 to 16:8, cut carbs further, and focused on whole foods. But this time felt different. No white-knuckling through cravings. No feeling deprived. Just clarity—both mental and nutritional.

The changes were immediate: sustained energy, zero cravings, mental clarity I hadn't felt in years.

The nutritionist that my cardiologist referred me to couldn't see me until April. By then, I'd lost another 12 pounds. She still pushed Zepbound, a GLP-1 injection. I agreed to try it for six months—as a tool, not a crutch. I was already making progress with lifestyle changes, but figured it might accelerate the process.

As of this writing in August 2025, I'm 247 pounds. I've lost 63 pounds in 16 months. But more than that, I've gained something invaluable: the knowledge that makes healthy choices feel effortless rather than restrictive. For the first time in decades, I felt like myself again—not because I'd found another diet, but because I'd stopped poisoning myself with products disguised as food.

This is what this book offers you: not just the truth about nutritional myths, but the biological understanding that makes living the truth sustainable. When you know how your body actually works—how insulin drives fat storage, how processed foods trigger addiction pathways, how inflammation damages your arteries—you don't feel deprived when you avoid these things. You feel protected.

The Pattern Behind Every Myth

As I investigated further, a disturbing pattern emerged. Every major nutritional myth of the past century followed the same playbook:

Step 1: Find a correlation in observational studies, no matter how weak.
Step 2: Ignore confounding variables that might explain the correlation.
Step 3: Transform preliminary findings into definitive headlines.
Step 4: Create institutional consensus through industry funding and lobbying.

Step 5: Profit from the fear by selling solutions to manufactured problems.
Step 6: When people get sicker, blame their lack of willpower rather than the advice itself.

This pattern repeated across every topic we'll explore: the demonization of fat, the obsession with cholesterol, the fear of salt, the breakfast myth, the supplement scam, and the latest pharmaceutical promises. Each myth was born from the same corrupted process, sustained by the same financial interests, and protected by the same institutional inertia.

Why This Matters More Than Ever

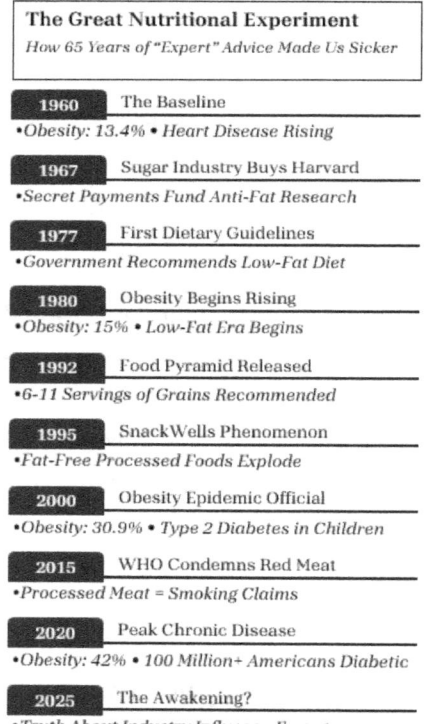

We're living through the consequences of the greatest nutritional experiment in human history. Never before had an entire civilization simultaneously abandoned the foods that sustained health for millennia and replaced them with factory-made alternatives designed for profit, not nourishment.

The results are measured not just in individual suffering, but in civilizational decline. We're raising the first generation expected to live shorter lives than their parents. Chronic diseases that were rare in 1960 now affect the majority of adults. Medical costs have skyrocketed to the point where health emergencies routinely destroy family finances.

But here's what gives me hope: once you see the pattern, you can't unsee it. Once you understand how nutritional myths are manufactured, you become immune to new ones. Once you reconnect with your body's wisdom, you remember that health isn't complicated—it's been deliberately confused.

What You'll Discover

This book is divided into three parts that build on each other:

Part I: Food Lies We Swallowed exposes the biggest nutritional myths of our time, revealing not just how each was created and who profited from promoting them, but exactly how these myths hijacked your biology to keep you sick, hungry, and dependent.

Part II: Medical Dogma and Systemic Failures examines how the healthcare system embraced and perpetuated these myths, creating a medical-industrial complex that profits from managing your symptoms rather than addressing their root causes.

The Great Nutritional Experiment
By the Numbers

- **3X** — Obesity Increase Since Low-Fat Guidelines
- **11X** — Type 2 Diabetes Increase Same Period
- **1/3** — Americans Now Have Fatty Liver Disease
- **#1** — Heart Disease Still Leading Killer Despite 60 Years of Low-Fat Advice
- **$4.1 T** — Annual Healthcare Costs for Chronic Diseases

Part III: The Way Forward provides practical strategies for reclaiming your health, building a supportive team, and creating lasting change that feels natural rather than forced—because you'll finally understand why it works.

A Personal Note on Credentials

I'm not a doctor, and I won't pretend to be one. What I am is an investigative researcher who spent years following medical advice that didn't work, then discovered why it was never designed to work in the first place. Sometimes the most valuable insights come from outside the institution—from people willing to ask uncomfortable questions and follow the evidence wherever it leads.

The medical establishment has a credibility problem that goes beyond individual competence. Most doctors receive virtually no training in clinical nutrition, yet they're expected to provide dietary guidance. They're taught to treat symptoms with medications, not to address root causes with lifestyle changes. This doesn't make them bad people—it makes them trapped people, operating within a system designed to generate revenue rather than create health.

The Choice Ahead

This book will challenge everything you've been taught about health. It will reveal uncomfortable truths about institutions you've trusted and profitable lies you've been sold. But this knowledge is also liberating. When you understand why the conventional approach failed you, you stop blaming yourself and start addressing the real problems.

You weren't broken. You weren't lacking willpower. You weren't genetically doomed to poor health. You were following advice designed to benefit industries rather than individuals, and you got exactly the results that advice was designed to produce.

The lies about food and health are powerful, but the truth is even more powerful. Your body knows the difference between real food and industrial products. It knows the difference between what feeds it and what confuses it. It's been trying to tell you this for years through symptoms, cravings, and energy crashes that no amount of medication could resolve.

It's time to listen.

We're not sick. We're being sold. But once you see the sales pitch for what it is, you can't be sold anymore. Your journey back to health starts with a simple realization: the foods that nourished human beings for thousands of years didn't suddenly become dangerous in 1977 with the food pyramid.

Welcome to your awakening. Let's begin.

Chapter Two

Part 1: Food Lies We Swallowed

How Industry Hijacked Our Plates, Rewrote Nutrition, and Made Us Sicker in the Name of Health

Important Note: This section examines nutrition research and industry influence on dietary guidelines. The information presented is for educational purposes and is not intended as medical advice. Individual nutritional needs vary, and readers should consult qualified healthcare professionals before making significant dietary changes, especially if they have existing health conditions or take medications.

We thought we were doing the right thing.

For decades, we gave up butter for margarine because we were told it would save our hearts. We swapped eggs for fortified cereals because experts said cholesterol was dangerous. We chose "heart-healthy" vegetable oils over animal fats, counted calories like a sacred ritual, and learned to fear the very foods our ancestors had thrived on for millennia. We embraced skim milk, low-fat yogurt, and fat-free cookies, believing we were making enlightened choices based on cutting-edge science.

We were told this was progress. We were told this was health. We were told to trust the experts, follow the guidelines, and ignore our instincts about what real food should look like, taste like, and make us feel like.

Instead of getting leaner, stronger, and healthier, we got sicker.

The Numbers Don't Lie—But They Do Tell a Story

The timeline is damning. In 1960, fewer than 13% of American adults were obese[1]. Today, that number has exploded to over 42%—and it's still climbing. Type 2 diabetes, once called "adult-onset" because it rarely affected young people, now strikes 1 in 5 adolescents with obesity[2]. Autoimmune diseases have more than tripled in the past 50 years[3]. Non-alcoholic fatty liver disease, virtually unknown before 1980, now affects roughly one in three American adults[4].

Despite spending more per capita on healthcare than any country in the world[5], the United States ranks near the bottom among developed nations for chronic disease rates and life expectancy. We followed the rules more faithfully than any generation in history—and became the sickest.

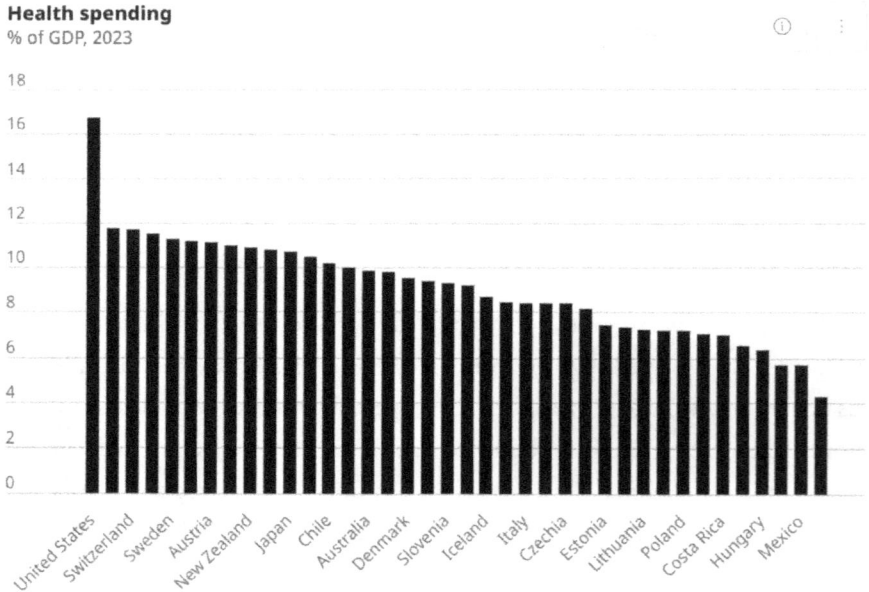

Health at a Glance: OECD Indicators. https://www.oecd.org/health/health-at-a-glance/

This wasn't supposed to happen. According to everything we'd been taught, replacing traditional foods with "scientifically improved" alternatives should have ushered in an era of unprecedented health and longevity. Low-fat diets should have eliminated heart disease. Vegetable oils should have cleared our arteries. Breakfast cereals fortified with vitamins should have optimized our nutrition. Plant-based alternatives should have extended our lives while saving the planet.

Instead, we created the most metabolically dysfunctional population in human history.

The Great Nutritional Experiment

What happened over the past sixty years represents the largest uncontrolled experiment in human history. Never before had an entire civilization simultaneously abandoned the foods that had sustained human health for thousands of years and replaced them with products designed in laboratories and manufactured in factories.

This wasn't gradual cultural evolution—it was orchestrated transformation. Between 1970 and 2000, the American food supply was fundamentally restructured. Traditional fats like butter, lard, and tallow were systematically replaced with industrial seed oils that had never existed in meaningful quantities in the human diet. Sugar consumption soared as it was added to products that had never contained sweeteners. Processed foods multiplied exponentially, filling supermarket aisles with products that required paragraphs of ingredients to describe their contents.

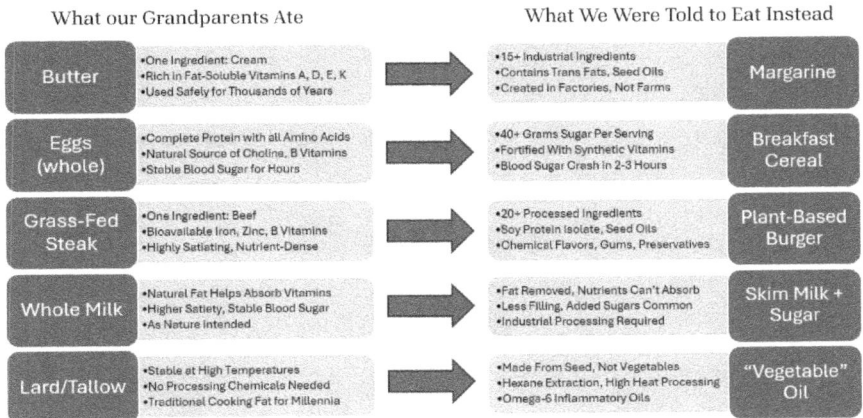

What We Swapped
Traditional Foods vs. "Healthy" Alternatives

The Result: Following Expert Advice Made Us Sicker
Obesity Tripled • Diabetes Epidemic • Heart Disease Still #1 Killer

Most remarkably, this transformation was sold as health improvement. The same foods that had nourished our grandparents were rebranded as dangerous, while factory-made alternatives were marketed as modern, scientific, and superior. Traditional whole milk became a liability; processed skim milk became virtuous. Real butter became a heart attack risk; artificial margarine became heart-healthy. Fresh eggs became cholesterol bombs; sugary cereals became the foundation of a balanced breakfast.

We didn't just change what we ate—we changed how we thought about food itself. Nutrition became about numbers rather than nourishment, labels rather than ingredients, marketing claims rather than traditional wisdom. Food stopped being something that connected us to the earth, the seasons, and our cultural heritage. It became fuel to optimize, numbers to calculate, and problems to solve through better chemistry.

How Fear Replaced Instinct

The transformation of our food supply required more than just new products—it required new beliefs. People needed to be convinced that their instincts about food were wrong, that traditional foods were dangerous, and that only experts could guide them toward proper nutrition.

This psychological shift was achieved through a sophisticated campaign that weaponized our natural concern for health and turned it into fear. Heart disease was rising in the mid-20th century, and people desperately wanted explanations and solutions. Into this anxiety stepped a collection of researchers, institutions, and companies ready to provide both—for a price.

Fear became the primary marketing tool. Fear of fat clogging arteries. Fear of cholesterol causing heart attacks. Fear of red meat causing cancer. Fear of salt raising blood pressure. Fear of skipping breakfast and destroying metabolism. Each fear created demand for alternative products that promised safety, health, and peace of mind.

The marketing was brilliant because it felt scientific. Complex studies with impressive statistics were cited. Prestigious institutions lent their credibility. Government agencies provided official endorsements. The message seemed to come from everywhere at once, creating the illusion of consensus when there was actually coordination.

Traditional food wisdom—the accumulated knowledge of cultures that had successfully fed their populations for generations—was systematically dismantled and replaced with laboratory theories that had never been tested in real-world populations over meaningful timeframes.

Corporate Profits Rewrote Common Sense

Behind the transformation of our food beliefs lay a simple economic reality: processed foods were far more profitable than whole foods. A farmer could sell a bushel of wheat for a few dollars, but that same wheat could be transformed into dozens of boxes of breakfast cereal selling for hundreds of dollars. Soybeans worth pennies per pound could become protein isolates, vegetable oils, and meat substitutes commanding premium prices.

The profit margins were irresistible, but they required consumer acceptance of fundamentally new categories of food. This acceptance was achieved through a combination of convenience marketing, health claims, and the systematic demonization of traditional alternatives.

Margarine manufacturers didn't just promote the benefits of their product—they funded research designed to make butter look dangerous. Cereal companies didn't just advertise their breakfast products—they created educational materials teaching children that traditional breakfast foods were unhealthy. Vegetable oil producers didn't just market their products as cooking oils—they positioned them as lifesaving alternatives to animal fats.

The strategy worked because it aligned the financial interests of food manufacturers with the genuine health concerns of consumers. People wanted to eat healthier, and companies provided products that claimed to deliver better health—along with greater convenience, longer shelf life, and lower preparation time.

The financial transformation was nothing short of spectacular. In just seventy years, the food industry evolved from a collection of small-scale operations selling basic commodities into a trillion-dollar empire built on processed products. The numbers tell the story of how dramatically our food system changed—and reveal where the real money was made.

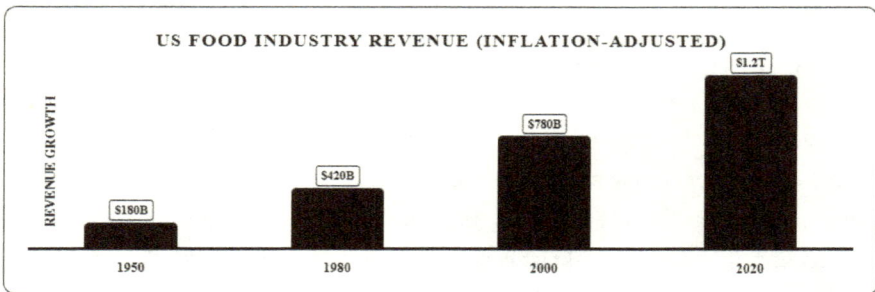

FOOD INDUSTRY REVENUE GROWTH

The Rise of Processed Foods

What consumers didn't realize was that these benefits came at a cost that wouldn't become apparent for decades: the systematic removal of essential nutrients and the introduction of novel compounds that human physiology was never designed to process.

"Evidence-Based" Became Code for "Sponsored"

Before we explore how the nutrition myth-making machine operates, you need to understand how to evaluate the "evidence" it produces. Not all scientific studies are created equal, and the nutrition industry has exploited this fact to devastating effect.

The Hierarchy of Evidence

Real scientific evidence follows a clear hierarchy. At the top sit systematic reviews and meta-analyses that synthesize multiple high-quality studies. Below them are randomized controlled trials (RCTs) that can actually prove causation by controlling variables and testing interventions. Further down are observational studies that can only show correlations, followed by cross-sectional surveys that provide mere snapshots in time.

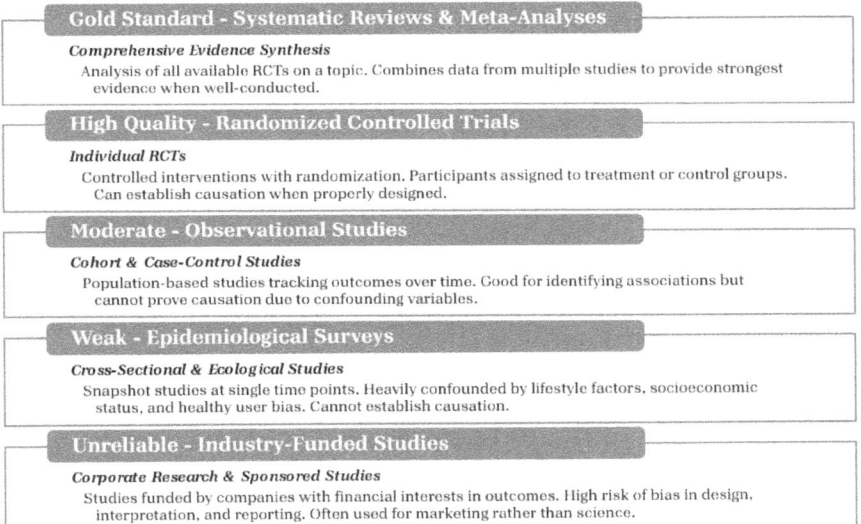

The critical insight is that most nutrition "science" you see in headlines comes from the bottom of this pyramid. High-quality systematic reviews and RCT's often contradict popular dietary advice, but receive little media attention. The industry-funded studies are not necessarily designed to discover truth, but to manufacture marketing claims.

The Corporate Takeover of Science

The transformation of nutrition science from observation-based wisdom to corporate-funded research represents one of the most successful examples of regulatory capture in modern history. Companies with predetermined conclusions began funding researchers willing to design studies that would support those conclusions. The sugar industry funded studies that blamed fat for heart disease.

Vegetable oil manufacturers sponsored research that demonized saturated fat. Cereal companies supported studies promoting breakfast consumption while using the weakest forms of evidence—observational studies that could only show correlations—and presenting them as if they proved causation.

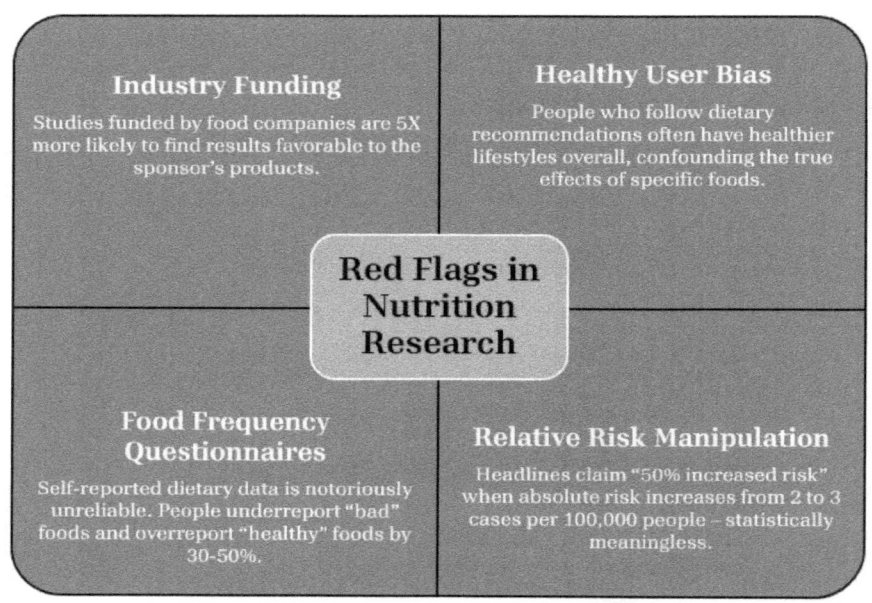

Red Flags of Nutritional Research

Here's the critical flaw: these studies systematically ignored confounding variables that might explain their correlations. When people who ate more red meat also smoked more, exercised less, and consumed more processed foods, researchers blamed the meat while ignoring everything else.

The Silencing of Dissent

When contradictory evidence emerged from independent researchers using higher-quality study designs, it was marginalized, discredited, or simply ignored. Scientists who questioned the prevailing orthodoxy found their funding dried up, their papers rejected, and their reputations attacked.

The scientific process, which should have been self-correcting, became self-reinforcing of predetermined conclusions. The institutions responsible for protecting public health became advocates for the industries they were supposed to regulate.

This systematically distorted process created the perfect environment for the nutrition myth-making machine to operate. Step one of this machine: find a correlation, no matter how weak or confounded...

The Myth-Making Machine

Each nutritional myth examined in the following chapters followed the same basic pattern of creation and promotion. Understanding this pattern is crucial because it's still being used today to manufacture health scares and sell solutions to problems that were created by previous solutions.

Step One: Identify a correlation. Find an observational study showing that people who consume a particular food have higher rates of some disease. The correlation doesn't need to be strong, and it certainly doesn't need to prove causation. It just needs to exist on paper.

Step Two: Ignore confounding variables. Don't account for the fact that people who eat certain foods often have different lifestyles, incomes, education levels, and health behaviors than people who don't. Blame the food rather than the broader pattern of choices it represents.

Step Three: Amplify through media. Transform preliminary correlations into definitive headlines. "Study Shows X Food Causes Y Disease" generates more clicks and fear than "Weak Correlation Found Between X Food and Y Disease After Failing to Control for Z Variables."

Step Four: Create institutional consensus. Get health organizations, government agencies, and medical associations to repeat the message. When multiple prestigious institutions say the same thing, it creates the appearance of scientific consensus even when the underlying evidence is weak.

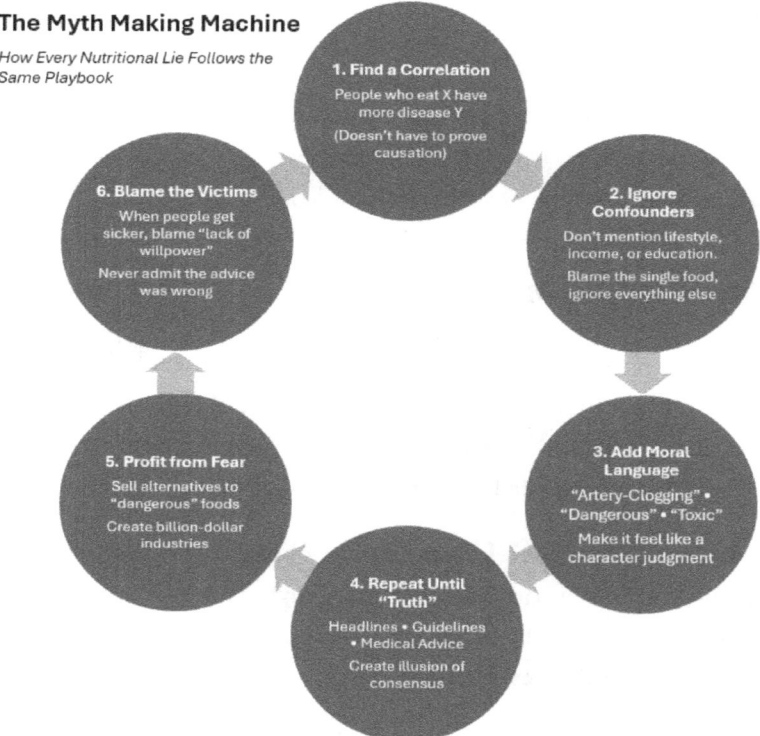

Step Five: Profit from the fear. Market alternative products as solutions to the newly identified problem. Create entire industries around avoiding the demonized food and replacing it with processed alternatives.

Step Six: Double down when problems emerge. When the alternative products create new health problems, blame other factors or create new fears that require additional products. Never admit that the original advice was wrong.

This pattern repeated across decades and multiple food categories, creating a web of interconnected myths that reinforced each other and made the entire system resistant to correction.

Once You See This Pattern, You Can't Unsee It
The same playbook is still being used today to sell new fears and solutions

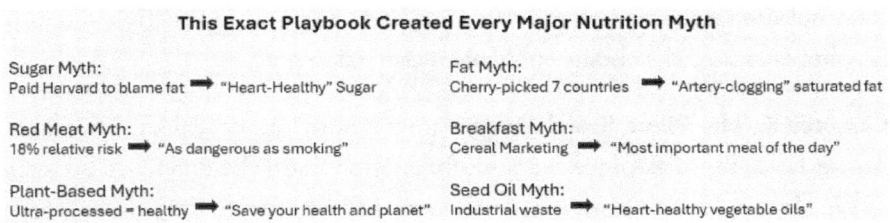

What You'll Discover in Part 1

The chapters that follow will systematically dismantle the biggest nutritional lies of the past century. You'll discover how each myth was created, who benefited from its promotion, and what the real science actually shows when examined critically.

Chapter 3: The Sugar Myth reveals how the sugar industry bought scientific conclusions and shifted blame to fat for diseases that sugar actually causes. You'll learn why your body requires exactly zero dietary sugar to function optimally and how artificial sweeteners create the same metabolic problems as regular sugar.

Chapter 4: The Fat Myth exposes how Ancel Keys' flawed research launched a sixty-year war against one of the most essential macronutrients. You'll understand why saturated fat doesn't cause heart disease and how the low-fat movement actually made us fatter and sicker.

Chapter 5: The Seed Oil Myth uncovers how industrial waste products were transformed into "heart-healthy" cooking oils through marketing rather than science. You'll learn why these oils promote inflammation and metabolic dysfunction while traditional animal fats support health.

Chapter 6: The Calorie Myth demolishes the "calories in, calories out" model that has frustrated millions of dieters. You'll discover why hormones trump calories in determining body composition and why the foods you eat matter more than the amounts you consume.

Chapter 7: The Low-Fat Myth shows how the demonization of fat created a market for processed alternatives that were far more harmful than the foods they replaced. You'll understand why your body needs fat to function and how fat-phobia created the obesity epidemic it claimed to prevent.

Chapter 8: The Plant-Based Myth examines how "eat more plants" became a Trojan horse for ultra-processed junk food. You'll learn the difference between whole plant foods and plant-based products, and why eliminating animal foods creates nutritional deficiencies that supplements cannot adequately address.

Chapter 9: The Red Meat Myth reveals how one of nature's most nutrient-dense foods became a scapegoat for diseases it doesn't cause. You'll discover why the studies linking red meat to cancer and heart disease are fundamentally flawed and how grass-fed meat can be part of an optimal diet.

Chapter 10: The Breakfast Myth traces how a cereal marketing slogan became nutritional dogma. You'll learn why "the most important meal of the day" is important mainly to breakfast food manufacturers and how meal timing flexibility can improve rather than harm metabolic health.

Each chapter follows the same structure: examining the dogma we've been taught, tracing its origins, documenting the consequences of following it, presenting what the science actually shows, and providing practical guidance for making better choices.

This Isn't About Perfection—It's About Truth

The goal of Part 1 isn't to create new dietary rules or promote a specific eating plan. It's to restore your ability to think critically about nutrition advice and make decisions based on evidence rather than marketing.

You'll discover that many of the foods you've been taught to fear are actually beneficial, while many of the products you've been encouraged to embrace are actively harmful. This knowledge is liberating because it means you can stop fighting your biology and start working with it.

The human body evolved over millions of years eating whole, unprocessed foods. For 99.975% of human history, our ancestors consumed wild game, seasonal plants, and natural fats—never encountering processed foods, refined sugar, vegetable oils, or artificial additives. The radical dietary experiment of the past sixty years ignored this evolutionary context, replacing foods your body recognizes with industrial products it struggles to process. Today's American diet consists of 73% ultra-processed foods—a complete inversion of our evolutionary blueprint.

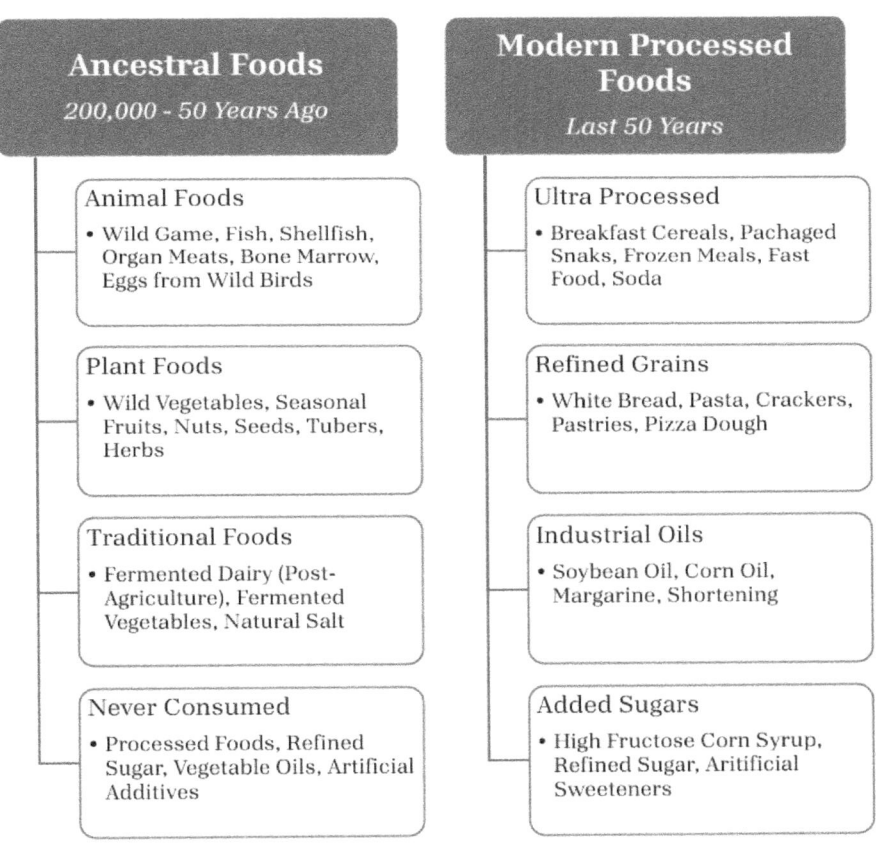

In that same brief snapshot of human history, our health has deteriorated into a full-blown crisis. While our ancestors maintained virtually no obesity, strong bones, excellent physical fitness, sharp mental acuity, and robust immune systems—with no type 2 diabetes, heart disease, or autoimmune disorders—we now face unprecedented rates of chronic disease. Today, 73% of Americans are overweight or obese, 37 million have diabetes, and metabolic dysfunction, mental health crises, and autoimmune diseases have become normalized. What took millions of years of evolution to perfect, we've managed to destroy in just five decades through our radical departure from ancestral eating patterns.

Returning to traditional foods doesn't mean abandoning all modern conveniences or embracing a romanticized past. It means understanding that some aspects of traditional food wisdom deserve preservation and that newer isn't always better when it comes to nourishment.

The Path Back to Real Food

Throughout Part 1, you'll notice that the solutions to our nutritional confusion aren't complex or expensive. They don't require supplements, special products, or complicated calculations. They require returning to foods that humans have eaten successfully for thousands of years and trusting your body's ability to regulate itself when provided with proper nourishment.

Real food doesn't need health claims because its benefits are self-evident. It doesn't require marketing campaigns because its value has been proven through millennia of human experience. It doesn't need to be fortified with synthetic nutrients because it naturally contains what your body needs in bioavailable forms.

The journey back to real food begins with understanding how we were led away from it in the first place. Once you see the pattern of how nutritional myths are created and promoted, you can't unsee it. You become immune to the marketing disguised as science and confident in your ability to distinguish between nourishment and manipulation.

Your Body Knows the Difference

Perhaps the most important realization you'll gain from Part 1 is that your body has always known the difference between real food and processed alternatives. The cravings, energy crashes, weight gain, and health problems you may have experienced weren't signs of personal failure—they were your body's attempt to communicate that something was wrong with what you were feeding it.

When you eat foods your body recognizes and can efficiently process, everything changes. Energy stabilizes. Cravings diminish. Weight normalizes. Health markers improve. This isn't magic—it's biology working as designed when provided with appropriate inputs.

The nutritional establishment spent decades convincing you that your instincts about food were wrong and that only experts could guide you toward proper nutrition. Part 1 will restore your confidence in your body's wisdom while giving you the knowledge to evaluate expert advice critically.

Ready to Reclaim Your Health

The chapters ahead will challenge everything you've been taught about nutrition. They'll reveal uncomfortable truths about institutions you've trusted and profitable lies you've been sold. They'll show you how good intentions were manipulated by commercial interests and how fear replaced wisdom in guiding our food choices.

This knowledge might initially feel overwhelming or even depressing. Learning that you've been systematically misled for decades can shake your confidence in other areas of health and medicine. But this knowledge is also empowering because it provides the tools to make better decisions moving forward.

You weren't the problem. You weren't lacking willpower, knowledge, or commitment. You were following advice that was designed to benefit industries rather than individuals. The weight gain, energy problems, and health issues that may have followed weren't personal failures—they were predictable consequences of systematically flawed guidance.

Now you can stop blaming yourself and start understanding the real causes of our nutritional confusion. You can stop fighting your biology and start working with it. You can stop fearing real food and start embracing the nourishment your body actually needs.

The lies about food were powerful, but the truth is more powerful still. And once you understand the truth about how we were misled about nutrition, you'll be prepared to recognize similar patterns in other areas of health and medicine.

Your journey back to real health starts with real food. And real food starts with real truth about how we lost our way in the first place.

References

1. Centers for Disease Control and Prevention. "Adult Obesity Facts." Updated May 17, 2023. https://www.cdc.gov/obesity/data/adult.html

2. Lawrence JM, et al. "Trends in incidence of type 1 and type 2 diabetes among youths — United States, 2002–2015." *NEJM*. 2021;384(15):1481-1484.

3. Cooper GS, Bynum MLK, Somers EC. "Recent insights in the epidemiology of autoimmune diseases: Improved prevalence estimates and understanding of clustering." Journal of Autoimmunity. 2009;33(3-4):197-207.

4. Younossi ZM, Koenig AB, Abdelatif D, Fazel Y, Henry L, Wymer M. Global epidemiology of nonalcoholic fatty liver disease-Meta-analytic assessment of prevalence, incidence, and outcomes. Hepatology. 2016 Jul;64(1):73-84. doi: 10.1002/hep.28431. Epub 2016 Feb 22. PMID: 26707365.

5. Organization for Economic Co-operation and Development Health Statistics 2023. "Health at a Glance: OECD Indicators." https://www.oecd.org/health/health-at-a-glance/

Chapter Three

The Sugar Myth

How Science Was Bought and Sold

The Lie That Shaped a Nation

In 1967, three Harvard scientists published a review in the prestigious *New England Journal of Medicine* that would shape American health policy for decades. The review blamed dietary fat for heart disease and largely exonerated sugar. What readers didn't know---what remained hidden for nearly fifty years---was that the sugar industry had paid these scientists to reach that exact conclusion[4,5]. The funding was never disclosed. The manipulation was never revealed. The lie became official government policy.

You're still living with the consequences.

This wasn't an isolated incident or honest mistake---it was the culmination of a deliberate campaign to rewrite nutritional science. The sugar industry didn't just influence research; they bought it, shaped it, and used it to convince an entire population that their product was harmless while demonizing the foods humans had thrived on for millennia.

Today, that same false narrative persists: sugar is just empty calories that, consumed in moderation alongside an active lifestyle, poses no real threat. Fat remains the villain, sugar the innocent bystander that simply provides energy.

The truth is far more sinister. Sugar isn't just empty calories---it's a metabolic saboteur that was never meant to flood our food supply in the quantities we see today.

The Corruption: How Sugar Bought Science

The story begins in the early 20th century when heart disease rates began climbing in industrialized nations. Scientists scrambled for explanations, and two competing theories emerged. The first blamed dietary fat, particularly saturated fat and cholesterol, for clogging arteries and killing hearts. The second pointed to sugar and refined carbohydrates as the true culprits behind rising chronic disease.

The fate of these theories---and the scientists who championed them---would determine the course of public health policy for generations.

The Battle of Two Scientists

By the 1950s, two men embodied these rival explanations, and their personal clash would echo through American kitchens for decades.

Ancel Keys was everything a public health crusader appeared to need: charismatic, politically connected, and utterly convinced of his mission. A physiologist with a gift for memorable sound bites, Keys became obsessed with the idea that dietary fat---especially saturated fat---was murdering Americans en masse. He led high-profile research including the famous Seven Countries Study[1] and landed on the cover of *Time* magazine in 1961, broadcasting his anti-fat gospel to millions of American families.

But Keys' science was compromised from the start. His Seven Countries Study, which seemed to prove that saturated fat caused heart disease, was built on cherry-picked data. Keys had access to information from 22 countries but chose to include only seven---conveniently omitting nations like France and Germany where people consumed massive amounts of saturated fat yet enjoyed remarkably low rates of heart disease. When critics pointed out these glaring omissions, Keys became combative and dismissive, using his powerful connections within the American Heart Association to silence opposition and push his hypothesis into mainstream policy.

On the other side stood John Yudkin, a British scientist who couldn't have been more different. Where Keys was bombastic, Yudkin was measured. Where Keys was politically savvy, Yudkin was academically focused. A trained physiologist, medical doctor, PhD, and founding professor of nutrition at Queen Elizabeth College London, Yudkin had noticed something Keys ignored: a striking correlation between rising sugar consumption and the chronic diseases plaguing modern society.

In 1972, Yudkin published *Pure, White, and Deadly*[3], a meticulously researched warning that sugar was fundamentally rewiring human metabolism and driving epidemics of obesity, diabetes, and heart disease. His evidence was compelling, his logic sound, his conclusions prophetic.

But in the battle for public attention, logic doesn't always win. Where Keys was aggressive and well-connected, Yudkin was reserved and lacked political clout. Industry-funded experts dismissed his work as alarmist scaremongering. Keys himself publicly ridiculed Yudkin's research, calling it unscientific nonsense. The media, hungry for simple narratives, embraced Keys' clear villain story while ignoring Yudkin's complex metabolic arguments.

The Sugar Industry's Secret War

Behind the scenes, however, the sugar industry was panicking. Yudkin's book represented something they couldn't tolerate: a credible threat to their profits delivered by a respected scientist to a public audience. Internal company memos, discovered decades later, reveal the industry's response was swift and ruthless. They launched a coordinated campaign to destroy Yudkin's credibility, referring to his life's work as "science fiction" and funding research specifically designed to contradict his findings.

The crown jewel of this campaign came in 1967, when the Sugar Research Foundation---now known as the Sugar Association---paid Harvard scientists including Dr. Mark Hegsted, who would later help write America's first official Dietary Guidelines, to publish that influential review in the *New England Journal of Medicine*. The review did exactly what the sugar industry paid for: it blamed fat for heart disease while treating sugar as a harmless source of energy.

The conflict of interest that compromised this research remained buried until 2016, when investigators published their findings in *JAMA Internal Medicine*[4]. By then, the damage was incalculable. That fraudulent review had shaped public understanding for nearly half a century. Yudkin died marginalized and largely forgotten. Keys' anti-fat message had become nutritional gospel. When the United States government issued its first Dietary Guidelines in 1977, the war on fat became official policy---and sugar flooded the American food supply virtually unchallenged.

I was consuming 'heart-healthy' cereals and low-fat products loaded with sugar, believing I was protecting my heart while unknowingly feeding the exact metabolic dysfunction that was filling my arteries with plaque.

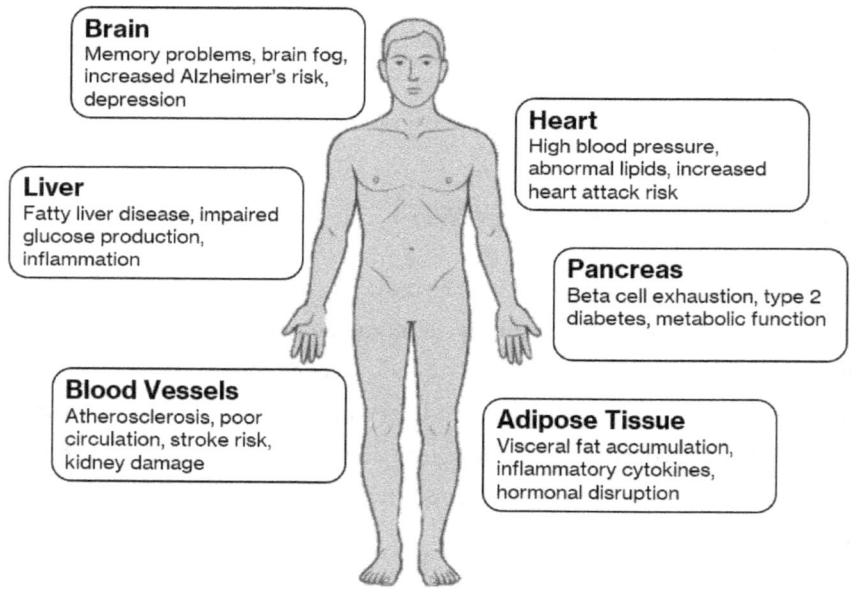

The Reality: Sugar Is Metabolic Sabotage

Dr. Robert Lufkin, author of *Lies I Taught in Medical School*[8], puts it bluntly: "Sugar should come with a warning label." The more we understand about sugar's effects on human physiology, the more his assessment seems not just accurate but conservative.

Sugar isn't simply empty calories that make you gain weight if you eat too much. It's a metabolic saboteur that hijacks fundamental biological processes whether it comes with calories or not. Even more disturbing, your body requires exactly zero dietary sugar to function optimally because it can make all the glucose it needs through a process called gluconeogenesis, which we discuss a little later. The problem is that the amounts of added sugar in modern processed foods far exceed any biological requirement and actively harm metabolic health.

The Sweetness Trap: How Taste Alone Triggers Disease

The sugar industry's most carefully guarded secret isn't about calories---it's about taste. Even artificial sweeteners that provide zero calories trigger the same metabolic disruption as regular sugar, and the mechanism reveals just how profoundly sweetness interferes with human biology.

The moment sweetness touches your tongue, specialized taste receptors send signals throughout your body launching what scientists call the cephalic phase insulin response[7]. Your body, evolved to prepare for incoming sugar based purely on taste, begins releasing insulin before a single calorie enters your bloodstream. This isn't speculation---it's a measurable biological response that occurs every time you taste sweetness, regardless of whether actual sugar follows.

When you consume artificial sweeteners, you create a cruel biochemical deception. Your body prepares for sugar that never arrives, leaving you in a state of metabolic confusion. Repeated exposure to this false alarm leads inexorably to insulin resistance, increased fat storage, and intense cravings for the calories your body was promised but never received.

The research proving this mechanism is extensive and unambiguous. A landmark 1999 study published in the *American Journal of Clinical Nutrition* by Teff and colleagues[7] demonstrated that simply tasting sweetness triggers insulin release even when no glucose enters the bloodstream. A 2014 study in *Nature* by Suez and colleagues[6] showed that artificial sweeteners like saccharin, sucralose, and aspartame don't just affect blood sugar---they actively disrupt the beneficial bacteria in your gut microbiome, leading to glucose intolerance in both laboratory animals and human subjects.

Whether the sweetness comes from cane sugar, high-fructose corn syrup, aspartame, sucralose, stevia, or monk fruit makes little difference to your metabolism. Sweetness itself triggers metabolic reactions that promote disease. Your brain gets fooled, your pancreas gets activated, your gut bacteria get disrupted, and long-term damage accumulates with every sweet taste you experience.

Individual tolerance varies somewhat---people who are highly active may handle occasional sugar intake better due to increased insulin sensitivity and faster glucose disposal---but this doesn't eliminate the fundamental risks of chronic exposure. The real problem isn't an athlete having a spoonful of honey after an intense workout; it's the relentless tsunami of hidden sugar flooding processed foods that most people never consciously chose to consume.

From Food to Drug: The Industrial Transformation of Sugar

Understanding modern sugar requires recognizing that our ancestors never encountered anything resembling what we call sugar today. Before the 1600s, humans experienced sweetness only in tiny quantities from seasonal fruits or the occasional dangerous raid on a wild beehive[9]. These natural sources came packaged with fiber, vitamins, minerals, and other compounds that slowed sugar absorption and provided actual nutrition.

Modern sugar represents something entirely different: an industrial product created through intensive processing that strips away everything natural about the original plant[3]. Manufacturers crush sugar cane or sugar beets, extract the juice, boil it down, purify it with chemicals, crystallize it, and refine it into pure sucrose---removing every trace of fiber, vitamin, mineral, and protective compound that existed in the living plant.

What remains isn't food in any meaningful sense. It's an isolated chemical compound that delivers a concentrated hit of glucose and fructose directly into your bloodstream faster than your body can process it safely. When you take a plant's most potent chemical component, isolate it through industrial processing, and remove all the natural factors that once moderated its effects, you're no longer eating nourishment---you're consuming what amounts to a drug.

Today, that drug permeates the food supply in ways that would have been unimaginable to previous generations. It's hidden in tomato sauce, salad dressing, bread, yogurt, and foods marketed as healthy. It's aggressively advertised to children whose developing brains are most vulnerable to its addictive properties. It's served in hospitals to sick patients whose bodies are least equipped to handle the metabolic stress. Most disturbing of all, it's delivered in doses that no human physiology was ever designed to process---doses that would have required our ancestors to consume dozens of pieces of fruit daily to match what we now get from a single soft drink[13],[14].

The Metabolic Cascade: Understanding Sugar's Systematic Destruction

When you consume modern processed sugar, particularly the refined white sugar and high-fructose corn syrup that dominate our food supply, you trigger a cascade of metabolic dysfunction that extends far beyond simple weight gain.

The first domino to fall is insulin sensitivity. Constant spikes in blood glucose force your pancreas to pump out insulin repeatedly throughout the day, but your cells gradually become deaf to insulin's signals. This insulin resistance sets the foundation for type 2 diabetes[10],[16], but the damage spreads far beyond blood sugar control.

Simultaneously, the fructose component of sugar places an enormous burden on your liver, which is the only organ capable of processing fructose in significant quantities. Unlike glucose, which can be used by cells throughout your body, fructose gets shuttled directly to the liver where it's rapidly converted into fat[12]. This process leads to non-alcoholic fatty liver disease, a condition that was virtually unknown before the sugar epidemic but now affects roughly one in three American adults[12]. As fat accumulates in liver cells, inflammation develops, followed by scarring and progressive loss of liver function.

Throughout your body, sugar promotes chronic inflammation[17], creating the perfect environment for cancer cells to thrive, neurons to degenerate, joints to deteriorate, and arteries to develop dangerous plaques. This isn't the acute inflammation that helps you heal from injuries---it's the persistent, low-grade inflammation that slowly destroys healthy tissue over years and decades.

Perhaps most insidiously, sugar hijacks the reward pathways in your brain, activating dopamine systems in patterns remarkably similar to cocaine, nicotine, and opioid drugs[18],[19]. Neuroimaging studies show that sugar lights up the same brain regions associated with addiction, creating genuine physical dependence that makes quitting sugar as challenging as quitting cigarettes. I remember how a single cookie used to turn into three without me even realizing.

Sugar isn't just "bad for you" in some vague sense---it's specifically engineered to create biological dependence while systematically damaging the organs and systems your life depends on.

The Zero-Calorie Deception

When artificial sweeteners flooded the market promising "all the sweetness with none of the calories," they seemed to offer the perfect solution to sugar's problems. The reality is far more disturbing.

Artificial sweeteners trigger the same cephalic insulin response as regular sugar[7] because your body responds to sweetness itself, not calories. When your brain tastes something sweet, it doesn't pause to calculate whether calories will follow---it immediately begins the metabolic preparation for sugar arrival. This means diet sodas, sugar-free gum, and zero-calorie sweeteners in your coffee all trigger insulin release just like regular sugar.

The consequences extend beyond insulin. When your brain anticipates calories based on sweet taste but those calories never arrive, hunger signals intensify dramatically[20]. Studies consistently show that people who consume artificial sweeteners end up eating more food overall as their confused metabolism drives them to seek the energy it was promised. You think you're saving calories, but you're actually programming your body to crave more food.

The Zero-Calorie Deception

Why "Diet" Sweeteners Are Just as Harmful as Sugar

Regular Sugar
(Sucrose, High Fructose Corn Syrup)

Artificial Sweeteners
(Aspartame, Sucralose, Stevia, etc,..)

Regular Soda
150 Calories

- Sweet Taste Hits Tongue → Brain Prepares for Sugar
- Massive Insulin Spike → Fat Storage Mode ON
- Blood Sugar Crash → Energy Plummets
- Intense Cravings → Want More Sugar
- Gut Bacteria Damaged → Inflammation

Diet Soda
0 Calories

- Sweet Taste Hits Tongue → Brain Prepares for Sugar
- Massive Insulin Spike → But No Calories Arrive!
- Metabolic Confusion → Body Expect Energy
- Stronger Cravings → Eat More Food Later
- Gut Bacteria Damaged → Same As Regular Sugar

Long Term Result:
- Weight Gain and Metabolic Dysfunction
- Insulin Resistance and Diabetes Risk
- Sugar Addiction and Constant Cravings

Long Term Result:
- MORE Weight Gain Than Regular Soda Drinkers
- Same Insulin Resistance and Diabetes Risk
- Worse Sugar Cravings Due to Unfulfilled Promise

The Problem Isn't Calories - It's Sweetness Itself

Your brain & metabolism respond to sweet taste regardless of calories

Solution: Eliminate ALL forms of Sweetness and let your taste buds reset

Even more concerning is the growing evidence that artificial sweeteners devastate the beneficial bacteria living in your digestive system[6,21]. These microorganisms play crucial roles in metabolism, immune function, and even mood regulation. When artificial sweeteners damage this delicate ecosystem, the effects ripple throughout your entire body, weakening your ability to process real food and defend against disease.

The harsh truth is that your body doesn't care about "zero calories"---it cares that you lied to it with the promise of sweetness. You didn't outsmart your biology; you simply found a more sophisticated way to disrupt it.

Your Body's Sugar Independence

Here's perhaps the most important fact the sugar industry hopes you never learn: there is no biological requirement for dietary sugar. Not a single gram. Your body can function perfectly---in fact, optimally---without ever consuming refined sugar, artificial sweeteners, or any other form of added sweetness.

Through a process called gluconeogenesis, your liver can manufacture all the glucose your brain and muscles need using protein and fat as raw materials. This isn't some emergency backup system---it's how human metabolism was designed to work. Your ancestors built civilizations, explored continents, and conquered every climate on Earth fueled by real food, not candy bars and energy drinks.

The persistent myth that you "need" sugar for energy or brain function isn't based on biology---it's propaganda created by industries that profit from your dependence on their products. Every time you feel like you "need" something sweet, you're experiencing the artificial cravings created by previous sugar consumption, not a genuine nutritional requirement.

This means you have far more power over sugar than you've been led to believe. The industry wants you to think you're fundamentally broken, that you need their products to survive and thrive. The opposite is true: you need to avoid their products to reclaim the metabolic health that's your birthright.

Where It All Went Wrong: The Timeline of Systematic Deception

The distortion of nutritional science didn't happen overnight---it unfolded through a carefully orchestrated campaign spanning decades. In 1954, the Sugar Research Foundation began systematically funding nutrition research, always with the implicit understanding that findings should favor sugar industry interests. The 1967 Harvard review in the *New England Journal of Medicine* represented the culmination of this strategy, providing scientific cover for sugar while demonizing fat. When the USDA released its first Dietary Guidelines in 1977, low-fat eating became official government policy, inadvertently opening the floodgates for sugar to replace fat in processed foods.

Throughout the 1980s and 1990s, grocery store shelves filled with low-fat products that compensated for removed fat by adding unprecedented amounts of sugar. Foods that had never contained sweeteners---bread, crackers, sauces, even meat products---suddenly became vehicles for sugar delivery. By 2005, non-alcoholic fatty liver disease had become the most common form of liver disease in the United States, affecting people who had never consumed alcohol but had unknowingly consumed massive amounts of hidden sugar for decades.

The full scope of the deception remained hidden until 2016, when researchers finally exposed the sugar industry's manipulation of that pivotal 1967 Harvard review[4]. By then, the damage was almost incalculable: obesity rates had tripled since the 1970s[11], more than 100 million Americans were living with prediabetes or type 2 diabetes[10], fatty liver disease affected one in three adults[12], and children were consuming three to four times the recommended daily sugar intake[14,15].

This wasn't the natural evolution of dietary habits---it was the engineered result of corporate manipulation of scientific research and government policy.

Even today, sugar defenders attempt to muddy the waters by claiming that "context matters" and that sugar is harmless if you're healthy, active, and consume it in moderation. This argument ignores the reality that sugar is hidden throughout the food supply, aggressively marketed to children, and consumed in quantities that no amount of exercise can offset. The science condemning sugar isn't unclear or controversial---what's unclear is how long we'll continue pretending otherwise.

Breaking Free from the Sugar Matrix

The truth about sugar was hidden by design, not by accident, which means breaking free requires more than just willpower---it requires understanding what you're really fighting and why the battle feels so difficult.

Start by recognizing that sugar functions as a metabolic saboteur, not merely as "empty calories" that contribute to weight gain. This reframing helps you understand why moderation feels impossible and why "just a little bit" often leads to consuming far more than intended. Sugar creates genuine biochemical addiction that makes quitting a medical challenge, not a character flaw.

Learning to identify hidden sugar requires becoming a detective with food labels, since the industry disguises sugar under more than fifty different names including seemingly innocent terms like "evaporated cane juice," "rice syrup," and "maltodextrin." The goal isn't to memorize every alias but to become suspicious of processed foods in general, since manufacturers have powerful financial incentives to include sugar in products where consumers don't expect it.

Eliminating artificial sweeteners is equally important since they trigger the same metabolic disruption as regular sugar while creating additional problems with hunger regulation and gut health. The promise of "having your cake and eating it too" with zero-calorie sweeteners is fundamentally false---you're still consuming the taste that creates sugar addiction while adding new forms of biological confusion.

Instead of focusing on what to avoid, redirect your attention toward whole foods that naturally satisfy your body's actual nutritional needs. Foods rich in healthy fats, fiber, and protein don't just provide better nutrition---they actively retrain your taste buds and appetite regulation systems to prefer real food over artificial sweetness. This isn't about forcing yourself to eat foods you dislike; it's about rediscovering how good real food tastes when your palate isn't overwhelmed by artificial flavors.

Perhaps most importantly, remember that your taste preferences aren't fixed or genetic---they're learned responses that can be unlearned. The intense sweetness cravings that feel so compelling are the result of previous sugar consumption, not an inherent need for sweetness. As you eliminate sources of artificial sweetness from your diet, these cravings will diminish and eventually disappear, often within a matter of weeks. Once I started avoiding sugar and realized that I didn't have the familiar 3 PM energy crash, I knew something fundamental had shifted. For the first time in decades, my body was running on stored energy instead of constantly demanding more fuel.

The sugar industry has spent enormous resources convincing you that you're fundamentally broken and dependent on their products to function normally. This is perhaps their greatest lie. You possess the biological machinery to thrive without consuming a single gram of their refined products. Your ancestors proved this for millennia, and you can prove it again.

The power to reclaim your metabolic health has always been yours. Now you know how to use it.

References

1. Keys A, ed. *Coronary Heart Disease in Seven Countries. Circulation.* 1970;41(Suppl 1):1–211.

2. Teicholz N. *The Big Fat Surprise: Why Butter, Meat and Cheese Belong in a Healthy Diet.* New York, NY: Simon & Schuster; 2014.

3. Yudkin J. *Pure, White, and Deadly: How Sugar Is Killing Us and What We Can Do to Stop It.* London: Penguin Books; 2012. Originally published 1972.

4. Kearns CE, Schmidt LA, Glantz SA. Sugar industry and coronary heart disease research: a historical analysis of internal industry documents. *JAMA Intern Med.* 2016;176(11):1680–1685. doi:10.1001/jamainternmed.2016.5394

5. Hegsted DM, McGandy RB, Myers ML, Stare FJ. Dietary fats, carbohydrates and atherosclerotic vascular disease. *N Engl J Med*. 1967;277(4):186–192. doi:10.1056/NEJM196707272770405

6. Suez J, Korem T, Zilberman-Schapira G, et al. Artificial sweeteners induce glucose intolerance by altering the gut microbiota. *Nature*. 2014;514(7521):181–186. doi:10.1038/nature13793

7. Teff KL, Young SN, Blundell JE. Sweet taste: effect on cephalic phase insulin release in humans. *Am J Clin Nutr*. 1999;69(3):512–519. doi:10.1093/ajcn/69.3.512

8. Lufkin R. *Lies I Taught in Medical School: And the Truths That Can Save Your Life*. 2023.

9. Lustig RH. *Fat Chance: Beating the Odds Against Sugar, Processed Food, Obesity, and Disease*. New York, NY: Hudson Street Press; 2012.

10. Centers for Disease Control and Prevention. *National Diabetes Statistics Report, 2022*. Atlanta, GA: CDC, US Department of Health and Human Services; 2022.

11. Centers for Disease Control and Prevention. Prevalence of obesity and severe obesity among adults: United States, 2017–2020. *NCHS Data Brief*. 2020;(360):1–8.

12. Younossi ZM, Koenig AB, Abdelatif D, et al. Global epidemiology of nonalcoholic fatty liver disease—meta-analytic assessment of prevalence, incidence, and outcomes. *Hepatology*. 2016;64(1):73–84. doi:10.1002/hep.28431

13. Bray GA, Nielsen SJ, Popkin BM. Consumption of high-fructose corn syrup in beverages may play a role in the epidemic of obesity. *Am J Clin Nutr*. 2004;79(4):537–543. doi:10.1093/ajcn/79.4.537

14. Centers for Disease Control and Prevention. Get the facts: added sugars. Updated October 3, 2024. Accessed September 9, 2025. https://www

.cdc.gov/nutrition/php/data-research/added-sugars.html

15. Harvard T.H. Chan School of Public Health. Healthy kids "sweet enough" without added sugars. *The Nutrition Source.* Updated May 9, 2024. Accessed September 9, 2025. https://nutritionsource.hsph.harvard.edu/2016/08/23/aha-added-sugar-limits-children/

16. Taylor R, Holman RR. Normal weight individuals who develop type 2 diabetes: the personal fat threshold hypothesis. *Clin Sci (Lond).* 2015;128(7):405–410. doi:10.1042/CS20140553

17. Della Corte KW, Perrar I, Penczynski KJ, et al. Effect of dietary sugar intake on biomarkers of subclinical inflammation: a systematic review and meta-analysis of intervention studies. *Nutrients.* 2018;10(5):606. doi:10.3390/nu10050606

18. Avena NM, Rada P, Hoebel BG. Evidence for sugar addiction: behavioral and neurochemical effects of intermittent, excessive sugar intake. *Neurosci Biobehav Rev.* 2008;32(1):20–39. doi:10.1016/j.neubiorev.2007.04.019

19. Schulte EM, Avena NM, Gearhardt AN. Which foods may be addictive? The roles of processing, fat content, and glycemic load. *PLoS One.* 2015;10(2):e0117959. doi:10.1371/journal.pone.0117959

20. Rogers PJ, Appleton KM. The effects of low-calorie sweeteners on energy intake and body weight: a systematic review and meta-analyses of sustained intervention studies. *Int J Obes (Lond).* 2021;45(3):464–478. doi:10.1038/s41366-020-00774-y

21. Sun Y, Zhang W, Zeng Q, et al. A critical review on effects of artificial sweeteners on gut microbiota and gastrointestinal health. *J Sci Food Agric.* 2025;105(2):545–558. doi:10.1002/jsfa.13245

Chapter Four

The Fat Myth

How We Got It Wrong for 60 Years

The Dogma That Changed Everything

For over half a century, we've been told a story about fat that fundamentally reshaped how billions of people eat, how doctors practice medicine, and how governments create food policy. The narrative was simple and seemingly unassailable: fat, especially saturated fat, clogs your arteries and causes heart disease. To live a long, healthy life, you must eat low-fat foods, avoid butter, eggs, cheese, and red meat, and replace them with "heart-healthy" whole grains, vegetable oils, and processed alternatives.

This wasn't merely dietary advice—it became nutritional gospel. Medical schools taught it as established fact. Government agencies mandated it through official dietary guidelines. Food companies built billion-dollar empires around it, creating entire categories of products to satisfy our newfound fear of fat.

But here's what they didn't tell you: this belief was never built on solid science.

As we learned from the sugar chapter, it emerged from cherry-picked data, industry influence, and a public health establishment desperate for simple answers to complex problems. The result wasn't just misguided—it was one of the most consequential mistakes in modern medicine, with ramifications that continue to shape our health landscape today.

Consider the paradox: while we diligently eliminated fat from our diets, obesity rates increased from 13.4% in 1960 to 41.9% by 2020—more than tripling over sixty years[1]. While we chose margarine over butter, diabetes became epidemic.

While we feared eggs and embraced "heart-healthy" cereals, heart disease remained our leading killer. The war on fat didn't save lives—it may have cost them.

How Fat Became the Villain

The demonization of fat traces back to a singular figure: Ancel Keys, the same scientist whose influence we encountered in our examination of sugar. Keys was a man of deep convictions who genuinely believed he had identified the primary cause of America's heart disease epidemic. While simultaneously dismissing John Yudkin's research on sugar as irrelevant, Keys was methodically building what he considered an airtight case against dietary fat.

In the 1950s, Keys observed what seemed like a compelling pattern—countries that consumed more fat appeared to have higher rates of heart disease. His Seven Countries Study, published in 1970, became the cornerstone for decades of anti-fat policy that followed[2]. Keys possessed a rare combination of scientific credentials, passionate certainty, and media savvy that made him a formidable advocate for his position.

Keys' unwavering focus on fat as the singular dietary villain, combined with his dismissal of other potential culprits like sugar, created what would prove to be a perfect storm. Whether intentional or not, his laser focus on fat helped deflect attention from other dietary factors while providing politicians and public health officials with the simple, actionable narrative they desperately needed.

But Keys' research contained critical flaws that his critics identified from the very beginning—warnings that were largely ignored in the rush to embrace his conclusions.

The Scientific Shortcomings

The foundation of the fat-heart disease hypothesis rested on shaky ground from the start. Keys initially surveyed 22 countries for his landmark research, but published data from only seven—specifically, those that supported his predetermined hypothesis[3]. Countries like France, with high fat intake but low heart disease rates, and Chile, with low fat intake but high heart disease rates, were excluded without scientific justification. When statistician Jacob Yerushalmy re-analyzed the complete dataset in 1957, the supposedly clear correlation between fat consumption and heart disease largely disappeared[4].

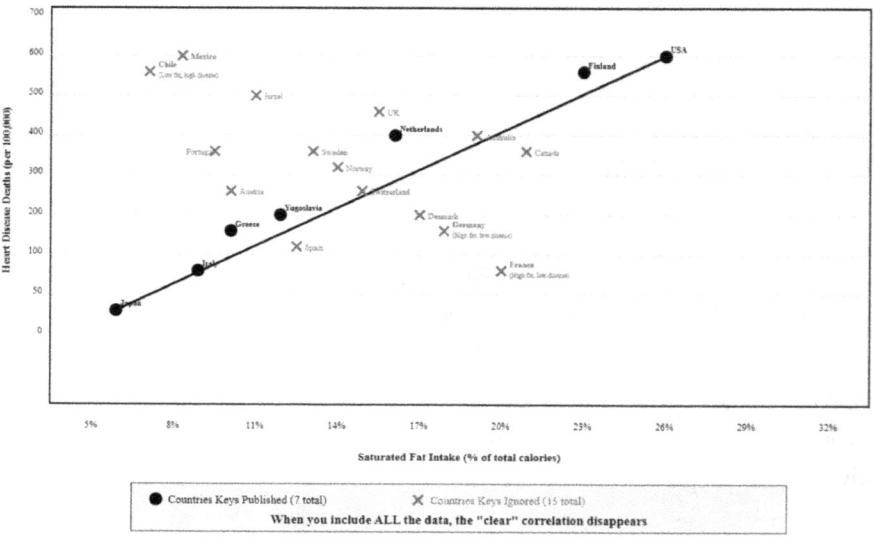

Even more troubling was Keys' failure to account for confounding variables that differed dramatically between the countries he studied. His research ignored crucial factors like smoking rates, sugar consumption, physical activity levels, stress, and overall dietary patterns. Mediterranean countries, for instance, consumed substantial amounts of fat but also ate more fish and vegetables, used olive oil rather than processed fats, and had different lifestyle patterns than the populations with higher heart disease rates.

Perhaps most significantly, Keys never established the actual mechanism by which dietary fat caused heart disease. His hypothesis relied on a theoretical pathway—that eating fat raised blood cholesterol, which then clogged arteries—but this connection was assumed rather than proven through his research.

The Institutional Steamroller

Despite legitimate scientific criticism, Keys' anti-fat message gained unstoppable institutional momentum. His charismatic personality, media connections, and ability to communicate complex ideas in simple terms made him a powerful advocate. In 1961, Time magazine featured him on its cover, cementing his status as America's nutrition authority[5].

The American Heart Association, swayed by Keys' persuasive advocacy and his growing media presence, officially recommended low-fat diets in 1961[6]. This endorsement from a respected medical organization lent credibility to Keys' position and helped silence dissenting voices within the scientific community.

The transformation from scientific theory to government policy happened with remarkable speed. By 1977, the U.S. Senate Select Committee on Nutrition published "Dietary Goals for the United States," which enshrined low-fat eating as federal policy[7]. The 1980 Dietary Guidelines for Americans made it official doctrine: Americans should reduce fat intake to 30% of calories or less[8].

This wasn't a unanimous scientific consensus. Prominent researchers like John Yudkin continued to argue that sugar, not fat, was the primary dietary culprit behind heart disease[9]. But their voices were systematically drowned out by institutional momentum, media messaging, and industry interests that had already aligned behind the low-fat narrative.

The Food Industry Gold Rush

Food manufacturers recognized the low-fat mandate as an unprecedented business opportunity. They quickly pivoted to create an entirely new category of processed products designed to satisfy Americans' newfound fear of fat while maintaining profitability and palatability.

SnackWells cookies became the poster child for this new era—marketed as guilt-free indulgence, they stripped away fat only to load products with sugar and refined flour[10]. Yogurt manufacturers followed a similar playbook, removing beneficial fats from their products while compensating with added sugars, artificial sweeteners, and thickeners to maintain the creamy texture and sweet taste consumers expected.

Even breakfast cereals heavy in sugar earned "heart-healthy" labels simply by virtue of their naturally low fat content. Margarine and vegetable shortening were aggressively promoted as healthy alternatives to butter, despite containing trans fats that we now know are genuinely harmful to cardiovascular health[11]. Salad dressing manufacturers replaced natural fats with high-fructose corn syrup and chemical additives, creating products that were technically low-fat but nutritionally problematic.

The fast food industry joined this transformation with calculated precision. McDonald's promoted its McLean Deluxe burger, which used seaweed extract to replace fat, while simultaneously supersizing french fry portions cooked in what they marketed as "healthier" vegetable oils. Subway built an empire around marketing "low-fat" sandwiches that were loaded with processed meats, refined bread, and sugary sauces as healthy alternatives to traditional fast food options.

The industry's genius lay in positioning themselves as part of the solution while actually accelerating the underlying problem. They replaced natural fats with refined carbohydrates, industrial oils, and hidden sugars while maintaining the massive portion sizes that drove profits. The irony was stark: in removing natural fats that humans had consumed safely for millennia, manufacturers added the very ingredients that would prove far more harmful to human health.

The Unintended Consequences

The timing of America's health crisis tells a story that should have raised immediate red flags. As Americans dutifully reduced their fat intake from 45% of calories in 1965 to 34% by 1995, something unexpected happened: instead of becoming healthier, we became dramatically sicker[12].

The obesity epidemic began in earnest during the height of the low-fat era. In 1960, 13.4% of American adults were obese. By 1980, as low-fat guidelines became entrenched, this figure had risen to 15.0%. But the real explosion came in the following decades: by 2000, 30.9% of adults were obese, and by 2020, a staggering 41.9% of American adults carried this classification[13].

Type 2 diabetes followed an eerily similar trajectory. In 1958, approximately 1% of adults had diagnosed diabetes[14]. By 1980, this had risen to 2.5%, by 2000 to 6.5%, and by 2020, 11.3% of American adults were living with diagnosed diabetes[15]. These weren't gradual increases—they represented an exponential explosion in metabolic dysfunction that coincided precisely with our embrace of low-fat, high-carbohydrate eating.

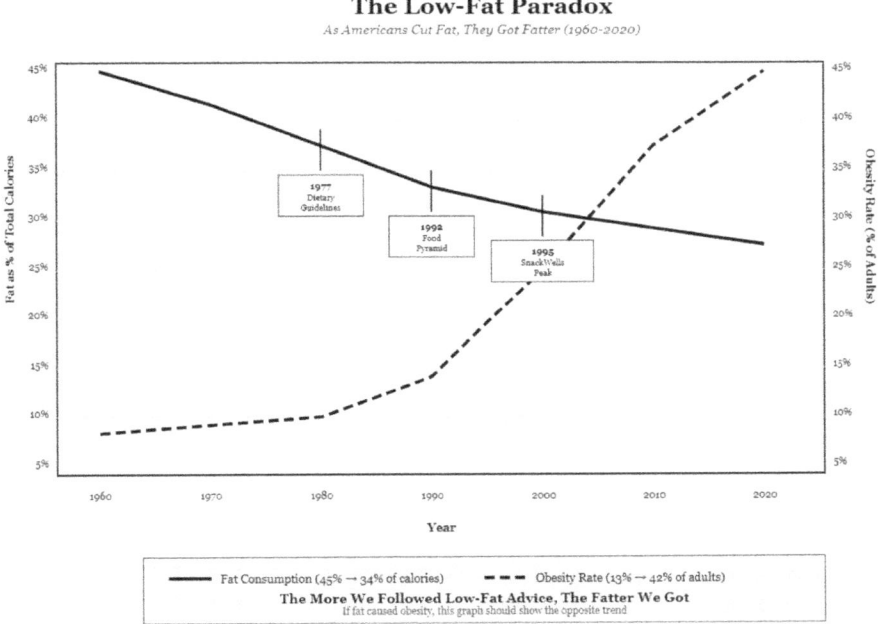

The Emergence of New Diseases

Perhaps most troubling was the appearance of diseases that had been virtually unknown before our war on fat began. Non-alcoholic fatty liver disease (NAFLD), a condition so rare before 1980 that it barely merited mention in medical textbooks, now affects approximately 32% of American adults[16]. Metabolic syndrome—a cluster of conditions including insulin resistance, high blood pressure, and abdominal obesity—became increasingly common as low-fat, high-carbohydrate diets became the standard recommendation.

The heart disease paradox was perhaps most damning of all. Despite six decades of low-fat recommendations, heart disease remains the leading cause of death in America, responsible for approximately 655,000 deaths annually[17]. If fat were truly the primary culprit, we should have seen dramatic improvements by now. Instead, we've witnessed the persistence of the very problem our dietary changes were supposed to solve.

For twenty years, I religiously avoided egg yolks, chose lean meats, and used margarine instead of butter. My reward? A calcium score that put me in the 92nd percentile for arterial plaque. The very foods I'd been taught to fear might have been protecting me from the condition I developed by avoiding them.

What the Science Actually Shows

Modern nutritional science has systematically dismantled the fat-heart disease hypothesis through large-scale, well-designed studies that Keys and his contemporaries could never have imagined. The evidence is now overwhelming: our fear of fat was not only misguided but potentially harmful.

The landmark PURE Study, published in 2017, followed 135,335 people across 18 countries for over seven years. Its findings directly contradicted decades of dietary dogma: higher saturated fat intake was associated with lower risk of stroke and total mortality, while higher carbohydrate intake was associated with higher risk of total mortality[18]. This wasn't a small study of a homogeneous population—it was a massive, diverse investigation that included people from different cultures, economic backgrounds, and dietary traditions.

Multiple comprehensive meta-analyses have reinforced these findings. In 2010, researchers analyzed 21 studies covering 347,747 people and found no association between saturated fat consumption and heart disease[19]. A 2014 review of 72 studies reached the same conclusion[20]. Most recently, a 2020 Cochrane review—the gold standard for medical evidence—found that reducing saturated fat intake had little effect on cardiovascular events[21].

2024 Research: The Final Vindication of Saturated Fat

The past year has brought even more definitive evidence that the war on saturated fat was fundamentally misguided. A comprehensive 2024 umbrella review published in *Frontiers in Public Health* examined the effect of reducing saturated fat intake on cardiovascular disease in adults[22]. The review's conclusions were unambiguous: reducing saturated fat intake showed no significant benefits for cardiovascular outcomes.

Even more significantly, a 2024 systematic review and meta-analysis published in the *Journal of the Medical Association of Japan* examined only randomized controlled trials—the gold standard for establishing causation[23]. After analyzing the highest quality evidence available, the researchers concluded that "saturated fat restriction for cardiovascular disease prevention showed no significant effect on cardiovascular disease mortality."

Perhaps most telling was a major 2024 review published in the *American Journal of Clinical Nutrition* that found the suggestion of benefits from reducing saturated fat in earlier meta-analyses was "due to the inclusion of inadequately controlled trials"[24]. When only properly designed studies were included, the benefits of avoiding saturated fat disappeared entirely.

These findings represent the final collapse of the diet-heart hypothesis that dominated nutrition policy for over sixty years. The evidence is now overwhelming: **natural** saturated fats don't cause heart disease, and avoiding them provides no cardiovascular benefits. This doesn't mean unlimited saturated fat consumption is optimal for everyone. Individual responses vary, and those with familial hypercholesterolemia or established heart disease may need different approaches under medical supervision.

The Cholesterol Revelation

For decades, the medical establishment taught that saturated fat raises "bad" LDL cholesterol, which then clogs arteries and causes heart attacks. This mechanistic explanation seemed logical and provided a clear pathway from dietary fat to heart disease. But this simplistic view missed crucial nuances that modern testing has revealed.

LDL cholesterol isn't a single, uniform substance. It comes in different sizes with dramatically different health implications. Large, buoyant LDL particles (Pattern A) are relatively benign—like beach balls floating harmlessly in your bloodstream. Small, dense LDL particles (Pattern B), however, are genuinely dangerous—like darts that can penetrate and damage arterial walls[25].

Here's where our understanding became inverted: saturated fats tend to raise the harmless large LDL particles, while refined carbohydrates and sugar promote the dangerous small, dense LDL particles. Carbohydrates also raise triglycerides and lower protective HDL cholesterol—a pattern that significantly increases cardiovascular risk[26].

Small, Dense LDL Particle

Causes Plaque

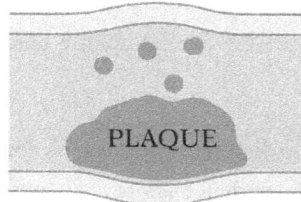

Small, dense LDL particles are more likely to penerrate the artery wall, leading to plaque fomation.

Large, Buoyant LDL Particle

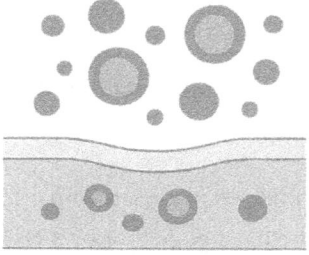

Large, buoyant LDL particles do not penetrate the artery wall and are less likely to cont ribute to plaque formation

Advanced lipid testing, including NMR LipoProfile and Ion Mobility analysis, can now measure LDL particle size and number directly, providing a much clearer picture of cardiovascular risk than total cholesterol measurements alone[27]. This technology has revealed that many people with "high" cholesterol actually have the beneficial large particle pattern, while others with "normal" cholesterol numbers carry the dangerous small particle pattern.

Learning from Traditional Populations

One of the most compelling arguments against the fat-heart disease hypothesis comes from studying populations that thrived on high-fat diets before the introduction of modern processed foods. These natural experiments provide insights that controlled studies cannot.

Inuit populations consuming 50-75% of their calories from fat, primarily from marine mammals, showed virtually no heart disease until Western processed foods were introduced to their communities[28]. Maasai warriors, whose traditional diet consisted largely of milk, blood, and meat from cattle, demonstrated excellent cardiovascular health and lean body composition despite consuming substantial amounts of saturated fat[29].

Mediterranean populations, ironically, provided some of the original data that Keys used to support his hypothesis. But these populations consumed high amounts of olive oil and other fats while maintaining lower heart disease rates than countries with lower fat intake[30]. The difference wasn't the presence or absence of fat—it was the type of fat and the overall dietary pattern.

Archaeological evidence suggests that heart disease was rare throughout human history before the agricultural revolution and the introduction of processed foods[31]. Our ancestors thrived on diets that would be considered dangerously high in fat by modern standards, yet they showed little evidence of the cardiovascular disease that plagues modern populations.

Why Fat Isn't the Enemy

Fat serves critical biological functions that low-fat diets compromise, often in ways that become apparent only after years of nutritional inadequacy. Understanding these functions helps explain why eliminating fat from our diets created more problems than it solved.

Cholesterol, the molecule we've been taught to fear, serves as the building block for essential hormones including testosterone, estrogen, cortisol, and vitamin D. Low-fat diets can suppress hormone production, leading to decreased libido, mood disorders, compromised stress response, and weakened bone health[34]. The brain, which is approximately 60% fat by dry weight, requires omega-3 fatty acids like DHA for optimal cognitive function, memory formation, and protection against neurodegenerative diseases[33].

Every cell in your body requires fatty acids to maintain membrane flexibility and function. Without adequate dietary fat, cellular communication breaks down, affecting everything from nutrient transport to waste removal[34]. The fat-soluble vitamins A, D, E, and K require dietary fat for proper absorption, meaning that low-fat diets can create deficiencies in these critical nutrients regardless of intake levels[34].

Perhaps most importantly from a practical standpoint, fat slows gastric emptying and blunts blood sugar spikes, promoting satiety and stable energy levels. Low-fat, high-carbohydrate meals create rapid blood sugar swings that trigger hunger and cravings, making weight management significantly more difficult[35,36].

The Real Dietary Villains

While we spent decades fearing butter and eggs, the actual culprits behind modern chronic disease were hiding in plain sight, often in the very foods we were told to eat instead of natural fats.

Refined carbohydrates—white flour, sugar, and high-fructose corn syrup—trigger dramatic insulin spikes that promote fat storage and contribute to insulin resistance over time[35,36]. These ingredients became ubiquitous in processed foods as manufacturers sought to replace the palatability and satiety that fat naturally provided.

Industrial seed oils, including soybean, corn, canola, and cottonseed oils, are high in omega-6 fatty acids and undergo extensive processing that creates inflammatory compounds. These oils were promoted as healthy alternatives to saturated fats despite their potential to promote inflammation and oxidative stress[37].

Trans fats, created through the partial hydrogenation of vegetable oils, were aggressively marketed as healthy alternatives to saturated fats despite being linked to increased heart disease risk. The irony is painful: we replaced natural fats that humans had consumed safely for millennia with industrially created fats that were genuinely harmful[11].

The rise of ultra-processed foods combined refined sugars, industrial oils, chemical additives, and artificial ingredients to create products that were hyperpalatable but nutritionally depleted. These foods hijacked our natural satiety mechanisms while providing empty calories that promoted weight gain and metabolic dysfunction[39].

Reclaiming Your Health – A Practical Approach to Eating Fat

The evidence is clear: natural fats aren't the enemy they've been portrayed as for the past six decades. But this doesn't mean all fats are created equal, nor does it suggest that individual optimization isn't important. The key is distinguishing between natural fats that support health and industrial fats that undermine it.

Embrace the natural fats that humans have consumed throughout history: grass-fed butter and ghee, which provide fat-soluble vitamins and beneficial fatty acids; pastured eggs including the nutrient-dense yolks; fatty fish like salmon, sardines, and mackerel that supply essential omega-3 fatty acids; avocados and extra virgin olive oil for their monounsaturated fats and antioxidants; coconut oil for cooking at higher temperatures; and nuts and seeds in moderation for their combination of healthy fats, protein, and minerals.

Simultaneously, eliminate the industrial products that emerged during the low-fat era: margarine and vegetable shortening that contain harmful trans fats; processed "vegetable" oils like soybean, corn, canola, and cottonseed oil that are high in inflammatory omega-6 fatty acids; low-fat processed foods that compensate for removed fat with added sugars and artificial ingredients; and any products containing trans fats or partially hydrogenated oils.

Focus your eating on whole, unprocessed foods: quality proteins from both animal and plant sources; non-starchy vegetables that provide fiber, vitamins, and minerals; full-fat dairy products from grass-fed sources when tolerated; fruits in moderation; and properly prepared grains and legumes if they agree with your digestive system.

Individual Considerations

While the general principle of embracing natural fats applies broadly, individual factors can influence optimal implementation. Some people carry genetic variants, such as ApoE4, that may require moderation of saturated fat intake while still avoiding processed alternatives[40]. Those with existing heart disease, familial hypercholesterolemia, or other medical conditions should work with knowledgeable healthcare providers to optimize their approach based on their specific circumstances.

Regular monitoring of comprehensive biomarkers can guide individual optimization. This includes advanced lipid panels that measure particle size and number rather than just total cholesterol, inflammatory markers like C-reactive protein and IL-6, and metabolic markers including fasting insulin, glucose, and HbA1c. These tests provide a much clearer picture of metabolic health than the simplistic cholesterol measurements that dominated previous decades.

The Path Forward

The fat myth wasn't just a scientific mistake—it was a cautionary tale about how institutional momentum, industry influence, and oversimplified public health messaging can override scientific rigor and common sense. We've spent six decades running from foods that sustained human health for millennia while embracing processed alternatives that contributed to unprecedented rates of chronic disease.

The evidence is now overwhelming: natural fats aren't the enemy we were taught to fear. They're essential components of a healthy diet that support hormone production, brain function, cellular health, and metabolic stability. The real threats to our health are the refined carbohydrates, industrial oils, and ultra-processed foods that filled the void when we removed natural fats from our diets.

This doesn't mean that all fats are identical in their health effects, or that individual optimization and medical supervision aren't important for some people. But it does mean we can stop fearing the butter, eggs, and fatty fish that our ancestors consumed while turning our attention to the genuinely problematic foods that emerged during the low-fat era.

The choice before us is clear: we can continue following dietary advice that coincided with the worst epidemic of chronic disease in human history, or we can return to the traditional foods that supported human health and vitality for generations. The science now supports what our great-grandparents knew intuitively—that natural, whole foods, including their natural fats, are the foundation of health.

Your body, your metabolism, and your long-term health will thank you for making the right choice.

The systematic demonization of natural fats didn't just eliminate butter and lard from American kitchens—it eliminated generations of nutritional wisdom. But your body still remembers what real nourishment feels like. When you eat natural fats, you feel satisfied. When you avoid them, you stay hungry no matter how much you eat.

Nature abhors a vacuum, and the food industry rushed to fill the void left by traditional fats with alternatives that would prove far more harmful than the foods they replaced. That story—and how those alternatives infiltrated every corner of our food supply—comes next.

References

1. Hales CM, Carroll MD, Fryar CD, Ogden CL. Prevalence of obesity and severe obesity among adults: United States, 2017–2018. *NCHS Data Brief*. 2020;(360):1–8.

2. Keys A, ed. *Coronary heart disease in seven countries.* Circulation. 1970;41(Suppl 1):1–211.

3. Teicholz N. *The Big Fat Surprise: Why Butter, Meat and Cheese Belong in a Healthy Diet.* New York, NY: Simon & Schuster; 2014.

4. Yerushalmy J, Hilleboe HE. Fat in the diet and mortality from heart disease; a methodologic note. *N Y State J Med*. 1957;57(14):2343–2354.

5. Time Magazine. Diet and Heart Disease: Eating to Live. Cover Story. January 13, 1961.

6. American Heart Association. Dietary fat and its relation to heart attacks and strokes. *Circulation*. 1961;23:133–136.

7. U.S. Senate Select Committee on Nutrition and Human Needs. *Dietary Goals for the United States.* 2nd ed. Washington, DC: U.S. Government Printing Office; 1977.

8. U.S. Department of Agriculture and U.S. Department of Health and Human Services. *Dietary Guidelines for Americans, 1980.* Washington,

DC: U.S. Government Printing Office; 1980.

9. Yudkin J. *Pure, White and Deadly*. London: Davis-Poynter; 1972.

10. Parker-Pope T. A high price for healthy food. *Wall Street Journal*. December 5, 2003.

11. Mozaffarian D, Katan MB, Ascherio A, et al. Trans fatty acids and cardiovascular disease. *N Engl J Med*. 2006;354(15):1601–1613. doi:10.1056/NEJMra054035

12. Austin GL, Ogden LG, Hill JO. Trends in carbohydrate, fat, and protein intakes and association with energy intake in normal-weight, overweight, and obese individuals: 1971–2006. *Am J Clin Nutr*. 2011;93(4):836–843. doi:10.3945/ajcn.110.005782

13. Centers for Disease Control and Prevention. Adult Obesity Facts. Updated September 30, 2022. Accessed September 9, 2025. https://www.cdc.gov/obesity/data/adult.html

14. National Commission on Diabetes. *The Long-Range Plan to Combat Diabetes*. Washington, DC: U.S. Department of Health, Education, and Welfare; 1975.

15. Centers for Disease Control and Prevention. *National Diabetes Statistics Report, 2022*. Atlanta, GA: CDC, US Department of Health and Human Services; 2022.

16. Younossi ZM, Koenig AB, Abdelatif D, et al. Global epidemiology of nonalcoholic fatty liver disease—meta-analytic assessment of prevalence, incidence, and outcomes. *Hepatology*. 2016;64(1):73–84. doi:10.1002/hep.28431

17. Centers for Disease Control and Prevention. Heart Disease Facts. Updated July 15, 2022. Accessed September 9, 2025. https://www.cdc.gov/heartdisease/facts.htm

18. Dehghan M, Mente A, Zhang X, et al. Associations of fats and carbo-

hydrate intake with cardiovascular disease and mortality in 18 countries from five continents (PURE): a prospective cohort study. *Lancet.* 2017;390(10107):2050–2062. doi:10.1016/S0140-6736(17)32252-3

19. Siri-Tarino PW, Sun Q, Hu FB, Krauss RM. Meta-analysis of prospective cohort studies evaluating the association of saturated fat with cardiovascular disease. *Am J Clin Nutr.* 2010;91(3):535–546. doi:10.3945/ajcn.2009.27725

20. Chowdhury R, Warnakula S, Kunutsor S, et al. Association of dietary, circulating, and supplement fatty acids with coronary risk: a systematic review and meta-analysis. *Ann Intern Med.* 2014;160(6):398–406. doi:10.7326/M13-1788

21. Hooper L, Martin N, Jimoh OF, Kirk C, Foster E, Abdelhamid AS. Reduction in saturated fat intake for cardiovascular disease. *Cochrane Database Syst Rev.* 2020;8(8):CD011737. doi:10.1002/14651858.CD011737.pub2

22. Aramburu A, Dolores-Maldonado G, Curi-Quinto K, et al. Effect of reducing saturated fat intake on cardiovascular disease in adults: an umbrella review. *Front Public Health.* 2024;12:1396576. doi:10.3389/fpubh.2024.1396576

23. Yamada T, Takeuchi M, Ishikawa Y, et al. Saturated fat restriction for cardiovascular disease prevention: a systematic review and meta-analysis of randomized controlled trials. *JMA J.* 2024;7(4):524–536. doi:10.31662/jmaj.2024-0324

24. Astrup A, Teicholz N, Magkos F, et al. Dietary saturated fats and health: are the U.S. guidelines evidence-based? *Am J Clin Nutr.* 2024;119(2):364–371. doi:10.3390/nu13103305

25. Krauss RM. Lipoprotein subfractions and cardiovascular disease risk. *Curr Opin Lipidol.* 2010;21(4):305–311. doi:10.1097/MOL.0b013e32833ac1e9

26. Siri-Tarino PW, Chiu S, Bergeron N, Krauss RM. Saturated fats versus polyunsaturated fats versus carbohydrates for cardiovascular disease prevention and treatment. *Annu Rev Nutr.* 2015;35:517–543. doi:10.1146/annurev-nutr-071714-034457

27. Cromwell WC, Otvos JD, Keyes MJ, et al. LDL particle number and risk of future cardiovascular disease in the Framingham Offspring Study—implications for LDL management. *J Clin Lipidol.* 2007;1(6):583–592. doi:10.1016/S1933-2874(15)00079-X

28. Ho KJ, Mikkelson B, Lewis LA, et al. Alaskan Arctic Eskimo: responses to a customary high fat diet. *Am J Clin Nutr.* 1972;25(8):737–745. doi:10.1093/ajcn/25.8.737

29. Mann GV, Shaffer RD, Anderson RS, Sandstead HH. Cardiovascular disease in the Masai. *J Atheroscler Res.* 1964;4:289–312. doi:10.1016/S0021-9150(64)80039-2

30. Keys A, Menotti A, Karvonen MJ, et al. The diet and 15-year death rate in the Seven Countries Study. *Am J Epidemiol.* 1986;124(6):903–915. doi:10.1093/oxfordjournals.aje.a114426

31. Thompson RC, Allam AH, Lombardi GP, et al. Atherosclerosis across 4000 years of human history: the Horus study of four ancient populations. *Lancet.* 2013;381(9873):1211–1212. doi:10.1016/S0140-6736(13)60534-X

32. Helms ER, Aragon AA, Fitschen PJ. Evidence-based recommendations for natural bodybuilding contest preparation: nutrition and supplementation. *J Int Soc Sports Nutr.* 2014;11:20. doi:10.1186/1550-2783-11-20

33. Freeman MP, Hibbeln JR, Wisner KL, et al. Omega-3 fatty acids: evidence basis for treatment and future research in psychiatry. *J Clin Psychiatry.* 2010;71(12):1397–1409. doi:10.4088/JCP.10r06149

34. Calder PC. Functional roles of fatty acids and their effects on human

health. *JPEN J Parenter Enteral Nutr.* 2015;39(1 Suppl):18S–32S. doi:10.1177/0148607114550188

35. Shearer MJ, Fu X, Booth SL. Vitamin K nutrition, metabolism, and requirements: current concepts and future research. *Adv Nutr.* 2012;3(2):182–195. doi:10.3945/an.111.001784

36. Acheson KJ, Flatt JP, Jéquier E. Glycogen synthesis versus lipogenesis after a 500 gram carbohydrate meal in man. *Metabolism.* 1982;31(12):1234–1240. doi:10.1016/0026-0495(82)90155-4

37. Ludwig DS, Hu FB, Tappy L, Brand-Miller J. Dietary carbohydrates: role of quality and quantity in chronic disease. *BMJ.* 2018;361:k2340. doi:10.1136/bmj.k2340

38. DiNicolantonio JJ, O'Keefe JH. Omega-6 vegetable oils as a driver of coronary heart disease: the oxidized linoleic acid hypothesis. *Open Heart.* 2018;5(2):e000898. doi:10.1136/openhrt-2018-000898

39. Monteiro CA, Cannon G, Moubarac JC, et al. Ultra-processed products are becoming dominant in the global food system. *Obes Rev.* 2013;14 Suppl 2:21–28. doi:10.1111/obr.12062

40. Corbo RM, Scacchi R. Apolipoprotein E (APOE) allele distribution in the world. Is APOE*4 a "thrifty" allele? *Ann Hum Genet.* 1999;63(Pt 4):301–310. doi:10.1046/j.1469-1809.1999.6340301.x

Chapter Five

The Seed Oil Myth

How Industrial Waste Became "Heart-Healthy" Food

Walk down any grocery aisle, and you'll find them everywhere---hidden in plain sight. Soybean oil in your salad dressing. Canola oil in your granola bars. Corn oil in your mayonnaise. These industrial seed oils have become so ubiquitous in our food supply that most people consume them multiple times daily without realizing it.

For decades, we've been told these oils are heart-healthy alternatives to saturated fats. Health authorities encouraged us to swap butter for margarine, replace lard with vegetable oil, and trust that these modern fats would protect our cardiovascular system. The messaging was consistent and persuasive: choose vegetable oils for better health.

But there's a problem with this story. These aren't traditional fats that humans have consumed for millennia. They're industrial products---byproducts of agriculture and manufacturing that were transformed through clever marketing into dietary staples. The rise of seed oils in our food supply represents one of the most dramatic nutritional experiments in human history, conducted without our informed consent.

The correlation is striking: as seed oil consumption has skyrocketed over the past century, so have rates of chronic diseases once considered rare. Heart disease, obesity, diabetes, autoimmune disorders, and neurodegenerative conditions have reached epidemic proportions in developed nations. While correlation doesn't prove causation, emerging research suggests these industrial oils may be far from the benign---or beneficial---substances we've been led to believe.

The Industrial Origins of Our "Vegetable" Oils

The story of seed oils begins not in a kitchen or a farm, but in the cotton fields and factories of the late 19th century. After cotton fibers were harvested, farmers faced a disposal problem: mountains of leftover cottonseeds that seemed to have no useful purpose. The oil extracted from these seeds was unstable, rancid-smelling, and unsuitable for human consumption. For years, cottonseed oil found its primary use in soap manufacturing and industrial lubricants.

Everything changed in 1907 when Procter & Gamble discovered how to chemically transform this industrial waste through hydrogenation. By forcing hydrogen atoms into the oil's molecular structure under high heat and pressure, they created a solid, shelf-stable fat that wouldn't spoil quickly. They called their invention Crisco---short for "crystallized cottonseed oil."[1]

The marketing campaign that followed was revolutionary. Rather than advertising an industrial byproduct, Procter & Gamble positioned Crisco as a modern, clean, and pure alternative to traditional animal fats. They hired nutritionists, published cookbooks, and even gave away free samples to housewives across America. By 1911, this former industrial waste was flying off grocery store shelves, and the seed oil revolution had begun.[1]

The success of Crisco opened the floodgates for other industrial oils. Wesson Oil, another cottonseed oil product, faced a marketing challenge---"cottonseed oil" didn't sound particularly appetizing to consumers. Their solution was brilliant in its simplicity: rebrand it as "vegetable oil." Never mind that cottonseed had nothing to do with vegetables people actually ate. The name stuck, and millions of consumers began purchasing what they believed were garden-fresh oils from factory production lines.[1]

How Seed Oils Are Made

1. Seed Collection & Cleaning
Seeds are harvested and cleaned of dirt and debris; agricultural **chemical residues may remain.**

2. Mechanical Pressing (Initial Extraction)
Seeds are crushed to squeeze out some oil; the leftover **oilcake** still holds a lot of oil.

3. Solvent Extraction (Chemical Stripping)
Oilcake is washed with **hexane** — *a petroleum-derived solvent used to dissolve oil from seed meal.* It's later boiled off, though **trace residues can remain.**

4. Degumming
Hot water/steam or acid removes **phospholipids, gums, and waxes** that make oil cloudy/unstable.

5. Neutralizing (Caustic Treatment)
Sodium hydroxide (lye) neutralizes free fatty acids to reduce rancidity.

6. Bleaching
Oil is filtered through **bleaching clay/activated carbon** to remove pigments and oxidation products — also strips natural antioxidants.

7. Deodorizing
Heated to **~450°F (232°C)** under vacuum to remove odors/tastes; this can form **some trans fats** and other **oxidation byproducts**.

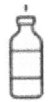
8. Packaging & Marketing
Clear, odorless liquid is bottled and marketed as "heart-healthy."

As industrial agriculture expanded throughout the 20th century, new sources of cheap oils emerged. Corn oil became a profitable byproduct of corn starch and syrup production. Soybean oil, once used primarily in paints, varnishes, and lubricants, found its way into the food supply during wartime shortages when traditional fats were rationed. Companies discovered they could extract oil from virtually any seed or grain, process it into a neutral-tasting liquid, and market it as a healthy cooking medium.

Perhaps the most audacious transformation was that of rapeseed oil. Traditional rapeseed contained high levels of erucic acid, a compound linked to heart damage in animal studies. In the 1970s, Canadian scientists developed a low-erucic variety and gave it a more appealing name: "canola," standing for "Canadian oil, low acid." Through selective breeding and clever marketing, a potentially toxic industrial oil became a kitchen staple promoted by nutritionists worldwide.

The pattern was consistent across all these oils: industrial waste or byproducts were refined, processed, deodorized, and marketed as modern improvements over traditional fats. None of these oils existed in meaningful quantities in the human diet before the 20th century. They were born from industrial convenience and economic opportunity, not nutritional wisdom.

The Perfect Marketing Storm

The transformation of industrial seed oils into dietary staples required more than just clever naming. It demanded a fundamental shift in how people thought about fat and health---a shift that would be orchestrated through decades of marketing campaigns, flawed research, and institutional endorsements.

The rise of margarine illustrates this process perfectly. Originally made from beef tallow, margarine was reformulated using hydrogenated seed oils to reduce costs. Early versions were so obviously artificial that laws in many states required it to be dyed pink to distinguish it from real butter---a warning to consumers about its unnatural origins. But as anti-saturated fat sentiment grew in the mid-20th century, margarine's industrial origins were forgotten, and it was rebranded as a heart-healthy alternative to butter.[1]

The food industry's timing was impeccable. As concerns about heart disease mounted in the 1950s and 1960s, seed oils were positioned as the solution. The hypothesis that saturated fats caused heart disease---though still debated among scientists---became nutritional dogma. Seed oils, being mostly unsaturated, were cast as the heroes in this narrative. Never mind that these oils underwent extensive industrial processing, contained novel fatty acid compositions, or had never been consumed by humans in significant quantities throughout evolutionary history.

Institutional endorsements followed. Medical associations, government agencies, and nutrition organizations began recommending vegetable oils as part of a heart-healthy diet. These recommendations carried tremendous weight with both healthcare providers and the public. When respected institutions spoke with one voice about the benefits of seed oils, few questioned the underlying evidence or the potential conflicts of interest.

The McDonald's french fry scandal of 1990 exemplifies how this narrative played out in practice. For decades, McDonald's had cooked their famous fries in beef tallow, which gave them their distinctive flavor and texture. But under pressure from activists warning about saturated fat, the company switched to hydrogenated vegetable oils. The irony was profound: in attempting to make their fries "healthier" by eliminating saturated fat, McDonald's introduced trans fats---industrial fats now recognized as far more dangerous than anything they replaced.[2]

Restaurant chains and food manufacturers embraced seed oils for reasons beyond health marketing. These oils were cheap, had long shelf lives, and could withstand the high-heat processing required for mass food production. The economic incentives aligned perfectly with the health messaging, creating a powerful force that would reshape the entire food system.

The Biochemical Reality

While marketing departments promoted seed oils as heart-healthy alternatives, researchers began uncovering troubling evidence about what these oils actually do inside the human body. The story they discovered bears little resemblance to the benign or beneficial narrative promoted by the food industry.

The primary concern centers on linoleic acid, an omega-6 fatty acid that comprises 50-80% of most seed oils. While linoleic acid is technically an essential fatty acid---meaning our bodies can't manufacture it and must obtain it from food---the amounts found in seed oils far exceed anything humans encountered throughout evolutionary history. Traditional diets contained linoleic acid in small quantities from nuts, seeds, and small amounts in animal products. Today's seed oil consumption provides 10-20 times these ancestral levels.

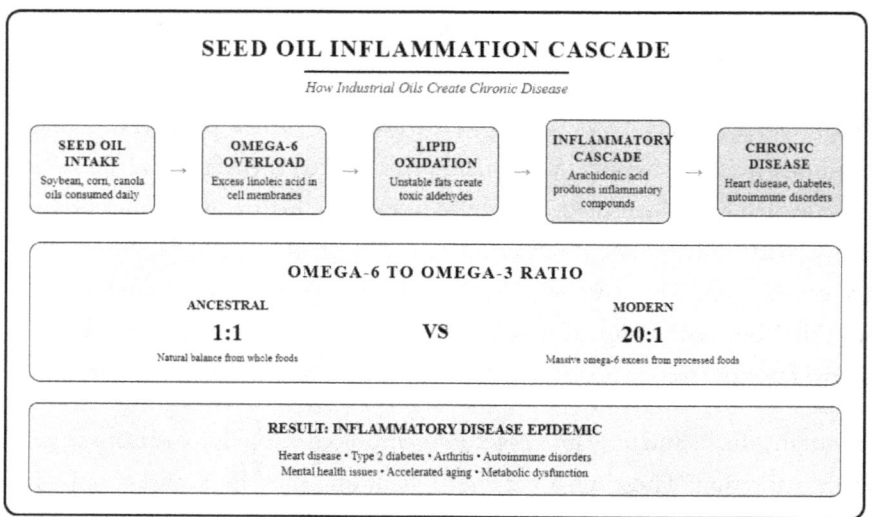

This massive increase in linoleic acid intake creates a cascade of biological problems. Unlike stable saturated fats, linoleic acid is highly susceptible to oxidation when exposed to heat, light, or oxygen---conditions routinely encountered during cooking and food processing. When linoleic acid oxidizes, it forms toxic compounds called aldehydes, including 4-hydroxynonenal (4-HNE), which has been linked to cellular damage, inflammation, and disease progression.[3,4]

The oxidation problem is compounded by how these oils are processed. Seed oil extraction involves high heat, chemical solvents, deodorization, and bleaching---processes that create oxidized fats before the oils even reach store shelves. Unlike traditional fat sources like butter or olive oil, which can be produced through simple mechanical pressing, seed oils require industrial processing to become edible.

Recent longitudinal research has strengthened concerns about seed oil consumption. The Sydney Diet Heart Study, a randomized controlled trial that followed participants for seven years, found that replacing saturated fats with linoleic acid-rich vegetable oils actually increased deaths from heart disease and all causes.[5] This finding directly contradicted the theoretical benefits that had been promoted for decades.

A 2019 analysis of the Framingham Heart Study data revealed that people with higher tissue levels of linoleic acid had increased rates of coronary artery disease, even after controlling for other cardiovascular risk factors.[6] The researchers noted that this association was independent of traditional risk factors like cholesterol levels, blood pressure, and smoking status.

More recently, a 2023 study published in *Circulation* examined the relationship between cooking oil consumption and cardiovascular outcomes in over 100,000 participants. The study found that frequent use of vegetable oils for cooking was associated with increased risk of cardiovascular events, while use of olive oil showed protective effects.[7]

Once consumed, excess linoleic acid becomes incorporated into cell membranes throughout the body, including those of vital organs like the heart and brain. This changes the physical properties of cellular membranes, making them more fragile and susceptible to damage.[8] When these linoleic acid-rich membranes are exposed to oxidative stress---which occurs constantly in normal metabolism---they produce inflammatory compounds that can trigger immune responses and tissue damage.

The mitochondria, often called the powerhouses of our cells, are particularly vulnerable to this process. These cellular structures are responsible for producing the energy that powers every biological function. When mitochondrial membranes become loaded with unstable fatty acids from seed oils, their efficiency declines, leading to reduced energy production and increased production of damaging free radicals.[9]

Research has also revealed how seed oils disrupt hormonal signaling, particularly the hormones that regulate hunger and satiety. Studies suggest that high linoleic acid intake can interfere with leptin sensitivity, making it harder for people to recognize when they're full and contributing to overeating and weight gain.[8] This may help explain why obesity rates have climbed alongside seed oil consumption.

Perhaps most concerning is the impact on the omega-6 to omega-3 fatty acid ratio. Traditional human diets maintained roughly equal amounts of these two fatty acid families, with ratios near 1:1 or 2:1. Today's seed oil-heavy diets can push this ratio to 10:1, 20:1, or even higher.[10] This imbalance promotes inflammation, as omega-6 fatty acids tend to produce pro-inflammatory compounds while omega-3s generate anti-inflammatory substances.[11]

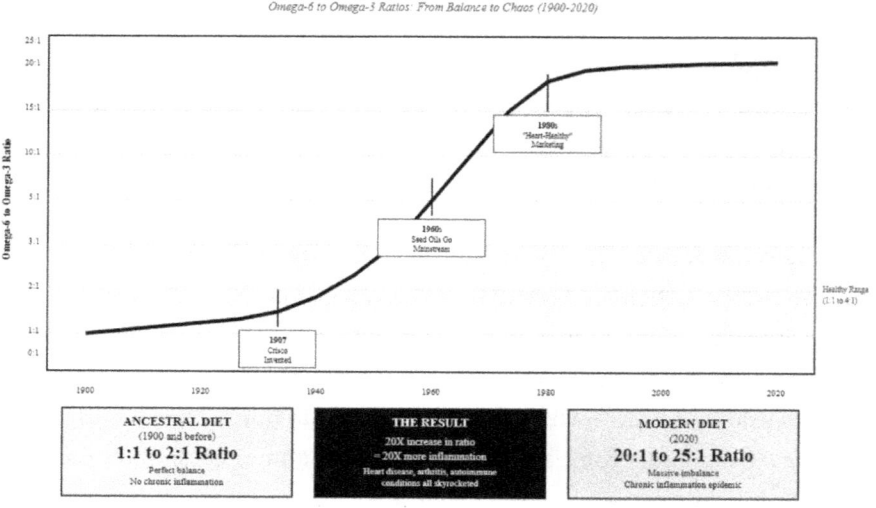

The Correlation We Can't Ignore

While establishing direct causation between dietary changes and disease patterns is challenging, the timeline of seed oil adoption and chronic disease emergence presents a compelling correlation that deserves serious consideration.

Heart disease provides perhaps the most striking example. Often called a "disease of civilization," heart attacks were so rare in the early 1900s that they barely appeared in medical literature. As seed oil consumption increased throughout the 20th century, heart disease rates climbed dramatically, eventually becoming the leading cause of death in developed nations. This occurred despite---or perhaps because of---widespread adoption of low-saturated fat, high-seed oil diets promoted as heart-healthy.

The obesity epidemic follows a similar pattern. Obesity rates remained relatively stable throughout most of human history, even during periods of abundance. The dramatic rise in obesity began in the 1970s and 1980s, coinciding with increased processed food consumption and the widespread replacement of traditional fats with seed oils in both home cooking and food manufacturing.

Diabetes rates tell a parallel story. Type 2 diabetes, once called "adult-onset diabetes" because it rarely occurred before middle age, now affects millions of children and young adults. The timeline of this epidemic corresponds closely with the industrialization of the food supply and the dominance of seed oil-based processed foods.

Perhaps most troubling is the rise in neurodegenerative diseases. Alzheimer's disease, sometimes called "type 3 diabetes" due to its association with insulin resistance, has become increasingly common as populations have aged. The brain, composed largely of fatty acids, may be particularly vulnerable to the oxidative damage caused by excess linoleic acid consumption.[12]

Autoimmune diseases present another concerning pattern. Conditions like multiple sclerosis, rheumatoid arthritis, and inflammatory bowel disease have increased dramatically in developed nations while remaining rare in populations consuming traditional diets low in processed foods and seed oils.[13]

These correlations don't prove that seed oils directly cause these diseases---chronic conditions typically result from multiple factors including genetics, lifestyle, environmental exposures, but also acknowledging that multiple dietary and lifestyle factors changed simultaneously during this period. However, the consistency of these patterns across different diseases and populations suggests that our massive dietary experiment with industrial oils may have unintended consequences that we're only beginning to understand.

The Path Forward

Recognizing the potential problems with seed oils is only the first step. The challenge lies in navigating a food system that has been built around these industrial oils over the past century. They're not just in obviously processed foods---they're hidden in restaurant meals, salad dressings, supposedly healthy snacks, and even baby formulas.

The most effective strategy begins with returning to traditional fats that humans have consumed safely for millennia. Butter, ghee, tallow, lard, and coconut oil all have long histories of human consumption and remain stable when heated. Extra virgin olive oil, while more susceptible to heat damage than saturated fats, has been consumed for thousands of years and offers well-documented health benefits when used appropriately.

How Traditional Fats Are Made

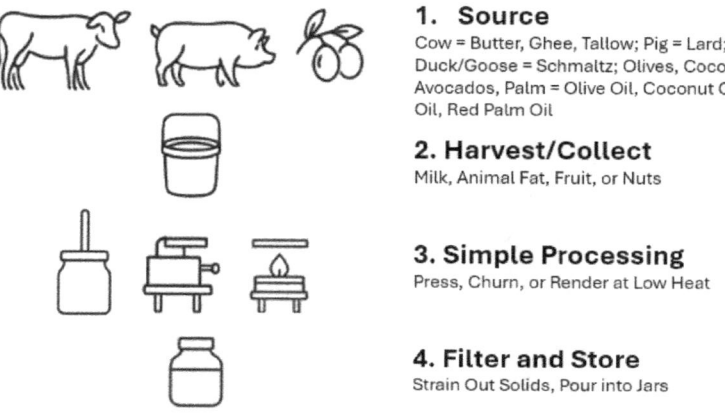

1. Source
Cow = Butter, Ghee, Tallow; Pig = Lard; Duck/Goose = Schmaltz; Olives, Coconuts, Avocados, Palm = Olive Oil, Coconut Oil, Avocado Oil, Red Palm Oil

2. Harvest/Collect
Milk, Animal Fat, Fruit, or Nuts

3. Simple Processing
Press, Churn, or Render at Low Heat

4. Filter and Store
Strain Out Solids, Pour into Jars

No Chemicals. No bleaching. No Extreme Heat. Just Food.

Reading ingredient labels becomes crucial in a seed oil-saturated food environment. Terms like "vegetable oil," "canola oil," "soybean oil," "corn oil," "cottonseed oil," "safflower oil," and "sunflower oil" indicate the presence of these industrial products. Even foods marketed as healthy---organic crackers, protein bars, salad dressings---often contain seed oils as primary ingredients.

Restaurant dining presents particular challenges, as most commercial kitchens rely heavily on seed oils for cost and convenience reasons. Some establishments will accommodate requests to cook food in butter or olive oil, but this requires asking specifically. Fast-casual and fine dining restaurants are generally more flexible than fast food chains, which typically have standardized cooking procedures that rely on seed oils.

Home cooking becomes an act of empowerment in this context. When you prepare meals from whole ingredients using traditional fats, you regain control over what enters your body. This doesn't require elaborate culinary skills---simple preparations using quality ingredients often produce the most nourishing and satisfying results.

The transition away from seed oils often brings unexpected benefits that extend beyond avoiding potential harm. Many people report improved energy levels, better skin health, reduced joint inflammation, and easier weight management when they eliminate these industrial oils from their diets. While individual experiences vary, these reports suggest that our bodies may indeed be poorly adapted to processing large quantities of these modern fats.

Reclaiming Food Wisdom

The seed oil story reveals something profound about how quickly fundamental aspects of human nutrition can change when industrial interests align with flawed scientific theories and aggressive marketing. In just a few generations, foods that had never existed in human diets became dietary staples, promoted by the very institutions people trusted to protect their health.

This transformation occurred not because new research revealed the superiority of industrial oils, but because they solved problems for food manufacturers: they were cheap, shelf-stable, and could be produced in massive quantities. The health narrative came later, built on preliminary research and theoretical frameworks that subsequent decades of investigation have called into question.

Traditional food cultures developed over thousands of years, refined through countless generations of trial and error. They emerged from the accumulated wisdom of people who understood that food is medicine, and that what we eat directly impacts how we feel, how we age, and how we die. These cultures didn't have randomized controlled trials or biochemical analyses, but they had something perhaps more valuable: time and evolutionary pressure to identify what truly nourished human health.

The industrialization of our food supply has brought many benefits---improved food safety, reduced spoilage, greater convenience, and lower costs. But it has also introduced novel substances into human diets on a scale and timeline that makes careful evaluation difficult. We are, in effect, conducting a massive uncontrolled experiment on ourselves and our children.

Questioning the safety and benefits of seed oils doesn't require rejecting all aspects of food technology or returning to a romanticized pre-industrial past. It simply means applying appropriate skepticism to dramatic dietary changes that occurred for primarily economic rather than nutritional reasons. It means recognizing that the human body evolved consuming certain types of fats and may not be well-adapted to processing the large quantities of highly processed oils that now dominate our food supply.

The power to change this situation lies not with government agencies, medical institutions, or food companies, but with individual consumers making informed choices about what they purchase and consume. Every meal represents an opportunity to vote with your fork for the kind of food system you want to support.

The path forward isn't about perfect adherence to any particular dietary doctrine, but rather about awareness, gradual change, and rediscovering the nourishing power of traditional foods prepared with care and attention. It's about recognizing that the most fundamental act of self-care may be choosing foods that have sustained human health for millennia over industrial products that have existed for barely a century.

In a food environment dominated by marketing messages and conflicting nutrition advice, perhaps the wisest approach is the simplest: eat foods that your great-grandmother would recognize, prepared in ways that humans have used for thousands of years. This isn't about nostalgia---it's about biological reality and the recognition that some aspects of traditional wisdom deserve preservation in our modern world.

The Future of Fat

The tide is slowly turning against seed oils as more researchers, physicians, and consumers recognize the mounting evidence of their potential harm. Some restaurants are beginning to advertise "cooked in beef tallow" or "prepared with real butter" as selling points. Health-conscious consumers are seeking out products made with traditional fats. Even some food manufacturers are quietly reformulating products to remove the most problematic oils.

But institutional change is slow, and economic incentives remain powerful. Seed oils are still cheap, shelf-stable, and profitable. The infrastructure built around them over the past century won't disappear overnight. Changing course requires consumer demand, regulatory updates, and a fundamental shift in how we think about fat and health.

The encouraging news is that individual change is immediate and powerful. You don't need to wait for institutions to catch up or for regulations to change. You can start making different choices today, and your body will respond accordingly. Many people notice improvements in energy, skin health, joint comfort, and overall well-being within weeks of eliminating seed oils and returning to traditional fats.

Making the Transition

If you're ready to reduce or eliminate seed oils from your diet, here's a practical approach:

Start by reading labels obsessively. Seed oils hide in unexpected places: packaged nuts, protein bars, salad dressings, mayonnaise, crackers, and even products labeled "natural" or "organic." The only way to avoid them is to know where they lurk.

Clean out your pantry gradually. Replace seed oil-containing products as you run out, rather than throwing everything away at once. This makes the transition more affordable and less overwhelming.

Learn to cook with traditional fats. Butter, ghee, coconut oil, and olive oil each have different properties and optimal uses. Experiment with them to discover your preferences and learn their cooking characteristics.

Find restaurants that accommodate your preferences. Many establishments will cook your food in butter or olive oil if you ask. Build relationships with restaurants that understand and respect your dietary choices.

Prepare for social situations. When eating at friends' houses or attending events, offer to bring a dish prepared with traditional fats, or eat beforehand and focus on socializing rather than the food.

Be patient with your taste buds. If you've been consuming seed oils for years, your palate may need time to adjust to the flavors of traditional fats. What might taste strange initially often becomes preferred with time.

Focus on whole foods. The easiest way to avoid seed oils is to eat foods that don't come in packages: fresh vegetables, fruits, quality meats, fish, eggs, and dairy. When most of your diet consists of whole foods, the occasional seed oil exposure becomes much less significant.

The Bigger Picture: Food as Medicine

The seed oil story is really a story about how we've forgotten that food is medicine. Every meal is an opportunity to either nourish or harm your body. The industrial food system has convinced us that convenience, shelf life, and cost are more important than the biological effects of what we consume.

Traditional cultures understood intuitively what we're now proving scientifically: that the quality and source of our food matters enormously for health. They didn't choose fats based on marketing claims or laboratory theories. They used what was available locally, what had sustained their ancestors, and what made them feel strong and healthy.

Returning to traditional fats isn't about rejecting all aspects of modernity or embracing a romanticized past. It's about recognizing that some innovations represent genuine improvements while others are steps backward disguised as progress. Seed oils fall firmly in the latter category: they solved problems for food manufacturers while creating new problems for human health.

The choice before us is clear: we can continue supporting a food system that prioritizes profit over health, or we can reclaim our right to nourishing food that supports our biological needs. We can accept the industrial oils that were never meant for human consumption, or we can return to the traditional fats that sustained our ancestors for thousands of years.

Your body knows the difference between industrial seed oils and traditional fats, even if your conscious mind has been convinced they're equivalent. When you eliminate the inflammatory, oxidized fats and replace them with stable, nourishing alternatives, your cells respond with improved function, reduced inflammation, and better overall health.

The seed oil experiment has been running for over a century now, and the results are clear: it failed. Rates of heart disease, obesity, diabetes, and inflammatory conditions have skyrocketed alongside seed oil consumption. It's time to end this experiment and return to the foods that actually support human health.

The power to make this change lies in your hands, in your shopping cart, and on your plate. Every meal is a choice between industrial manipulation and ancestral wisdom, between corporate profits and personal health, between continuing the failed experiment and reclaiming your biological birthright.

Choose wisely. Your body will thank you.

References

1. Minger D. Death by Food Pyramid. Malibu, CA: Primal Blueprint Publishing; 2014.

2. Enig MG. *Know Your Fats.* Silver Spring, MD: Bethesda Press; 2000.

3. Ramsden CE, Zamora D, Leelarthaepin B, et al. Use of dietary linoleic acid for secondary prevention of coronary heart disease and death: evaluation of recovered data from the Sydney Diet Heart Study and updated meta-analysis. *BMJ.* 2013;346:e8707. doi:10.1136/bmj.e8707

4. Zárate R, El Jaber-Vazdekis N, Tejera N, Pérez JA, Rodríguez C. 4-Hydroxynonenal: a marker of oxidative stress in neurodegenerative diseases. *Curr Alzheimer Res.* 2017;14(5):474-479. doi:10.2174/1567205013666160930110553

5. Ramsden CE, Zamora D, Majchrzak-Hong S, et al. Re-evaluation of the traditional diet-heart hypothesis: analysis of recovered data from the Minnesota Coronary Experiment (1968-73). *BMJ.* 2016;353:i1246. doi:10.1136/bmj.i1246

6. Harris WS, Tintle NL, Imamura F, et al. Blood n-3 fatty acid levels

and total and cause-specific mortality from 17 prospective studies. *Nat Commun.* 2021;12(1):2329. doi:10.1038/s41467-021-22370-2

7. Guasch-Ferré M, Li Y, Willett WC, et al. Consumption of olive oil and risk of total and cause-specific mortality among US adults. *J Am Coll Cardiol.* 2022;79(2):101-112. doi:10.1016/j.jacc.2021.10.041

8. Hulbert AJ. Membrane fatty acids as pacemakers of animal metabolism. *Lipids.* 2007;42(9):811-819. doi:10.1007/s11745-007-3058-0

9. Wallace DC. A mitochondrial paradigm of metabolic and degenerative diseases, aging, and cancer: a dawn for evolutionary medicine. *Annu Rev Genet.* 2005;39:359-407. doi:10.1146/annurev.genet.39.110304.095751

10. Simopoulos AP. The importance of the omega-6/omega-3 fatty acid ratio in cardiovascular disease and inflammatory diseases. *Exp Biol Med (Maywood).* 2008;233(6):674-688. doi:10.3181/0711-MR-311

11. Bazinet RP, Layé S. Polyunsaturated fatty acids and their metabolites in brain function and disease. *Nat Rev Neurosci.* 2014;15(12):771-785. doi:10.1038/nrn3820

12. Morris MC, Evans DA, Bienias JL, et al. Dietary fats and the risk of incident Alzheimer disease. *Arch Neurol.* 2003;60(2):194-200. doi:10.1001/archneur.60.2.194

13. Hotamisligil GS. Inflammation and metabolic disorders. *Nature.* 2006;444(7121):860-867. doi:10.1038/nature05485

Chapter Six

The Calorie Myth

How We Got It All Wrong

The Simple Story That Failed Spectacularly

For decades, we've been told a simple story about weight and health that sounds scientific, feels logical, and promises easy solutions. The story goes like this: calories are calories, weight is simple math, and if you want to lose weight, you just need to burn more than you eat. It doesn't matter whether those calories come from sugar, fat, protein, vegetables, soda, or donuts—your body supposedly treats them all the same. Energy in, energy out.

This message has been hammered into us by doctors, dietitians, governments, and weight loss companies for generations. We've been told to track our calories, eat "low calorie" foods, and exercise more to "burn it off." Count every bite, measure every portion, and calculate your way to health. The approach feels scientific because it involves numbers, and it sounds simple because it reduces the complexity of human metabolism to basic arithmetic.

And it failed spectacularly.

The calorie-counting model of health and weight loss didn't save us from obesity and metabolic disease. Instead, it made us heavier, sicker, hungrier, and more confused about how our bodies actually work. We weren't dealing with an energy math problem, as we'd been led to believe. We were dealing with a hormonal and metabolic problem—and decades of well-intentioned but fundamentally flawed science led us astray.

The most devastating aspect of the calorie myth wasn't just that it didn't work—it was that it blamed individuals for the failure of the system. When people followed calorie-restricted diets and failed to maintain weight loss, they were told they lacked willpower, discipline, or commitment. The possibility that the fundamental approach was wrong was never seriously considered by the mainstream health establishment.

The Birth of an Obsession

To understand how we became trapped in this numerical prison, we need to go back to where it all began. The idea of "calories in, calories out" traces its roots to the 19th century, when early scientists began studying heat and energy in food using the principles of thermodynamics.

In 1890, American chemist Wilbur Atwater developed what became known as the "Atwater system," which estimated the energy content of food based on how much heat it produced when burned in a device called a bomb calorimeter[1]. This approach worked well for understanding combustion in machines and laboratory settings, but it contained a fundamental flaw: human beings are not machines, and eating is not combustion.

Atwater himself was trying to help laborers and the poor maximize energy from food during a time of economic hardship—a noble goal that had nothing to do with creating a weight-loss dogma. He was interested in ensuring adequate nutrition, not restricting it. But decades later, his reductionist model would be weaponized in ways he never intended.

The cultural shift from eating for nourishment to eating by numbers began in earnest in 1918, when Dr. Lulu Hunt Peters, a pediatrician and early diet guru, published "Diet and Health: With Key to the Calories"[2]. The book sold over 2 million copies and became the first mainstream calorie-counting diet manual. Peters didn't just teach people how to count calories—she made calorie control a moral imperative and a sign of modern sophistication.

"Hereafter you are going to eat calories of food," she wrote, "instead of food." This single sentence captured the essence of what would become a century-long obsession: the transformation of nourishment into mathematics, of meals into equations, of food into fuel to be calculated rather than enjoyed.

Meanwhile, processed food manufacturers discovered that the calorie model was a perfect partner for their business interests. They could now market their products as "healthy" as long as the number on the label was low, regardless of what was actually inside the package. A 100-calorie pack of cookies could be positioned as healthier than a handful of nuts with twice the calories, despite the vastly different nutritional and metabolic impacts of these foods.

World War II accelerated the adoption of calorie tracking through military rations and civilian rationing programs, and after the war, the practice became deeply entrenched in American culture. Government programs, school lunches, hospital diets, and workplace wellness initiatives all began using calorie math as the gold standard for nutrition planning.

The commercialization of calorie obsession reached new heights in the 1960s when Weight Watchers built a global business around a calorie-based points system, adding social accountability and group support to make dieting feel achievable and sustainable. The program's success spawned countless imitators and established calorie counting as the default approach to weight management.

By the 1980s and 1990s, brands like SnackWell's flooded grocery stores with low-calorie, high-sugar processed foods[3]. These products were loaded with preservatives, refined carbohydrates, and industrial seed oils, but they were marketed as "healthy" because their calorie counts were low. The actual ingredients—and their effects on hormones, blood sugar, and metabolism—were considered irrelevant as long as the numbers added up.

The Government Seal of Approval

The transformation of calorie counting from commercial gimmick to official policy reached its culmination in 1992 with the release of the USDA Food Guide Pyramid[4]. This dietary guideline enshrined calorie-focused eating into federal policy, with the base of the pyramid recommending 6 to 11 servings of bread, rice, and pasta per day—a recommendation that bore the clear influence of grain industry lobbying rather than nutritional science.

The pyramid told Americans that as long as they kept their calories in check, they were on the right track. Fat was relegated to the tiny tip of the pyramid, suggesting it should be eaten sparingly, while sugar was barely mentioned at all. The complexity of human metabolism, the hormonal effects of different foods, and the importance of nutrient density were all sacrificed on the altar of caloric simplicity.

Despite mounting evidence of metabolic health problems across the population, government agencies doubled down on the calorie model. Food labels were mandated to display calorie information prominently, while other crucial information about processing methods, ingredient quality, and nutrient density remained hidden or absent entirely.

Calories appeared everywhere—on every food label, in every diet app, in every health guideline, in every medical recommendation. The complexity of human metabolism had been reduced to a simple calculator, and what was inside the food mattered less than the number on the package.

We had turned nutrition into accounting, and it didn't work. Your body isn't a bank account—it's a hormone-regulated, adaptive, dynamic biological system that treats 500 calories of broccoli very differently than 500 calories of soda. The calorie myth became nutritional law not because it was effective, but because it was easy to measure, easy to market, and easy to monetize.

The Devastating Consequences

The obsession with calories has done far more than simply confuse the public—it has actively harmed metabolic health, distorted food choices, and shifted blame from industry practices to individual failings. The damage is visible everywhere you look, yet the calorie paradigm remains so entrenched that questioning it feels almost heretical.

Consider the SnackWell's phenomenon of the 1990s, which perfectly illustrates how the calorie model corrupted our understanding of nutrition. These fat-free cookies exploded in popularity, marketed as "guilt-free" indulgence because of their reduced calorie count compared to regular cookies. Dietitians recommended them, health-conscious consumers embraced them enthusiastically, and the media celebrated them as proof that you could have your cake and eat it too.

But these cookies were packed with sugar, refined flour, and chemical additives designed to replace the fat that had been removed. They triggered blood sugar spikes, intense cravings, and metabolic disruption that regular cookies with higher calorie counts might not have caused. People didn't stop at one or two cookies—they ate half the box, thinking they were making healthy choices. Hunger rebounded stronger than before, metabolism suffered, and weight gain often followed.

This wasn't because people failed to count properly—it was because they were counting the wrong thing entirely. The calorie model had taught them to ignore the biological effects of food in favor of numerical abstractions that bore no relationship to how their bodies actually responded to what they ate.

Meanwhile, the food industry profited enormously from this confusion. They could create products that were technically "low calorie" while being metabolically disruptive, nutritionally bankrupt, and designed to promote overconsumption. When people gained weight despite following calorie guidelines, the blame landed squarely on the consumer for supposedly lacking willpower or discipline.

This pattern repeated itself across the entire food landscape. When calories became the only metric that mattered, food companies responded with a flood of low-calorie, nutrient-deficient products that satisfied the numerical requirements while ignoring biological reality. Fat, which is calorie-dense but biologically essential for hormone production and satiety, was systematically stripped out of foods. What replaced it? Sugar, industrial seed oils, and processed starches—ingredients that were calorie-light on paper but inflammatory and metabolically devastating in practice.

The calorie model also created a devastating victim-blaming culture that persists to this day. By reducing health to simple mathematics, the paradigm implied that anyone who gained weight simply lacked discipline and self-control. Obesity, diabetes, and chronic disease were framed as personal moral failures rather than predictable outcomes of hormonal dysregulation and toxic food environments created by following official dietary advice.

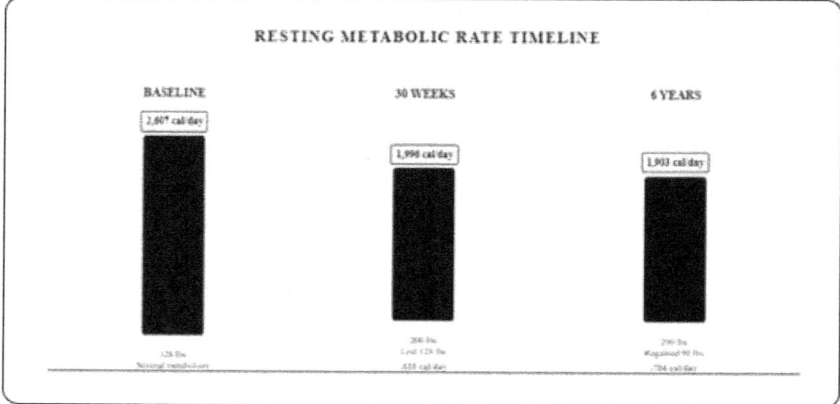

Television shows like "The Biggest Loser" reinforced this cruel mentality, celebrating dramatic weight loss achieved through extreme calorie restriction and punishing exercise regimens[5]. The show's contestants became living experiments in the calorie model, and the results were both predictable and tragic. A landmark 2016 study following former contestants revealed that nearly all had regained their weight within six years, and their metabolisms remained permanently damaged[6].

One contestant had to eat 800 fewer calories per day than someone of similar size just to maintain his weight. His body had gone into defensive shutdown mode and never fully recovered. This wasn't a failure of willpower—it was the predictable result of treating the human body like a simple machine rather than a complex adaptive system.

The Metabolic Adaptation Reality

The calorie model's most fundamental flaw lies in its assumption that the human body is a passive machine that burns energy at a fixed rate regardless of how much food it receives. In reality, your metabolism is a dynamic system that adapts to calorie restriction by slowing down energy expenditure and increasing hunger signals—a survival mechanism that evolved to protect us from starvation.

When you dramatically reduce calorie intake, your body doesn't just burn stored fat and maintain its normal metabolic rate. Instead, it begins a coordinated defense response designed to preserve life during what it perceives as a famine. Metabolic rate slows, hunger hormones increase, satiety hormones decrease, and the body becomes more efficient at extracting energy from whatever food is available[7].

This adaptation served our ancestors well during actual famines, but it makes voluntary calorie restriction a losing battle for most people. The harder you restrict calories, the more your body fights back with increased hunger, reduced energy expenditure, and metabolic changes that promote weight regain when normal eating resumes.

The research on this phenomenon is overwhelming and consistent. Studies of people on calorie-restricted diets show that metabolic rate can decrease by 20-40% within weeks of starting a diet[8]. This isn't just due to weighing less—it represents a genuine slowing of cellular metabolism that can persist for months or years after the diet ends.

Even more troubling, repeated cycles of calorie restriction and weight regain—the yo-yo dieting pattern that characterizes most people's weight loss attempts—can progressively damage metabolic function. Each cycle tends to result in more fat regain and less muscle recovery, leaving people with higher body fat percentages and lower metabolic rates than when they started[9].

The Hormonal Reality: What Actually Controls Body Weight

Understanding why the calorie model fails requires recognizing that body weight and composition are primarily controlled by hormones, not by conscious calorie calculations. The foods you eat send powerful signals to your endocrine system that determine whether you store fat or burn it, feel hungry or satisfied, and maintain stable energy or experience crashes and cravings.

Insulin stands at the center of this hormonal orchestra. When you eat, especially carbohydrates, insulin rises to help move glucose from your bloodstream into your cells for energy or storage. Occasional insulin spikes after meals are completely normal and healthy. But constant, prolonged elevation—known as hyperinsulinemia—leads to insulin resistance, fat gain, and eventually type 2 diabetes[10].

Here's the crucial point that the calorie model completely misses: insulin is primarily a storage hormone. When insulin levels are high, fat burning essentially shuts down and fat storage becomes the body's default mode. You become biochemically locked into storing rather than burning energy, regardless of how many calories you're consuming or burning through exercise.

Carbohydrates, particularly refined ones like sugar, bread, pasta, and processed cereals, cause dramatic spikes in blood sugar and trigger large insulin releases[11]. When insulin is constantly elevated due to frequent intake of these foods, your body remains in fat-storage mode most of the time. You can eat fewer calories, exercise more, and still struggle to lose weight because the hormonal environment prevents your body from accessing stored fat for energy.

Fat and protein, by contrast, have minimal effects on insulin while stimulating powerful satiety hormones like leptin, which signals fullness, and peptide YY, which helps control appetite and reduces overeating[12]. Fat provides essential building blocks for hormone production and helps you absorb crucial fat-soluble vitamins. Protein preserves muscle mass during weight loss, increases satiety, and requires significant energy to digest and process—a phenomenon known as the thermic effect of food[13].

This hormonal difference explains why two meals with identical calories can have completely opposite effects on your metabolism, hunger, and body composition:

Scenario A: 500 calories from a large soda and a donut creates a massive blood sugar spike, followed by an insulin surge, leading to fat storage and hunger rebound within 2-3 hours.

Scenario B: 500 calories from grilled salmon with roasted vegetables maintains stable blood sugar, promotes satiety, and allows your body to continue accessing stored fat for energy for 4-6 hours.

The calorie model treats these meals as equivalent. Your hormones know better.

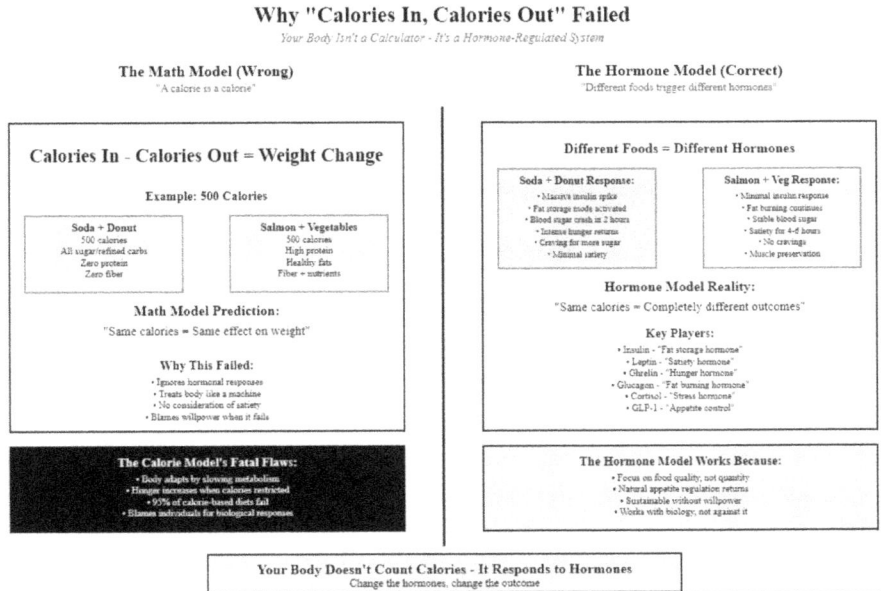

I had spent years tracking calories, weighing portions, and following the 'calories in, calories out' gospel. I remember standing in my kitchen, weighing out exactly 28 grams of almonds because I had 160 calories 'left' for the day, wondering why I was hungry again an hour after dinner. I'd calculated everything perfectly, followed every rule, and still felt like a failure when the scale wouldn't budge. Yet I kept gaining weight and losing energy. It wasn't until I stopped counting calories and started paying attention to insulin that everything changed. The math I'd been taught was wrong because it ignored the most important variable: what those calories were doing to my hormones.

The Context That Calories Miss

The calorie paradigm also ignores crucial context factors that profoundly influence how your body responds to food. Meal timing, sleep quality, stress levels, and activity patterns all affect metabolic function in ways that simple calorie calculations cannot capture.

Circadian rhythms play a crucial role in metabolic health, with insulin sensitivity naturally declining as evening approaches[14]. This means eating refined carbohydrates at night is far more likely to promote fat storage than eating the same foods in the morning, even if the calorie content is identical.

Sleep quality affects every hormone involved in appetite regulation and energy metabolism. Poor sleep raises ghrelin, your hunger hormone, while suppressing leptin, your satiety hormone[15]. Chronic sleep deprivation can make weight loss nearly impossible regardless of calorie intake, yet this factor is completely ignored by calorie-focused approaches.

Chronic stress keeps cortisol elevated, which promotes insulin resistance, triggers cravings for high-calorie comfort foods, and encourages fat storage around your midsection[16]. These hormonal disruptions can drive fat gain even when calorie intake remains low, yet stress management is rarely considered part of weight management in calorie-based approaches.

Exercise timing and type also influence how your body responds to food. Resistance training improves insulin sensitivity and increases muscle mass, which burns more calories at rest. High-intensity interval training can improve metabolic flexibility and fat oxidation. But these benefits have little to do with the calories burned during exercise and everything to do with the hormonal and metabolic adaptations that exercise creates.

The Protein Priority That Changes Everything

One of the most significant discoveries in modern nutrition research is the profound importance of protein adequacy for metabolic health, satiety, and body composition. Yet the calorie model treats protein as just another energy source rather than recognizing its unique biological functions.

Protein serves as the building blocks for muscle tissue, enzymes, hormones, and countless other biological molecules. When protein intake is inadequate, your body begins breaking down its own muscle tissue to obtain necessary amino acids, leading to a lower metabolic rate and decreased functional capacity[17].

Research consistently shows that diets containing 25-30% of calories from protein produce dramatically different outcomes compared to lower-protein diets with the same calorie content[18]. High-protein diets increase satiety, reduce spontaneous calorie intake, preserve muscle mass during weight loss, and increase the thermic effect of food—meaning your body burns more calories just digesting and processing the protein.

Perhaps most importantly, adequate protein intake helps regulate appetite and reduce cravings for processed foods. Many people who struggle with constant hunger and food obsession find that increasing protein intake to appropriate levels naturally reduces their desire to overeat, without requiring conscious calorie restriction.

The Quality Revolution: Why What Matters More Than How Much

The failure of the calorie model has led to a growing recognition that food quality matters more than food quantity for long-term health and weight management. This shift represents a fundamental change in how we think about nutrition—from a reductionist focus on isolated nutrients and energy content to a holistic understanding of how whole foods affect our biology.

Whole foods—vegetables, fruits, meats, fish, eggs, nuts, and seeds—come packaged with fiber, vitamins, minerals, antioxidants, and countless other compounds that work together to nourish your body and regulate your appetite. These foods naturally tend to be more filling, less likely to promote overeating, and more likely to support optimal metabolic function.

Processed foods, regardless of their calorie content, are designed to be hyperpalatable and easy to overconsume. They often lack the fiber, protein, and micronutrients that signal satiety to your brain, leading to a disconnect between calories consumed and feelings of satisfaction. Many processed foods also contain additives, preservatives, and novel compounds that may disrupt metabolic function in ways we're only beginning to understand.

Ultra-processed foods represent the extreme end of this spectrum—products that bear little resemblance to any whole food and are engineered to override your natural appetite regulation mechanisms[19]. These foods can trigger addictive-like eating behaviors and make it nearly impossible to regulate food intake naturally, regardless of calorie awareness or willpower.

The Exercise Myth Within the Calorie Myth

The calorie model has also distorted our understanding of exercise by reducing it to a simple "calories out" calculation. This perspective treats exercise primarily as a way to burn calories and create a larger deficit for weight loss, missing the far more important metabolic and hormonal benefits of physical activity.

While exercise does burn calories, the number is often much smaller than people expect, and the body tends to compensate for increased activity by reducing energy expenditure in other areas[20]. A typical 30-minute gym session might burn 200-400 calories—the equivalent of a small snack that can be eaten in minutes.

The real benefits of exercise are hormonal and metabolic, not just caloric. Regular physical activity improves insulin sensitivity, allowing your cells to respond better to insulin and reducing the amount needed to manage blood sugar. Exercise also stimulates growth hormone and other anabolic hormones that preserve muscle mass and promote fat burning. Strength training, in particular, builds metabolically active muscle tissue that continues burning energy long after your workout ends.

However, exercise alone cannot overcome a poor diet or dysfunctional hormonal environment. You cannot out-train a metabolically damaging way of eating, no matter how many calories you burn in the gym. The hormonal environment created by your food choices will always be the primary driver of your body composition and metabolic health.

Breaking Free from Calorie Prison

Understanding the truth behind the calorie myth is profoundly liberating because it points toward real solutions that work with your biology rather than against it. Instead of fighting your body with restriction and willpower, you can create the hormonal and metabolic conditions that allow your body to naturally regulate its weight and energy levels.

The first step is shifting your focus from calorie quantity to food quality. Choose whole, unprocessed foods that humans have eaten for thousands of years: high-quality proteins, healthy fats, and fiber-rich vegetables. These foods naturally regulate your hormones and appetite without requiring constant calculation and measurement.

Prioritize protein at every meal to support muscle mass, hormone production, and satiety. Aim for 25-30 grams of high-quality protein from sources like meat, fish, eggs, or dairy at each meal. This isn't about restricting other foods—it's about ensuring your body has the building blocks it needs to function optimally.

Don't fear natural fats from sources like olive oil, butter, avocados, nuts, and fatty fish. These fats help regulate hormones, keep you satisfied between meals, and provide essential nutrients your body cannot make on its own. The fear of fat that drove the low-calorie obsession has been thoroughly debunked by modern research.

Focus on eliminating or dramatically reducing refined carbohydrates that spike insulin and trigger fat storage. This means cutting back on bread, pasta, crackers, baked goods, sugary drinks, and breakfast cereals. These foods are metabolically harmful regardless of their calorie content, and removing them will help restore your insulin sensitivity and metabolic flexibility.

The Meal Timing Revolution

Give your digestive system regular breaks from food through approaches like intermittent fasting or time-restricted eating that work for your lifestyle. When you're not constantly eating, insulin levels can fall naturally, allowing your body to access stored fat for energy. This isn't about starvation—it's about giving your metabolic machinery time to reset and repair.

Start simply by eating your meals within a 12-hour window (such as 7 AM to 7 PM) and avoiding snacking between meals. As your metabolism improves and your hunger regulation normalizes, you may naturally find yourself comfortable going longer periods without food.

Many people discover that when they stop forcing themselves to eat every few hours and instead eat when genuinely hungry, their bodies naturally settle into patterns that support optimal weight and energy levels. This might mean eating two larger meals instead of three smaller ones, or having dinner earlier and breakfast later.

Address the Lifestyle Factors

Address the lifestyle factors that profoundly impact your hormones and metabolism, even though they have nothing to do with calories. Chronic stress wreaks havoc on your metabolic health by keeping cortisol elevated, which drives insulin resistance and promotes fat storage around your midsection. Find sustainable ways to manage stress through regular movement, meditation, time in nature, or whatever helps you feel grounded and calm.

Sleep quality might be even more important than diet for metabolic health. Poor sleep disrupts every hormone involved in appetite regulation and energy metabolism. Prioritize getting 7-9 hours of quality sleep each night in a cool, dark environment, and consider this as essential as any dietary change.

Measure What Matters

Finally, change how you measure progress and success. Instead of obsessing over calories consumed or pounds on the scale, pay attention to how you feel and function:

Energy levels: Do you have steady energy throughout the day, or do you experience crashes and need stimulants?

Hunger patterns: Are you naturally hungry at meal times, or do you experience constant cravings and need to snack frequently?

Mental clarity: Is your thinking sharp and focused, or do you experience brain fog and difficulty concentrating?

Sleep quality: Do you fall asleep easily and wake up refreshed, or do you toss and turn and wake up tired?

Mood stability: Do you feel emotionally balanced, or do you experience irritability and mood swings related to food?

Body composition: How do your clothes fit? Do you notice changes in your shape and muscle tone?

Physical performance: Are you getting stronger, more flexible, or more enduring?

These markers of health and vitality are far more meaningful than calorie counts or scale weight, and they reflect the true state of your metabolic health rather than arbitrary numerical targets.

The Path Forward: From Calculation to Intuition

The calorie myth represented everything wrong with modern nutrition advice: reductionism masquerading as science, oversimplification of complex biological systems, and the transformation of eating from a natural, intuitive process into a calculated, anxious exercise in self-control.

The truth is far more encouraging: your body is remarkably intelligent and will naturally regulate your weight when you provide the right inputs and remove the metabolic obstacles that interfere with normal function. You don't need superhuman willpower or perfect calculations—you need to work with your biology instead of fighting against it.

This doesn't mean that energy balance is irrelevant—you cannot create energy from nothing, and consuming vastly more energy than you expend will eventually lead to weight gain. But energy balance is the result of metabolic health, not the cause of it. When your hormones are functioning properly and your metabolism is flexible, your appetite naturally aligns with your energy needs without conscious effort.

The calorie myth taught us to distrust our bodies and rely on external calculations to determine how much we should eat. The truth is that your body provides more reliable feedback about food intake than any app, formula, or guideline when it's functioning properly. Hunger, satiety, energy levels, and cravings are sophisticated signals that can guide you toward optimal health—but only when they're not being disrupted by processed foods, chronic stress, poor sleep, and metabolic dysfunction.

Recovering your natural ability to self-regulate requires patience, as years of calorie restriction and processed food consumption may have damaged the very systems that should guide your eating. But this capacity can be restored through consistent choices that support rather than undermine your metabolic health.

The calorie myth provided the perfect cover for the food industry's next great deception. With people focused on numbers rather than nourishment, manufacturers could create an entire category of "healthy" foods that were anything but healthy. The low-fat movement would transform the calorie obsession from a personal struggle into a cultural mandate, turning the fear of fat into the foundation of a trillion-dollar industry built on processed alternatives.

References

1. Atwater WO. *Foods: Nutritive Value and Cost.* Washington, DC: U.S. Government Printing Office; 1894.

2. Peters LH. *Diet and Health: With Key to the Calories.* Chicago, IL: Reilly & Britton Co; 1918.

3. O'Connor A. How the fat-free craze fueled America's obesity epidemic. *The New York Times.* February 20, 2016.

4. US Department of Agriculture. *The Food Guide Pyramid.* Washington, DC: US Government Printing Office; 1992.

5. Kolata G. After "The Biggest Loser," their bodies fought to regain weight. *The New York Times.* May 2, 2016.

6. Fothergill E, Guo J, Howard L, et al. Persistent metabolic adaptation 6 years after "The Biggest Loser" competition. *Obesity (Silver Spring).* 2016;24(8):1612-1619. doi:10.1002/oby.21538

7. Leibel RL, Rosenbaum M, Hirsch J. Changes in energy expenditure resulting from altered body weight. *N Engl J Med.* 1995;332(10):621-628. doi:10.1056/NEJM199503093321001

8. Knuth ND, Johannsen DL, Tamboli RA, et al. Metabolic adaptation following massive weight loss is related to the degree of energy imbalance and changes in circulating leptin. *Obesity (Silver Spring).* 2014;22(12):2563-2569. doi:10.1002/oby.20900

9. Dulloo AG, Jacquet J, Montani JP, Schutz Y. How dieting makes the lean fatter: from a perspective of body composition autoregulation through adipostats and proteinstats awaiting discovery. *Obes Rev.* 2015;16(Suppl 1):25-35. doi:10.1111/obr.12246

10. Corkey BE. Hyperinsulinemia: cause or consequence? *Nat Rev Endocrinol.* 2012;8(10):585-590. doi:10.1038/nrendo.2012.98

11. Ludwig DS, Ebbeling CB. The carbohydrate-insulin model of obesity: beyond "calories in, calories out." *JAMA Intern Med.* 2018;178(8):1098-1103. doi:10.1001/jamainternmed.2018.2933

12. Weigle DS, Breen PA, Matthys CC, et al. A high-protein diet induces sustained reductions in appetite, ad libitum caloric intake, and body weight despite compensatory changes in diurnal plasma leptin and ghre-

lin concentrations. *Am J Clin Nutr.* 2005;82(1):41-48. doi:10.1093/ajcn.82.1.41

13. Westerterp KR. Diet induced thermogenesis. *Nutr Metab (Lond).* 2004;1(1):5. doi:10.1186/1743-7075-1-5

14. Scheer FA, Hilton MF, Mantzoros CS, Shea SA. Adverse metabolic and cardiovascular consequences of circadian misalignment. *Proc Natl Acad Sci USA.* 2009;106(11):4453-4458. doi:10.1073/pnas.0808180106

15. Spiegel K, Tasali E, Penev P, Van Cauter E. Sleep curtailment in healthy young men is associated with decreased leptin levels, elevated ghrelin levels, and increased hunger and appetite. *Ann Intern Med.* 2004;141(11):846-850. doi:10.7326/0003-4819-141-11-200412070-00008

16. Drapeau S, Poirier P, Moorjani S, et al. Waist circumference, visceral obesity, and cardiovascular risk. *J Cardiopulm Rehabil.* 2003;23(3):161-169. doi:10.1097/00008483-200305000-00008

17. Phillips SM, van Loon LJ. Dietary protein for athletes: from requirements to optimum adaptation. *J Sports Sci.* 2011;29(Suppl 1):S29-S38. doi:10.1080/02640414.2011.619204

18. Leidy HJ, Clifton PM, Astrup A, et al. The role of protein in weight loss and maintenance. *Am J Clin Nutr.* 2015;101(6):1320S-1329S. doi:10.3945/ajcn.114.084038

19. Monteiro CA, Cannon G, Moubarac JC, et al. Ultra-processed products are becoming dominant in the global food system. *Obes Rev.* 2013;14(Suppl 2):21-28. doi:10.1111/obr.12107

20. Pontzer H, Durazo-Arvizu R, Dugas LR, et al. Constrained total energy expenditure and metabolic adaptation to physical activity in adult humans. *Curr Biol.* 2016;26(3):410-417. doi:10.1016/j.cub.2015.12.046

Chapter Seven

The Low-Fat Myth

How We Were Fooled Into Fearing Food

The Dogma That Defined a Generation

Sarah thought she was doing everything right. Every morning, she poured skim milk over her bowl of high-fiber cereal, spread fat-free cream cheese on her whole wheat bagel, and packed a lunch of turkey breast on low-fat bread with fat-free mayo. Her snacks were carefully chosen: fat-free yogurt, baked chips, and those revolutionary new fat-free cookies that promised guilt-free indulgence. She followed every guideline, read every label, and avoided fat like her life depended on it.

Twenty years later, Sarah was 40 pounds heavier, pre-diabetic, and constantly hungry. Her cholesterol was higher than when she started. Her energy crashed every afternoon. The promise of low-fat living had become a prison of processed food and perpetual craving.

Sarah's story isn't unique—it's the story of an entire generation that followed three simple statements that shaped how we thought about food: Fat makes you fat. Fat clogs your arteries. Fat causes heart disease. These weren't whispered suggestions—they were shouted from every corner of the health establishment, proclaimed with the certainty of gospel truth.

From the 1970s through the early 2000s, "low-fat" became more than a dietary recommendation; it became a moral imperative. Doctors prescribed it. Dietitians preached it. Government agencies mandated it. The media amplified it. The message was clear and uncompromising: if we wanted to lose weight, protect our hearts, and live healthy lives, we had to cut the fat.

So we did exactly what we were told. We abandoned butter for margarine, swapped whole milk for skim, and filled our shopping carts with an endless parade of "fat-free" and "low-fat" alternatives. The grocery store became our battlefield against fat: SnackWell's Devil's Food Cookie Cakes promised "fat-free" indulgence, Entenmann's fat-free pastries flew off the shelves, and Olestra-laden chips carried the bold claim "Bet you can't eat just one"—and we couldn't, because they never satisfied us.

Our grandparents had eaten eggs fried in butter, steaks grilled in their own fat, and vegetables sautéed in lard. They drank whole milk, ate full-fat cheese, and used real cream in their coffee. But we knew better—or so we thought. We replaced their simple, traditional foods with products that required paragraphs of ingredients and carried health claims louder than carnival barkers.

The promise was seductive: follow the guidelines, cut the fat, and watch the pounds melt away while your heart grew stronger. It was simple. It was logical. It was wrong.

The result of this massive dietary experiment wasn't the health renaissance we'd been promised. Instead, we got fatter. We got sicker. Heart disease remained stubbornly persistent as the leading killer[1]. Diabetes exploded across the population. Obesity rates didn't just rise—they increased 2.4-fold[2]. The low-fat movement, heralded as our salvation, had become our downfall.

This wasn't merely a case of misguided advice or innocent error. The low-fat crusade represented one of the most destructive health myths of the last century, a dogma that wrecked our metabolism, distorted our relationship with food, and left us terrified of the very nutrients our bodies desperately needed.

The Birth of a Lie: How Bad Science Became Public Policy

To understand how an entire nation was led astray, we need to trace the origins of the low-fat mythology back to its flawed foundation. The roots of this movement grew from the same contaminated soil that nurtured the war on saturated fat and cholesterol: Ancel Keys' infamous Seven Countries Study. Despite its cherry-picked data and glaring methodological flaws, Keys' work wielded enormous influence in shaping the narrative that fat—particularly saturated fat—was public enemy number one.

By the early 1970s, this anti-fat sentiment had moved beyond academic circles and into the halls of political power. The pivotal moment came in 1977, when the U.S. Senate Select Committee on Nutrition and Human Needs, chaired by Senator George McGovern, released the first federal dietary guidelines[3]. These weren't merely suggestions—they were official government recommendations that would shape American eating habits for generations.

The process that led to these guidelines reveals everything wrong with how nutrition policy is made. Several distinguished scientists, including Dr. Robert Olson and Dr. Pete Ahrens, appeared before the committee to voice serious concerns about the anti-fat recommendations[4]. The evidence linking fat to heart disease was preliminary at best, they argued, built on weak assumptions and incomplete research. Dr. Olson's testimony was particularly prescient: "I plead in my report and will plead again orally here for more research on the problem before we make announcements to the American public"[4].

These weren't fringe voices or industry shills—these were respected researchers urging caution, asking for more time to understand the complex relationship between diet and disease. But their warnings fell on deaf ears. The committee was under pressure to act, driven by rising heart disease rates and public demand for guidance. Political expediency trumped scientific rigor. As McGovern's aides later admitted with startling candor, "Senators don't have the luxury of waiting for every last shred of evidence"[5].

This single statement encapsulates the fundamental problem: major public health policy was being driven not by scientific certainty, but by political urgency. The guidelines that emerged urged Americans to reduce fat intake—especially saturated fat—while increasing carbohydrate consumption. These recommendations weren't based on rock-solid science; they were educated guesses dressed up as established fact[6].

The SnackWell's Phenomenon: A Case Study in Deception

Nothing embodied the absurdity of the low-fat era quite like SnackWell's cookies. Launched by Nabisco in 1992, these "fat-free" treats became the poster child for everything wrong with low-fat thinking. The Devil's Food Cookie Cakes contained no fat but were loaded with sugar, corn syrup, and a cocktail of chemicals designed to create the texture that fat normally provided.

People bought them by the case, convinced they were making healthy choices. The cookies flew off grocery store shelves so quickly that rationing became common. Meanwhile, each "fat-free" cookie contained as many calories as a regular cookie, sometimes more, but without any of the satiety that fat provides. People found themselves eating entire boxes in one sitting, then wondering why they couldn't stop.

SnackWell's had cracked the code: remove the nutrient that makes you feel full, add more of the ingredients that make you crave more, then market it as healthy. It was food engineering masquerading as nutrition science, and it worked perfectly—for the company's bottom line, if not for America's waistline.

The food industry watched this unfolding drama with keen interest, quickly recognizing a golden opportunity. If fat was now the enemy, they could reformulate their products to remove it, creating an entirely new category of "healthy" processed foods. The economics were irresistible: stripping fat from products and replacing it with cheaper ingredients like sugar, starches, gums, and emulsifiers didn't just reduce production costs—it allowed companies to market these reformulated foods as premium health products.

I was the target market for every low-fat product of the 1990s and 2000s. I chose fat-free salad dressings, low-fat yogurts, and baked chips, believing I was making smart choices. Each 'healthy' substitution moved me further from real food and closer to the metabolic dysfunction that would eventually require a calcium scan to reveal.

Real fats like butter, cream, and lard were expensive to produce and store, with limited shelf life and complex supply chains. Refined carbohydrates, sugar, and industrial seed oils, by contrast, were cheap, shelf-stable, and could be mass-produced with industrial efficiency. The "low-fat" revolution wasn't just a health message—it was an economic gold rush that transformed the entire food landscape.

These new "low-fat" foods could carry health claims, command higher prices, and tap into consumer fear of fat. By the 1980s and 1990s, grocery stores had become shrines to fat-phobia. Entire aisles were dedicated to fat-free cookies, sugar-laden yogurts, and highly processed diet snacks, all bearing health claims and commanding premium prices. The USDA food pyramid, released in 1992, provided the visual blueprint for this new nutritional orthodoxy[7]. Grains formed the foundation, to be consumed in abundance. Fats were relegated to the tiny apex, to be used "sparingly" like some dangerous condiment.

The messaging was everywhere and inescapable. Cereal commercials proclaimed the heart-healthy benefits of oat bran. School lunch programs eliminated whole milk. Butter became a dirty word, replaced by spreads that bore little resemblance to food. An entire generation grew up believing that avoiding fat was the key to health, even as they consumed unprecedented amounts of sugar and processed carbohydrates.

The Great Cheese Glut: An Unintended Consequence

One of the most bizarre and revealing side effects of the low-fat campaign emerged from an unexpected source: the dairy industry's surplus problem. When the government began promoting low-fat and skim milk as heart-healthy alternatives to whole milk, dairy producers faced a logistical nightmare. Whole milk naturally contains only about 3.25% fat, but when that fat was removed to create skim milk, producers were left with enormous quantities of unwanted milk fat.

Rather than waste this byproduct, the government intervened with a solution that would seem absurd if it weren't so tragically real. They subsidized the production of butter, cheese, and powdered milk, creating massive surpluses that were stockpiled in government storage facilities—underground caves that became known, with dark humor, as "cheese caves." At the height of this program, the U.S. government owned over 500 million pounds of surplus cheese.

Eventually, this mountain of dairy had to go somewhere. Government programs began inserting subsidized cheese and dairy products into school lunches, food assistance programs, and fast food promotions. Advertising campaigns like "Got Milk?" received government support, while partnerships with chains like Domino's and Taco Bell pushed cheesy, calorie-dense foods with unprecedented marketing muscle.

The irony was breathtaking: Americans were being told to fear butter and whole milk while government programs actively promoted processed cheese consumption. This contradiction perfectly illustrated the fundamental flaw in nutrient-focused policy—when you try to manipulate isolated components of the food system without understanding the whole, unintended consequences ripple through every aspect of what we eat.

But Wait! There's More

The cheese cave debacle wasn't an isolated incident—it was a symptom of a much larger problem with how government subsidies shape what Americans eat. While the dairy industry was creating mountains of surplus cheese, an even more consequential subsidy program was quietly transforming the entire food landscape.

For decades, agricultural subsidies have created a bizarre economic reality where the government pays farmers to grow the exact ingredients that form the foundation of our most harmful processed foods, while providing virtually no support for the foods we're told to eat more of.

The numbers reveal a system working completely backwards from public health goals. Corn receives the largest subsidies—over $7 billion annually—not because corn on the cob is a dietary staple, but because corn becomes high fructose corn syrup, cornstarch, and feed for factory-farmed animals. Soybeans, heavily subsidized at over $4 billion per year, don't end up as whole soybeans on dinner plates but as soybean oil—the industrial cooking oil that has become ubiquitous in processed foods.

GOVERNMENT SUBSIDY ALLOCATION

Supporting the Wrong Foods

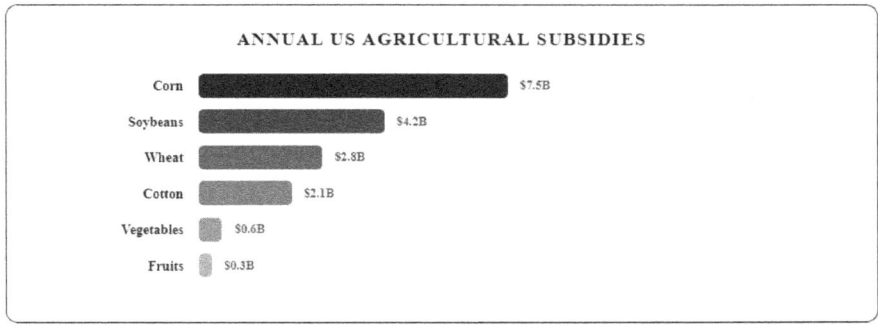

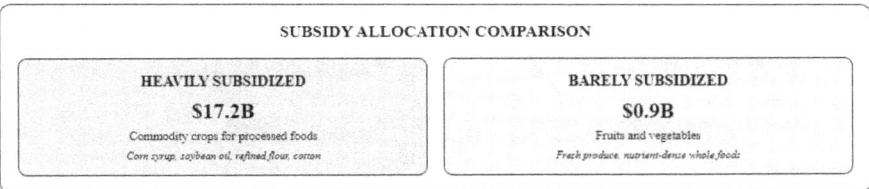

Meanwhile, the fruits and vegetables that nutrition guidelines tell us should fill half our plates receive less than $1 billion in combined subsidies. The government spends nearly twenty times more supporting the production of ingredients for junk food than supporting the production of actual healthy food.

This isn't accidental—it's the result of decades of agricultural policy written by and for industrial food processors, not public health advocates.

The Wreckage: What the Low-Fat Era Cost Us

The low-fat crusade had promised a health revolution: weight loss, heart protection, and disease prevention. Instead, it delivered a public health catastrophe that we're still struggling to understand and reverse.

The Hunger That Never Ended

By stripping fat from foods and replacing it with refined carbohydrates and sugar, the low-fat reformulation fundamentally altered how our bodies responded to meals. Fat provides satiety—the feeling of fullness and satisfaction that naturally regulates appetite. Sugar and refined carbs do the opposite, creating insulin spikes that lead to rapid blood sugar drops, triggering renewed hunger within hours of eating.

FULL-FAT VS LOW-FAT FOODS
Comprehensive Nutrient Density & Satiety Analysis

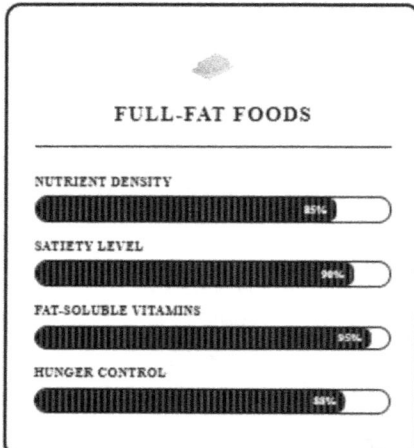 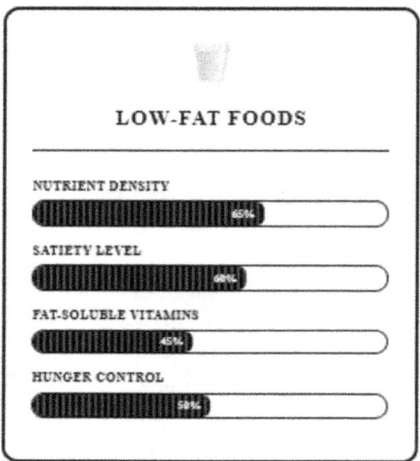

The result was a population caught in a metabolic trap. The more "light" and "low-fat" products people consumed, the hungrier they became. Meals that should have satisfied for hours left people reaching for snacks within minutes. The food industry had inadvertently created products that increased consumption while claiming to promote health.

The Obesity Paradox by the Numbers

From the 1980s to today, as grocery stores filled with low-fat options and fat-phobia reached its peak, obesity rates didn't just rise—they more than doubled[2]. This wasn't supposed to happen. According to the low-fat hypothesis, removing fat should have led to weight loss. Instead, the era of fat-free cookies and diet sodas coincided with the sharpest rise in metabolic disease in modern history.

The timeline is damning: Low-fat product sales peaked in the 1990s, reaching $15.9 billion annually by 1998. During this exact same period, obesity rates climbed from 15% to 23% of the adult population. The more low-fat products

Americans bought, the fatter they became. It wasn't correlation—it was causation wrapped in a cruel irony.

The explanation lies in understanding what actually replaced the fat. Food manufacturers discovered that removing fat made products taste like cardboard, so they compensated with sugar, salt, and a cocktail of chemical additives designed to create palatability. These reformulated foods were often more calorie-dense than their full-fat predecessors, but they completely bypassed the body's natural satiety mechanisms.

The Fear of Real Food

Perhaps the most tragic consequence of the low-fat era was how it severed our connection to traditional, nourishing foods. People began to view whole eggs with suspicion, despite their status as one of nature's most complete proteins. Steak became a guilty pleasure rather than a source of essential nutrients. Butter was banished from kitchens, replaced by industrial margarine made from seed oils and chemical stabilizers. Avocados, rich in heart-healthy monounsaturated fats, were treated like dietary land mines.

Meanwhile, engineered substitutes proliferated. Fat-free cheese that bore no resemblance to actual cheese. Yogurt so loaded with sugar it rivaled ice cream in sweetness. Salad dressings that contained more chemicals than a chemistry lab. We had learned to fear foods that had nourished humans for millennia while embracing products that couldn't exist outside of industrial food processing.

The Rise of Ultra-Processed Foods

The low-fat movement didn't just change individual food choices; it transformed the entire food supply. With fat removed, processed food manufacturers faced a palatability crisis. Their solution created an entirely new category of edible products: ultra-processed foods designed in laboratories rather than grown on farms.

These products relied on starches, gums, emulsifiers, and sweeteners to create texture and taste. They were calorie-dense but nutrient-poor, designed for shelf stability rather than human nutrition. They inflamed the body, disrupted hormones, and undermined metabolism while carrying health claims and government endorsements.

The Scientific Stagnation

By focusing obsessively on fat as the dietary villain, the medical establishment missed the real drivers of heart disease and metabolic dysfunction. Sugar consumption, particularly in the form of high fructose corn syrup, exploded during the low-fat era. Industrial seed oils, never before consumed by humans in significant quantities, became dietary staples. Insulin resistance, inflammation, and metabolic syndrome—now recognized as key factors in chronic disease—were barely understood because attention was fixated on the fat content of foods.

Generations of dietitians, doctors, and patients were steered away from the truth, trained to focus on macronutrient ratios rather than food quality, on eliminating nutrients rather than addressing the root causes of disease.

The human cost of this misdirection is measurable and heartbreaking. Obesity rates increased 2.4-fold since 1980[2]. Type 2 diabetes, once called "adult-onset" diabetes, now affects children as young as elementary school age[8]. Non-alcoholic fatty liver disease has become common even among people who follow conventional "healthy" eating guidelines[9]. Despite decades of fat-phobia and billions spent on low-fat products, heart disease remains the number one killer in America[1].

We didn't ignore the advice—we followed it religiously. And it made us sicker than we'd ever been.

The Vindication: Science Discovers What Our Bodies Always Knew

The fat myth is finally crumbling under the weight of better science and mounting evidence. What we're discovering is both vindicating for those who questioned the orthodoxy and devastating for those who built their careers on promoting it.

Fat doesn't make you fat. It doesn't clog your arteries. It doesn't poison your heart. These aren't contrarian opinions or wishful thinking—they're conclusions supported by large-scale studies, meta-analyses, and decades of research that actually followed scientific method rather than political expediency.

Your body needs fat not just to survive, but to thrive. Every cell membrane in your body is built from fatty acids. Your brain, composed of nearly 60% fat, requires dietary fat for optimal function. Hormones like testosterone, estrogen, and cortisol are synthesized from cholesterol and fat. The fat-soluble vitamins A, D, E, and K can't be absorbed without dietary fat. Your immune system relies on specific fatty acids to regulate inflammation and fight infection.

When we stripped fat from our diets, we didn't remove disease—we removed the very nutrients our bodies needed to maintain health and metabolic balance. What we replaced them with was far more dangerous: more sugar, more processed carbohydrates, more chemical additives, and more confusion about what constitutes real food.

Even saturated fat, the most demonized form of dietary fat, has been largely vindicated by modern research. The 2010 meta-analysis by Siri-Tarino et al. in the American Journal of Clinical Nutrition, examining 21 studies and nearly 348,000 subjects, found no association between saturated fat intake and heart disease risk[10]. A 2015 systematic review by de Souza et al. in the BMJ reached similar conclusions, analyzing data from 73 studies involving over 600,000 people[11].

These weren't small studies or industry-funded research—these were comprehensive analyses of the best available evidence, published in the most prestigious medical journals. The verdict was clear: the war on saturated fat had been based on flawed assumptions and cherry-picked data. Meanwhile, diets high in refined carbohydrates and ultra-processed foods show strong, consistent associations with metabolic syndrome, inflammation, cardiovascular disease, and early death[12].

The evidence is clear: fat wasn't the villain—it was the scapegoat. The low-fat experiment didn't fail because Americans cheated or lacked willpower. It failed because it was built on bad science, driven by political pressure, and sustained by economic interests that profited from our confusion and fear.

Key Scientific Insights

Hormone Response	Nutrient Absorption
• Full-fat foods trigger stronger CCK and GLP-1 release, leading to better appetite control and reduced calorie intake at subsequent meals.	• Fat-soluble vitamins (A, D, E, K) require dietary fat for optimal absorption. Low-fat versions may impair nutrient utilization. |//

Processing Effects	Metabolic Impact
• Many low-fat products contain added sugars and artificial ingredients to compensate for full flavor and texture loss during fat removal.	• Studies show full-fat diary consumption is associated with lower risk of obesity and metabolic syndrome compared to low-fat alternatives.

The Low-Fat Mindset Still Lives: How It Looks Today

Think you've escaped the low-fat trap? Think again. The low-fat mindset didn't disappear when the food pyramid was replaced—it just got more sophisticated. Today's version of fat-phobia hides behind new buzzwords and health trends, but the underlying fear remains the same.

Walk through any grocery store and you'll see it everywhere: Greek yogurt with fruit on the bottom (loaded with added sugar), egg white omelets (throwing away the most nutritious part), skinless chicken breast (the driest, least satisfying cut), turkey bacon (a processed imitation of real food), and plant-based meat alternatives that contain more ingredients than a chemistry set.

The modern low-fat believer shops the perimeter of the store, chooses lean proteins, and still reads labels looking for fat content. They order dressing on the side, remove the skin from chicken, and feel guilty about eating nuts because they're "high in fat." They've been convinced that avocados are healthy but still limit their portions because of the calories from fat.

This is the insidious nature of the low-fat myth—it doesn't just change what we eat, it changes how we think about food. Even people who intellectually understand that fat isn't evil still carry behavioral patterns programmed by decades of fat-phobia.

Signs You're Still Trapped by Low-Fat Thinking

- You automatically choose the lowest-fat option when shopping

THE LOW-FAT MYTH 105

- You feel guilty eating foods high in saturated fat, even natural ones

- You remove egg yolks or eat only egg whites

- You choose turkey over beef primarily because it's "leaner"

- You limit nuts and avocados because they're "high in fat"

- You buy products specifically labeled "low-fat" or "reduced fat"

- You drain ground beef after cooking to remove fat

- You choose skim or low-fat dairy over full-fat versions

- You avoid cooking with butter or coconut oil

- You think eating fat will make you gain weight faster than eating carbs

If any of these behaviors sound familiar, you're still operating under low-fat programming, even if you've rejected the diet consciously. The myth runs deeper than knowledge—it's embedded in our daily habits and automatic choices.

Reclaiming Your Relationship with Real Food

You've been lied to for long enough. The path forward isn't about finding the next dietary trend or waiting for permission from health authorities who have already been wrong for decades. It's about reconnecting with the wisdom of real food and trusting your body's innate ability to recognize what nourishes it.

Stop fearing fat. Natural fats like butter, eggs, olive oil, avocados, and grass-fed meats aren't your enemies—they're essential partners in your health. These foods provide the building blocks for hormones, support brain function, regulate inflammation, and help your body absorb critical nutrients. They also provide something that no low-fat substitute can: genuine satiety that helps you naturally regulate your appetite.

The key is shifting your focus from quantity to quality. Instead of obsessing over fat grams and macronutrient ratios, focus on the source and processing of your food. Real, whole foods don't need health claims or marketing campaigns—their nutritional value speaks for itself.

This means abandoning the products that defined the low-fat era and still crowd our grocery stores today. If a label screams "low-fat," "reduced fat," or "fat-free," ask yourself a simple question: what did they add instead? The answer is usually sugar, starch, gums, emulsifiers, and artificial flavors—ingredients that create more metabolic damage than the original fat ever could.

When you see "low-fat" on a package, think of it as a warning label. It's telling you that this product has been stripped of nutrients and satisfaction, then engineered to make you want more. These products exist not because they're healthier, but because they're more profitable and create repeat customers through manufactured cravings.

Return to cooking with real fats that humans have used for thousands of years: butter, ghee, olive oil, coconut oil, and animal fats like tallow and lard. These traditional fats are not only safe but beneficial, providing unique nutrients and flavor profiles that industrial seed oils can never match. Ditch the margarine, canola oil, soybean oil, and other industrial products that didn't exist before the 20th century.

Build your meals around foods that don't require labels or health claims. Choose foods that could have been available to your great-grandmother: vegetables, fruits, meats, fish, eggs, nuts, and dairy from healthy animals. These foods carry their own inherent wisdom, providing nutrients in forms and combinations that your body has evolved to recognize and utilize.

Focus on protein, healthy fats, and fiber rather than refined carbohydrates and engineered substitutes. This combination naturally regulates appetite, stabilizes blood sugar, and provides sustained energy without the hunger cycles that characterize the low-fat, high-carb approach.

Most importantly, relearn to trust your body's signals. When you eat real food that includes adequate fat and protein, you'll find yourself naturally eating less while feeling satisfied longer. The constant hunger, cravings, and food obsession that characterize the low-fat trap will fade as your metabolism heals and your hormones rebalance.

You don't need to fear real food. You need to fear the lies that have kept you sick, confused, and separated from the nourishment your body craves. Fat isn't your enemy—it's part of your biological design, essential for health, vitality, and the kind of deep satisfaction that comes from truly nourishing your body.

The fat myth has ruled long enough. It's time to reclaim your right to real food, real health, and real satisfaction. Your body has been waiting.

The low-fat movement's spectacular failure left millions of people searching for answers. They had followed the guidelines, avoided traditional fats, and embraced processed alternatives—only to become sicker than ever. Into this confusion stepped a new message that seemed to offer redemption: eat more plants. It sounded pure, natural, and scientifically grounded. But this seemingly innocent advice would become a Trojan horse for an entirely new generation of ultra-processed foods, proving that the industry had learned to weaponize our desire for health itself.

References

1. Centers for Disease Control and Prevention. (2023). *Leading Causes of Death*. National Center for Health Statistics. Updated 2023. Accessed September 9, 2025. https://www.cdc.gov/nchs/fastats/leading-causes-of-death.htm

2. Fryar CD, Carroll MD, Afful J. Prevalence of overweight, obesity, and severe obesity among adults aged 20 and over: United States, 1960–1962 through 2017–2018. *NCHS Health E-Stats*. 2020. Accessed September 9, 2025. https://www.cdc.gov/nchs/data/hestat/obesity-adult-17-18/obesity-adult.htm

3. U.S. Senate Select Committee on Nutrition and Human Needs. *Dietary Goals for the United States*. Washington, DC: U.S. Government Printing Office; 1977.

4. Olson RE. Testimony before the US Senate Select Committee on Nutrition and Human Needs. In: *Dietary Goals for the United States.* Washington, DC: US Government Printing Office; 1977. Cited in: Oppenheimer GM, Benrubi ID. McGovern's Senate Select Committee on Nutrition and Human Needs versus the meat industry on the diet-heart question (1976–1977). *Am J Public Health.* 2014;104(1):59–69. doi:10.2105/AJPH.2013.301464

5. Oppenheimer GM, Benrubi ID. McGovern's Senate Select Committee on Nutrition and Human Needs versus the meat industry on the diet-heart question (1976–1977). *Am J Public Health.* 2014;104(1):59–69. doi:10.2105/AJPH.2013.301464

6. US Senate Select Committee on Nutrition and Human Needs. *Dietary Goals for the United States.* 2nd ed. Washington, DC: US Government Printing Office; 1977.

7. US Department of Agriculture. *The Food Guide Pyramid.* Washington, DC: US Government Printing Office; 1992.

8. Dabelea D, Mayer-Davis EJ, Saydah S, et al. Prevalence of type 1 and type 2 diabetes among children and adolescents from 2001 to 2009. *JAMA.* 2014;311(17):1778–1786. doi:10.1001/jama.2014.3201

9. Younossi ZM, Koenig AB, Abdelatif D, Fazel Y, Henry L, Wymer M. Global epidemiology of nonalcoholic fatty liver disease—meta-analytic assessment of prevalence, incidence, and outcomes. *Hepatology.* 2016;64(1):73–84. doi:10.1002/hep.28431

10. Siri-Tarino PW, Sun Q, Hu FB, Krauss RM. Meta-analysis of prospective cohort studies evaluating the association of saturated fat with cardiovascular disease. *Am J Clin Nutr.* 2010;91(3):535–546. doi:10.3945/ajcn.2009.27725

11. de Souza RJ, Mente A, Maroleanu A, et al. Intake of saturated and trans unsaturated fatty acids and risk of all cause mortality, cardiovascular disease, and type 2 diabetes: systematic review and meta-analysis of ob-

servational studies. *BMJ.* 2015;351:h3978. doi:10.1136/bmj.h3978

12. Micha R, Shulkin ML, Peñalvo JL, et al. Etiologic effects and optimal intakes of foods and nutrients for risk of cardiovascular diseases and diabetes: systematic reviews and meta-analyses from the Global Burden of Disease Study 2013. *PLoS One.* 2017;12(4):e0175149. doi:10.1371/journal.pone.0175149

Chapter Eight

The Plant-Based Myth

How "Eat More Plants" Became a Trojan Horse for Ultra-Processed Junk

The Dogma That Conquered the World

Plants are healthy. Plants are clean. Plants are the future.

From documentaries and doctors to dietitians and influencers, the message is everywhere: the best diet is a plant-based one. Walk into any grocery store and you'll see the evidence—entire aisles dedicated to "plant-based" alternatives that promise to save your health and the planet simultaneously. Oat milk lattes have replaced dairy in coffee shops across America. Impossible Burgers sizzle on grills that once exclusively cooked beef. Even fast food chains now offer "plant-based" options as premium, health-conscious choices.

The messaging feels inescapable and morally urgent. Major health organizations have thrown their weight behind plant-based eating. The American Heart Association promotes plant-based diets to reduce cardiovascular disease risk[1]. Harvard Health highlights plant-based eating as a strategy to lower blood pressure, cholesterol, and diabetes risk[2]. Environmental reports from the UN and journals like Nature Communications advocate plant-based diets as a key solution to reduce greenhouse gas emissions, land use, and water consumption[3].

The institutional support is overwhelming. A 2023 study in *Circulation* showed that those following the Portfolio Diet—a plant-based approach—had up to 30% lower risk of heart disease and stroke[4]. Harvard T.H. Chan School of Public Health highlights that healthy plant-based diets generate fewer greenhouse gas emissions and require fewer resources[5]. A 2024 *Nature Communications* meta-analysis found that shifting toward plant-based diets can cut emissions up to 52% and drastically reduce land and water use[6].

The narrative is simple, compelling, and seemingly unassailable: meat is bad, fat is dangerous, and if you care about your heart, your health, or the planet—you should eat more plants.

What began as commonsense advice—"eat your vegetables"—has morphed into a moral, medical, and environmental crusade to eliminate animal foods entirely. Schools removed animal products from lunch lines. Doctors began prescribing meatless diets for heart health. Governments introduced food pyramids and climate guidelines that prioritize plant calories over animal nutrition. Corporations rushed to capitalize, backing plant-based brands that use synthetic ingredients, industrial oils, and ultra-processing to mimic meat.

And people listened. The plant-based food market exploded from $3.1 billion in 2010 to over $15 billion by 2023[7]. Venture capital poured billions into companies promising to revolutionize food through technology and chemistry rather than agriculture.

But here's the problem that nobody wants to acknowledge: "plant-based" doesn't mean whole foods anymore. It means marketable. It means processed. It means anything that isn't animal-based—even if it's loaded with seed oils, starches, gums, emulsifiers, additives, and sugar.

While we've tried to eat greener, our health has gotten redder. We are more obese, more diabetic, and more chronically inflamed than ever before[8]. Paradoxically, we're also more nutrient deficient despite consuming more fortified and supplemented foods than any generation in history[9].

We were told to eat more plants to save ourselves. Instead, we got sold a myth—wrapped in ideology, funded by industry, and flavored like bacon.

The Ideological Roots: From Religion to Revenue

The push for plant-based eating didn't start with science. It started with belief, moral conviction, and a peculiar blend of religious doctrine and dietary reform that has shaped American nutrition policy for over a century.

In the late 1800s, Dr. John Harvey Kellogg ran a sanitarium in Battle Creek, Michigan, where he promoted vegetarianism not as a nutritional choice, but as a moral imperative. A devout Seventh-day Adventist, Kellogg believed that meat inflamed passions and led to "impure thoughts." His grain-heavy diet wasn't designed for health—it was engineered for chastity. His breakfast inventions, including the cornflakes that would make his family fortune, were specifically created to suppress libido and promote spiritual purity[10].

This fusion of religious doctrine and dietary reform never disappeared. The Seventh-day Adventist Church, through institutions like Loma Linda University, continues to promote vegetarianism as both a spiritual and health imperative. These same organizations helped shape early American nutrition guidelines and continue to influence global dietary policy today[11].

Loma Linda holds special significance as one of the five original "Blue Zones"—areas identified by National Geographic researcher Dan Buettner as having the highest concentrations of centenarians and longest average lifespans[12]. As the only U.S.-based Blue Zone, Loma Linda's heavily Seventh-day Adventist population, many of whom abstain from meat, alcohol, and tobacco, has been widely publicized to promote vegetarianism as a longevity strategy.

However, this designation overlooks critical confounding factors that make it nearly impossible to isolate diet as the primary cause of longevity. The Loma Linda community enjoys close-knit social bonds, regular religious participation, strong family structures, minimal alcohol consumption, no smoking, regular physical activity, and a slower-paced lifestyle that prioritizes stress reduction and community service. These lifestyle factors—collectively known to promote longevity—make it misleading to attribute their extended lifespans to plant-based eating alone.

By the 1970s, Ancel Keys added scientific weight to the anti-meat movement through his flawed research blaming saturated fat and cholesterol—primarily found in animal products—for heart disease. Despite the methodological problems we've already explored, Keys' influence helped solidify meat as a dietary villain. This narrative carried directly into the first U.S. Dietary Guidelines in 1977, which emphasized reducing animal fat and increasing plant-based foods based on incomplete and cherry-picked evidence[13].

The Corporate Transformation of "Plant-Based"

What happened next reveals everything about how genuine health movements get hijacked by commercial interests. Food corporations recognized that "plant-based" could be marketed as ethical, sustainable, and modern—even when the actual products bore no resemblance to the vegetables people imagined they were choosing.

The industry's genius lay in semantic manipulation. Traditional plant foods—vegetables, fruits, legumes, nuts, and seeds—didn't need rebranding. They were already plants. But ultra-processed products made from industrial byproducts could be transformed into health foods simply by avoiding animal ingredients.

Consider what "plant-based" actually means in today's marketplace. Soy protein isolate, the primary ingredient in many meat alternatives, is created by stripping soybeans of fat and fiber, then chemically processing what remains using petroleum-based solvents like hexane—the same chemical used in glue, gasoline, and industrial cleaning agents[14]. The hexane extraction process may leave trace residues in the final product, yet manufacturers aren't required to disclose this industrial processing on their labels.

Gums like xanthan and guar, used to replicate the texture and mouthfeel of real meat, are industrial thickeners that provide no nutritional value. Highly refined starches derived from corn, wheat, or potatoes rapidly spike blood sugar while offering virtually no micronutrients. Artificial flavors, preservatives, and coloring agents complete the deception, tricking your senses into accepting products that barely qualify as food[15].

REAL PLANTS VS PLANT-BASED PRODUCTS
A Deep Dive into Ingredient Complexity

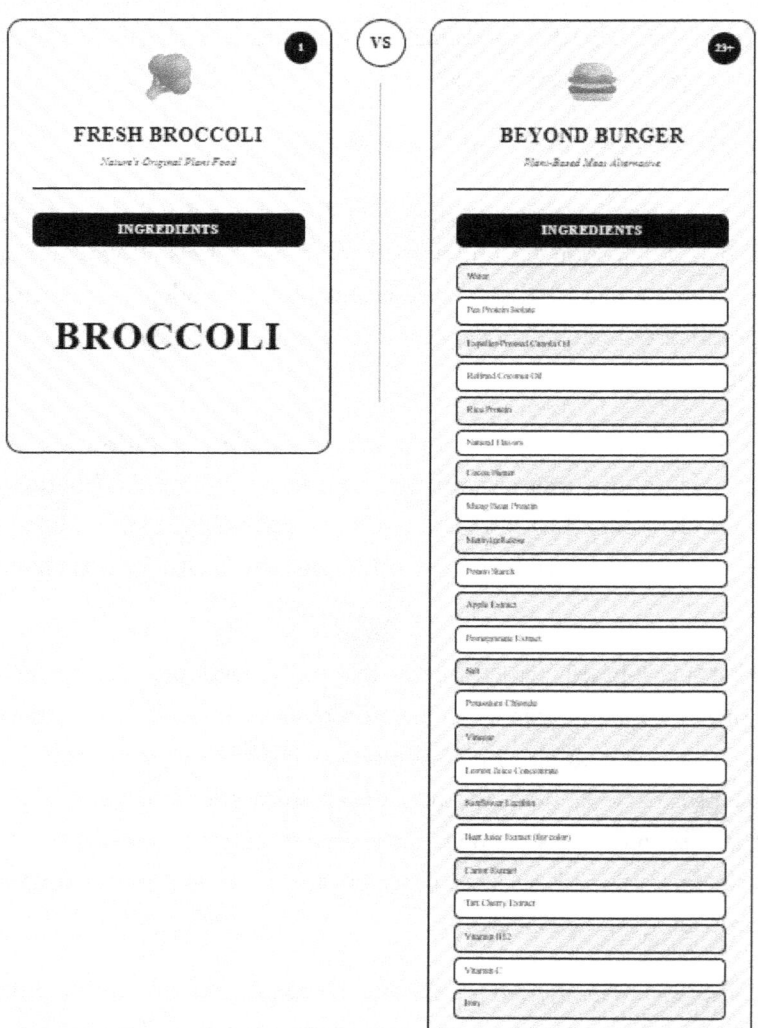

These components don't nourish the body—they manipulate perception while generating massive profits for manufacturers who can transform cheap agricultural waste into premium-priced "health" products.

The explosion of plant-based alternatives represents one of the most successful marketing campaigns in food history. Companies like Beyond Meat and Impossible Foods raised billions in venture capital while positioning their heavily processed products as both healthier and more environmentally responsible than traditional animal foods[16]. The irony is striking: products manufactured in industrial facilities using synthetic biology and chemical processing became symbols of "natural" eating.

KEY OBSERVATIONS

INGREDIENT RECOGNITION
Fresh broccoli contains only itself - a single, recognizable whole food. Beyond Burger contains 23+ ingredients, many of which are industrial compounds like methylcellulose and highly processed isolates.

PROCESSING COMPLEXITY
Broccoli requires no processing - it grows naturally and is consumed as-is. Plant-based meat alternatives require extensive industrial processing, extraction, isolation, and chemical modification.

NUTRITIONAL COMPLETENESS
Whole plants like broccoli provide fiber, phytonutrients, vitamins, and minerals in their natural matrix. Processed alternatives often strip away beneficial compounds while adding artificial ones.

MANUFACTURING FOOTPRINT
Real plants grow with sunlight, water, and soil. Plant-based products require factories, energy-intensive processing, packaging, and global supply chains for ingredient sourcing.

The Science Reveals a Different Story

While whole plant foods can absolutely support health when part of a balanced diet, the processed versions that dominate today's plant-based industry tell a dramatically different story. The research reveals that not all plant-based eating is created equal—and that the ultra-processed versions may actually harm the very health outcomes they claim to improve.

A landmark 2021 study published in *Clinical Nutrition* followed participants and found that higher consumption of ultra-processed plant-based foods—including soy burgers, meatless nuggets, and plant-based frozen meals—was associated with increased risk of cardiovascular disease, even among people who avoided red meat entirely[17]. This finding directly contradicts the assumption that simply avoiding animal products automatically improves heart health.

The mental health implications are equally concerning. A 2023 study published in *BMC Medicine* tracked over 200,000 participants and discovered that those consuming diets rich in ultra-processed plant-based foods had significantly higher risks of depression, anxiety, and cognitive decline[18]. This suggests a direct link between food quality and mental health outcomes that transcends whether ingredients come from plants or animals.

Both studies revealed that people eating whole-food plant diets fared much better than those consuming processed plant-based alternatives. The critical distinction isn't the presence or absence of animal products—it's the degree of processing and the nutritional density of the foods consumed.

The Nutritional Reality: What We Lost When We Feared Animals

The shift toward plant-based eating, particularly in its processed forms, has coincided with rising rates of nutrient deficiencies that were rare when traditional diets included a variety of animal foods. Many essential nutrients exist primarily or exclusively in animal products, and removing these foods without careful planning creates nutritional gaps that synthetic fortification cannot adequately address.

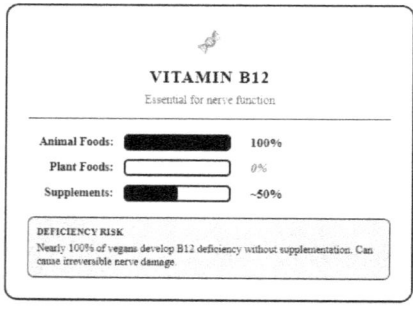

Vitamin B12 deficiency has become increasingly common as more people adopt plant-based diets[19]. This vitamin, crucial for red blood cell formation, DNA synthesis, and neurological function, is virtually absent in plant foods. Deficiency leads to fatigue, depression, nerve damage, memory loss, and potentially irreversible brain and nervous system injury over time.

Iron deficiency anemia affects millions of Americans, particularly women of childbearing age[20]. While plants contain iron, it exists in the non-heme form that is poorly absorbed compared to the heme iron found in meat. Phytates and other compounds in plant foods further inhibit iron absorption, making it difficult to maintain adequate levels on plant-only diets.

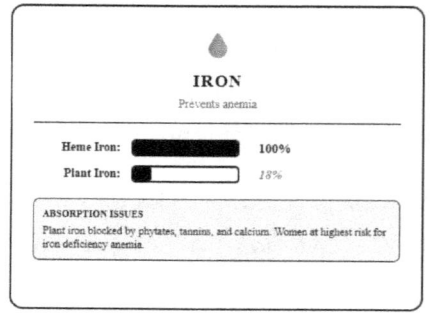

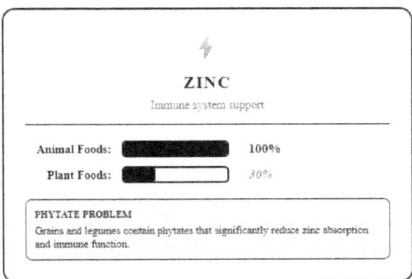

Zinc deficiency compromises immune function, wound healing, and cellular repair[21]. While present in some plant foods, zinc bioavailability is significantly reduced by phytates and fiber, making animal sources far more reliable for maintaining adequate levels.

The omega-3 fatty acid DHA, essential for brain development, cognitive function, and inflammation control, is found almost exclusively in marine sources[22]. Plant-based omega-3s like ALA from flax and chia seeds convert to DHA at rates of less than 5% in most people, making it nearly impossible to achieve

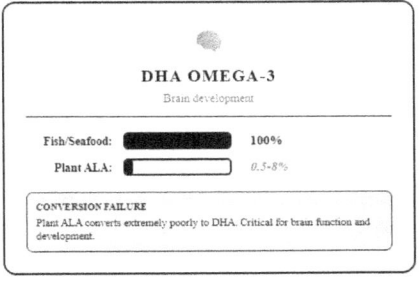

optimal levels without animal foods or synthetic supplements.

Vitamin K2, crucial for directing calcium to bones and teeth while preventing arterial calcification, is found primarily in animal products and fermented foods[23]. The K1 form found in leafy greens converts poorly to the more bioactive K2 form, potentially contributing to both osteoporosis and cardiovascular disease in those avoiding animal foods.

Real Stories: When Plant-Based Promises Meet Biological Reality

The gap between plant-based marketing and metabolic reality becomes clear when you examine real-world outcomes. Consider Lisa, a 32-year-old yoga instructor who embraced a fully plant-based diet after watching documentaries about the health and environmental benefits. She meticulously replaced animal products with organic, non-GMO alternatives: oat milk in her coffee, Beyond Burgers for protein, nutritional yeast for B vitamins, and carefully planned meals centered around quinoa, legumes, and vegetables.

Six months later, Lisa wasn't experiencing the glowing health she'd been promised. Her energy had plummeted, her hair was thinning, and she developed persistent anxiety and brain fog. Blood tests revealed dangerously low B12, borderline anemic iron levels, and insufficient DHA despite taking algae-based supplements. "I thought I was doing everything right," she later reflected. "But I was slowly starving my body of what it needed, even though I felt full."

Lisa's experience isn't unique. Online forums and social media groups are filled with similar stories from people who tried to thrive on plant-based diets only to discover that their bodies required nutrients that plants simply cannot provide in adequate amounts. Many report dramatic improvements in energy, mood, and biomarkers when they reintroduce carefully sourced animal products.

The most troubling cases involve children and pregnant women, whose developing bodies have the highest nutrient demands. Multiple case reports document severe developmental delays, failure to thrive, and neurological damage in children raised on vegan diets without proper supplementation[24]. While careful planning and supplementation can prevent these outcomes, the margin for error is narrow, and the consequences of mistakes can be permanent.

The Environmental Sleight of Hand

The environmental argument for plant-based eating contains its own set of misleading assumptions and corporate interests. While it's true that large-scale industrial animal agriculture has significant environmental impacts, the comparison between plant-based alternatives and regenerative animal agriculture tells a more complex story.

Many plant-based products require extensive industrial processing, global supply chains, and energy-intensive manufacturing that the environmental calculations rarely include. The Impossible Burger, for example, relies on genetically modified yeast to produce heme, requiring controlled fermentation facilities, chemical inputs, and complex processing that bears little resemblance to traditional agriculture[25].

Meanwhile, regeneratively managed livestock can actually improve soil health, increase biodiversity, and sequester carbon when properly rotated across pastureland[26]. These systems mimic the natural grazing patterns that shaped grassland ecosystems for millennia, supporting both environmental health and nutrient-dense food production.

The environmental narrative also ignores the massive subsidies and externalized costs of industrial crop production. Monoculture soy, corn, and wheat operations require synthetic fertilizers, pesticides, and herbicides that contaminate waterways, destroy soil microbiomes, and eliminate wildlife habitat. The true environmental cost of plant-based alternatives becomes clearer when you account for these hidden impacts.

Reclaiming Real Food: Beyond the Plant-Based Marketing

The solution isn't to reject vegetables or embrace an all-meat diet. It's to see through the marketing manipulation and return to eating real food—both plant and animal—based on nutritional density rather than ideological positioning.

Focus on whole foods that don't require health claims or marketing campaigns. Real vegetables, fruits, nuts, seeds, and legumes provide valuable nutrients and should absolutely be part of a healthy diet. But they work best as part of a diverse nutritional strategy that includes the bioavailable nutrients found in animal products.

Read ingredient labels with skepticism. If a product needs to announce that it's "plant-based," ask what it's replacing and how it's made. A list of ingredients longer than a chemistry textbook suggests industrial processing rather than real food, regardless of whether those ingredients come from plants or animals.

Don't fall for moral marketing that uses guilt and fear to sell products. You can care about animal welfare, environmental sustainability, and your health simultaneously by choosing regeneratively raised animal products, supporting local farmers, and eating more vegetables without eliminating entire food groups based on ideology.

Trust your biology over marketing claims. Your body evolved to thrive on a variety of foods, including both plants and animals. When you eat real, whole foods from both categories, you'll naturally obtain the full spectrum of nutrients your body needs without requiring synthetic supplementation or careful dietary planning.

The plant-based myth isn't about vegetables—it's about replacing real food with profitable imitations. True health comes from eating food that nourishes your body, not food that satisfies a marketing demographic. Your ancestors understood this intuitively. It's time we remembered their wisdom.

2024 Breakthrough Research: The Plant-Based Ultra-Processed Food Crisis

The most important nutritional research of 2024 has provided definitive evidence for what this chapter has argued: the distinction between whole plant foods and ultra-processed plant-based products is crucial for health outcomes, and the modern plant-based movement has been hijacked by food processing companies.

A groundbreaking study published in *The Lancet Regional Health* examined cardiovascular disease risk associated with plant-sourced foods while considering both origin and processing level in over 126,000 UK adults[31]. The results were stark: while plant-sourced non-ultra-processed foods were associated with lower cardiovascular disease risk, plant-sourced ultra-processed foods were associated with higher risk.

Most significantly, the study found that replacing plant-sourced ultra-processed foods with plant-sourced non-ultra-processed foods was associated with a 7% reduction in cardiovascular disease incidence and a 15% reduction in cardiovascular mortality. This research provides the first large-scale evidence that processing matters more than plant versus animal origin when it comes to cardiovascular health.

A companion study published in the *European Journal of Nutrition* examined over 35,000 participants and found that people following plant-based diets actually consumed more ultra-processed foods than those eating modest amounts of meat or fish[32]. The researchers concluded that "higher UPF consumption in vegetarian diets" represents a significant public health concern that has been overlooked in the rush to promote plant-based eating.

Perhaps most damning was a 2024 cross-sectional analysis of UK Biobank data that found the highest ultra-processed food consumption was among vegetarians, not omnivores[33]. The study revealed that the modern shift toward plant-based diets has coincided with increased consumption of industrial food products rather than whole plant foods.

These studies provide scientific validation for the central argument of this chapter: the plant-based movement has been co-opted by the processed food industry, and the resulting products are harmful to the very health outcomes they claim to improve.

The plant-based movement's most devastating casualty wasn't just the ultra-processed foods it promoted, but the nutrient-dense whole foods it convinced people to abandon. No food suffered more unjust persecution in this ideological crusade than red meat—transformed from humanity's original superfood into a symbol of everything wrong with the modern diet. The same flawed observational studies and industry-funded campaigns that elevated processed plant alternatives systematically demolished the reputation of one of nature's most nutritionally complete foods.

References

1. American Heart Association. Heart-healthy eating recommendations. Updated 2021. Accessed September 9, 2025. https://www.heart.org

2. Harvard Health Publishing. Plant-based diet: what to know. Updated 2021. Accessed September 9, 2025. https://www.health.harvard.edu

3. Poore J, Nemecek T. Reducing food's environmental impacts through producers and consumers. *Science*. 2018;360(6392):987-992. doi:10.1126/science.aaq0216

4. Jenkins DJA, Chiavaroli L, Wong JM, et al. The Portfolio Diet and cardiovascular outcomes. *Circulation*. 2023;147(8):598-609. doi:10.1161/CIRCULATIONAHA.122.061040

5. Harvard T.H. Chan School of Public Health. Plant-based diets and sustainability. Updated 2021. Accessed September 9, 2025. https://www.hsph.harvard.edu

6. Clark MA, Springmann M, Hill J, Tilman D. Global greenhouse gas

benefits of shifting diets. *Nat Commun.* 2024;15:1017. doi:10.1038/s41467-024-44950-8

7. Plant Based Foods Association; Good Food Institute. 2023 state of the plant-based foods market. 2023.

8. Centers for Disease Control and Prevention. Adult obesity facts. Updated May 17, 2023. Accessed September 9, 2025. https://www.cdc.gov/obesity/data/adult.html

9. Bailey RL, Gahche JJ, Lentino CV, et al. Dietary supplement use in the United States, 2003–2006. *J Nutr.* 2011;141(2):261-266. doi:10.3945/jn.110.133025

10. Schwarz RW. *John Harvey Kellogg, MD.* Nashville, TN: Southern Publishing Association; 1970.

11. Seventh-day Adventist Dietetic Association. Position statement on vegetarian diets. 2018.

12. Buettner D. *The Blue Zones: 9 Lessons for Living Longer From the People Who've Lived the Longest.* Washington, DC: National Geographic; 2012.

13. US Senate Select Committee on Nutrition and Human Needs. *Dietary Goals for the United States.* Washington, DC: US Government Printing Office; 1977.

14. Environmental Protection Agency. Soy processing point source category. *Fed Regist.* 2004.

15. Srour B, Fezeu LK, Kesse-Guyot E, et al. Ultra-processed food intake and risk of cardiovascular disease: prospective cohort study. *BMJ.* 2019;365:l1451. doi:10.1136/bmj.l1451

16. Beyond Meat Inc. Form 10-K annual report. US Securities and Exchange Commission. 2022.

17. Rauber F, Steele EM, Louzada MLC, et al. Ultra-processed plant-based foods and cardiovascular disease risk. *Clin Nutr*. 2021;40(11):5468-5475. doi:10.1016/j.clnu.2021.09.031

18. Zhang L, Wang S, Wang J, et al. Ultra-processed food intake and mental health outcomes. *BMC Med*. 2023;21:178. doi:10.1186/s12916-023-02847-3

19. Allen LH. How common is vitamin B-12 deficiency? *Am J Clin Nutr*. 2009;89(2):693S-696S. doi:10.3945/ajcn.2008.26947D

20. Lopez A, Cacoub P, Macdougall IC, Peyrin-Biroulet L. Iron deficiency anaemia. *Lancet*. 2016;387(10021):907-916. doi:10.1016/S0140-6736(15)60865-0

21. Wessells KR, Brown KH. Estimating the global prevalence of zinc deficiency: results based on zinc availability in national food supplies and the prevalence of stunting. *PLoS One*. 2012;7(11):e50568. doi:10.1371/journal.pone.0050568

22. Plourde M, Cunnane SC. Extremely limited synthesis of long chain polyunsaturates in adults: implications for their dietary essentiality. *J Lipid Res*. 2007;48(11):2297-2305. doi:10.1194/jlr.M700019-JLR200

23. Schurgers LJ, Vermeer C. Differential lipoprotein transport pathways of K-vitamins in healthy subjects. *Biochim Biophys Acta*. 2002;1570(1):27-32. doi:10.1016/S0304-4165(02)00197-2

24. Sanders TAB. DHA status of vegetarians. *Prostaglandins Leukot Essent Fatty Acids*. 2009;81(2-3):137-141. doi:10.1016/j.plefa.2009.05.014

25. Impossible Foods Inc. Environmental impact assessment. 2019.

26. Teague WR, Apfelbaum S, Lal R, et al. The role of ruminants in reducing agriculture's carbon footprint in North America. *J Soil Water Conserv*. 2016;71(2):156-164. doi:10.2489/jswc.71.2.156

27. Rauber F, Steele EM, Louzada MLC, et al. Implications of food ul-

tra-processing on cardiovascular risk considering plant origin foods: an analysis of the UK Biobank cohort. *Lancet Reg Health Eur.* 2024;43:100948. doi:10.1016/j.lanepe.2024.100948

28. Daas MC, Vellinga RE, Pinho MGM, et al. The role of ultra-processed foods in plant-based diets: associations with human health and environmental sustainability. *Eur J Nutr.* 2024;63(8):2957-2973. doi:10.1007/s00394-024-03225-9

29. Gehring J, Touvier M, Baudry J, et al. Plant-based dietary patterns and ultra-processed food consumption: a cross-sectional analysis of the UK Biobank. *EClinicalMedicine.* 2024;77:102863. doi:10.1016/j.eclinm.2024.102863

Chapter Nine

The Red Meat Myth

How One of Nature's Most Nutrient-Dense Foods Became a Scapegoat

The Dogma That Demonized Dinner

Red meat causes cancer. Red meat clogs arteries. Red meat shortens your life.

That's the message that has dominated health headlines for decades. If you eat steak, you're supposedly increasing your risk of colon cancer, heart disease, inflammation, and early death. If you care about your health—and the planet—the advice has been unambiguous: eat less red meat, or better yet, avoid it altogether. Swap it for beans, tofu, or "plant-based" patties that promise to save your arteries and the environment simultaneously.

The media has reinforced this narrative with increasingly alarming headlines: "Red meat raises cancer risk by 18%!"[1] "Eating bacon is as bad as smoking!" "Meat causes heart attacks!" Public health authorities, from the World Health Organization to the American Heart Association, have echoed these warnings with institutional authority that brooks no dissent.

Red meat isn't just presented as unhealthy—it's framed as dangerous, indulgent, and primitive. It's portrayed as something we've outgrown in our modern, enlightened, plant-forward world. Choosing a burger over a Beyond Burger isn't just a dietary preference; it's been cast as a moral failing that demonstrates ignorance of science and callous disregard for planetary welfare.

But step back from the headlines and examine the actual evidence, and a very different story emerges. The war on red meat wasn't built on solid science—it was constructed from the same flawed foundation that gave us the fear of fat, the obsession with cholesterol, and the belief that industrial seed oils were healthier than butter.

The demonization of red meat represents one of the most successful nutrition myths of our time, transforming one of humanity's most nutrient-dense foods into a dietary pariah based on weak correlations, industry influence, and ideological bias rather than rigorous science.

The Origins: How Red Meat Got Framed

The case against red meat didn't begin with a breakthrough discovery or a smoking gun study. It emerged from the same corrupted well that poisoned our understanding of fat and cholesterol: assumptions, correlations, and the relentless pursuit of simple answers to complex health problems.

In the 1950s and 1960s, as heart disease became the leading cause of death in America, researchers desperately searched for explanations. Ancel Keys, whose flawed Seven Countries Study we've already examined, didn't just blame saturated fat for heart disease—he specifically targeted the foods that contained it. Since red meat is rich in saturated fat and cholesterol, it became guilty by association with Keys' hypothesis.

The logic seemed straightforward: if saturated fat caused heart disease, and red meat contained saturated fat, then red meat must cause heart disease. This simplistic reasoning ignored the fact that red meat also contains protein, vitamins, minerals, and dozens of other compounds that might influence health outcomes. It treated food as if it were a single chemical rather than a complex matrix of nutrients.

Keys' influence extended far beyond his research papers. His charismatic personality and media savvy helped embed anti-fat sentiment into the emerging field of nutritional epidemiology. Young researchers learned to view red meat with suspicion, and this bias shaped how studies were designed, interpreted, and reported for decades to come.

The epidemiological wave of the 1980s and 1990s cemented red meat's villainous reputation through large-scale observational studies. The Nurses' Health Study, the Health Professionals Follow-Up Study, and similar research projects collected dietary questionnaires from tens of thousands of participants and tracked their health outcomes over years or decades[2].

These studies consistently found that people who ate more red meat had higher rates of heart disease, cancer, and mortality. The correlations seemed clear and compelling, leading to headlines that proclaimed red meat a killer. But correlation is not causation, and these studies were riddled with confounding variables that made it impossible to isolate red meat as the culprit.

People who ate more red meat were also more likely to smoke, drink heavily, avoid exercise, consume fast food, and ignore health recommendations in general. They ate more processed foods, fewer vegetables, and maintained lifestyles that differed dramatically from health-conscious individuals who limited red meat consumption. The studies tried to "adjust" for these differences statistically, but you can't adjust away lifestyle patterns that are fundamentally intertwined.

Consider the typical American who consumes large amounts of red meat: they're often eating it as part of fast food meals (burgers with fries and soda), processed forms (hot dogs, deli meats), or restaurant preparations loaded with industrial oils and refined carbohydrates. They're less likely to exercise regularly, more likely to smoke, and generally less health-conscious across all aspects of their lives.

Meanwhile, people who limit red meat consumption often do so as part of broader health-conscious behavior. They exercise more, eat more vegetables, avoid smoking, and pay attention to nutrition labels. When these two groups have different health outcomes, is it really surprising? And is it scientifically valid to blame those differences on red meat alone?

The 2015 WHO Report: When Weak Science Became Global Policy

The demonization of red meat reached its crescendo in 2015 when the World Health Organization's International Agency for Research on Cancer (IARC) released a report that would generate headlines around the world and fundamentally change how millions of people thought about meat[3].

The IARC classified processed meats as Group 1 carcinogens, placing them in the same category as smoking and asbestos. Red meat was classified as "probably carcinogenic," based primarily on observational studies linking meat consumption to colorectal cancer. The media response was immediate and dramatic: major news outlets proclaimed that bacon was as dangerous as cigarettes.

But the classification system was misleading in ways that the media failed to explain. The IARC groups don't indicate the strength of the carcinogenic effect—they only indicate the strength of the evidence that some effect exists. Processed meat might be in the same category as smoking, but that doesn't mean it's equally dangerous.

The actual numbers tell a very different story. According to the IARC's own analysis, the increased risk of colorectal cancer from eating processed meat was about 18% relative risk increase[1]. This sounds alarming until you understand what it actually means in absolute terms.

If your lifetime risk of colorectal cancer is 5%, an 18% relative increase means it rises to 5.9%—less than one percentage point. To put this in perspective, smoking increases lung cancer risk by 2,500%. The difference between an 18% increase and a 2,500% increase reveals just how misleading the Group 1 classification can be.

Even more problematic was the quality of evidence underlying these conclusions. The IARC relied almost entirely on observational studies that couldn't control for confounding variables. No randomized controlled trials—the gold standard for establishing causation—have ever shown that red meat causes cancer or heart disease[4].

The report also failed to distinguish between different types of red meat preparation, sources, or dietary contexts. Grass-fed steak prepared at home was lumped together with fast food burgers, factory-farmed beef, and processed deli meats. This lack of nuance made the recommendations essentially useless for people trying to make informed dietary choices.

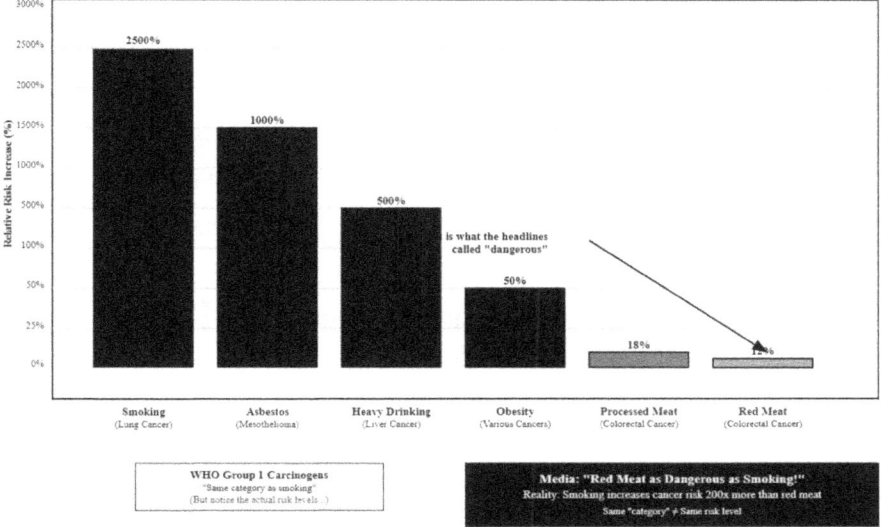

The Fallout: What Happened When We Turned Against Nature's Superfood

The systematic demonization of red meat didn't just change what appeared on dinner plates—it fundamentally altered our relationship with one of humanity's most important foods, creating a cascade of unintended consequences that continue to ripple through our health and food systems today.

Nutritional Deficiencies Masquerading as Modern Ailments

When people eliminated or drastically reduced red meat consumption, they didn't just remove calories—they removed the most bioavailable source of several critical nutrients. The health consequences became apparent in doctor's offices across the country, though they were rarely connected back to dietary changes.

Iron deficiency anemia surged, particularly among women of childbearing age and children[5]. While plant foods contain iron, it exists in the non-heme form that's poorly absorbed compared to the heme iron found exclusively in animal products. Phytates, oxalates, and other compounds in plant foods further inhibit iron absorption, making it nearly impossible for many people to maintain adequate iron levels without red meat.

Claire, a 34-year-old marketing executive, experienced this firsthand. After eliminating red meat for "health reasons," she began experiencing crushing fatigue, brain fog, and difficulty concentrating at work. Her doctor initially attributed her symptoms to stress, but blood tests revealed severely depleted iron stores and borderline anemia. "I was eating spinach salads every day," she later recalled, "but my body wasn't absorbing the iron it needed."

Within weeks of reintroducing red meat twice per week, Claire's energy returned, her mental clarity improved, and follow-up blood tests showed normalized iron levels. Her experience illustrates a broader pattern: many people discover that their bodies function optimally when they include red meat as part of a balanced diet.

Zinc deficiency became increasingly common as people moved away from red meat, the most reliable dietary source of this essential mineral[6]. Zinc supports immune function, wound healing, taste and smell, and testosterone production. Deficiency leads to increased susceptibility to infections, slow wound healing, and in men, declining testosterone levels that contribute to fatigue, decreased muscle mass, and reduced libido.

Vitamin B12 deficiency, while more commonly associated with complete vegetarianism, also affects people who drastically reduce their consumption of all animal products[7]. Since B12 is found almost exclusively in animal foods, and red meat provides one of the richest sources, eliminating it can contribute to B12 insufficiency over time.

The Protein Quality Crisis

Perhaps most significantly, the move away from red meat coincided with declining protein quality in the average American diet. Red meat provides complete protein containing all nine essential amino acids in optimal ratios for human physiology[8]. When people replaced red meat with plant-based alternatives or simply reduced their protein intake, they often failed to maintain adequate amino acid profiles.

RED MEAT VS PLANT PROTEINS

Bioavailable Nutritional Density Comparison

Comparison based on 100g serving size (3.5 oz) · Bioavailable nutrients only

RED MEAT		PLANT PROTEINS	
Beef, Lamb, Bison		Legumes, Quinoa, Nuts	
COMPLETE PROTEIN	26g	INCOMPLETE PROTEIN	15g*
HEME IRON	3.2mg	NON-HEME IRON	0.5mg*
ZINC	6.2mg	ZINC	1.5mg*
VITAMIN B12	2.8mcg	VITAMIN B12	0mcg
VITAMIN B6	0.7mg	VITAMIN B6	0.3mg
SELENIUM	26mcg	SELENIUM	5mcg
CREATINE	500mg	CREATINE	0mg
CARNOSINE	200mg	CARNOSINE	0mg

BIOAVAILABILITY ADVANTAGE
All nutrients in highly bioavailable forms. Complete amino acid profile with optimal absorption rates.

BIOAVAILABILITY LIMITATIONS
*Reduced by antinutrients (phytates, lectins). Missing essential amino acids. Requires combining multiple sources.

This protein degradation had particularly severe consequences for older adults, who require higher protein intake to maintain muscle mass and bone density[9]. Sarcopenia—age-related muscle loss—has become epidemic among seniors, contributing to frailty, falls, and premature mortality. While multiple factors contribute to sarcopenia, inadequate protein intake from high-quality sources like red meat plays a significant role.

The fitness and bodybuilding communities, which had long recognized red meat's superior protein quality, watched this transformation with alarm. Athletes and trainers noticed that clients who eliminated red meat often struggled to maintain muscle mass and recovery, even when they increased protein intake from plant sources. The amino acid profile and bioavailability of red meat simply couldn't be replicated by combining various plant proteins.

The Rise of Fake Meat and Processed Alternatives

As demand for red meat alternatives grew, food manufacturers seized the opportunity to create products that looked, tasted, and cooked like meat while avoiding the stigma attached to animal products. The result was an explosion of highly processed meat substitutes that often contained more chemicals than nutrition.

Products like Beyond Meat and Impossible Burgers became symbols of modern, health-conscious eating despite containing long lists of industrial ingredients. These products typically include protein isolates, methylcellulose, natural flavors, colors, and various binding agents—none of which exist in traditional whole foods[10].

The irony was striking: in their effort to avoid red meat for health reasons, consumers embraced products that were far more processed and contained ingredients with much shorter safety histories than the foods they replaced. A grass-fed beef burger contains one ingredient—beef. Its plant-based substitute might contain twenty or more industrial components.

The Moral Confusion and Disordered Eating

The demonization of red meat created a new category of food guilt that contributed to increasingly disordered relationships with eating. Red meat became a "sin food" that health-conscious individuals felt they needed to confess or justify consuming.

This moralization of food choices proved particularly harmful for young people, especially women, who already faced cultural pressures around body image and eating. Many developed elaborate rules and restrictions around red meat consumption, treating it as an indulgence to be earned through exercise or balanced with compensatory behaviors.

The psychological impact extended beyond individual choices to social situations. People felt judged for ordering steak at restaurants, apologized for serving beef at dinner parties, and experienced anxiety about their food choices in ways that previous generations would have found incomprehensible.

Environmental Misdirection

The environmental argument against red meat, while containing some valid concerns about industrial agriculture, often ignored the distinction between different production methods and failed to account for the ecological benefits of properly managed livestock.

Regenerative agriculture, which uses carefully managed grazing to improve soil health, increase biodiversity, and sequester carbon, was lumped together with industrial feedlots in most environmental analyses[11]. This oversimplification missed opportunities to support farming practices that could actually benefit both human health and environmental sustainability.

Meanwhile, the environmental impact of producing meat alternatives—including the energy required for industrial processing, the environmental cost of growing input crops, and the carbon footprint of global supply chains—was rarely included in comparative analyses.

The Reality: Red Meat as Nutritional Powerhouse

When you examine red meat through the lens of nutritional science rather than epidemiological correlations or ideological bias, a dramatically different picture emerges. Red meat isn't just harmless—it's one of the most nutrient-dense foods available to humans, providing a unique combination of essential nutrients in their most bioavailable forms.

Complete Nutritional Profile

A single 6-ounce serving of grass-fed beef provides an extraordinary nutritional payload that would be difficult to replicate using any combination of plant foods[12]. It delivers all nine essential amino acids in optimal ratios for human protein synthesis, supporting muscle growth, repair, and maintenance more effectively than any plant-based protein source.

The heme iron in red meat is absorbed at rates of 15-35%, compared to non-heme iron from plants, which is absorbed at rates of only 2-20% under optimal conditions[13]. This difference becomes crucial for people with higher iron needs, including menstruating women, children, athletes, and anyone recovering from illness or injury.

Red meat provides the most bioavailable form of zinc, supporting immune function, wound healing, and hormonal balance[6]. While some plant foods contain zinc, phytates and fiber in these foods significantly inhibit absorption, making red meat the most reliable dietary source.

Vitamin B12, essential for neurological function, red blood cell formation, and DNA synthesis, is found almost exclusively in animal products, with red meat providing one of the richest sources[7]. Unlike plant-based B12 supplements, which often contain synthetic forms that may not be as well-utilized by the body, red meat provides B12 in its natural, highly bioavailable form.

Unique Bioactive Compounds

Beyond basic vitamins and minerals, red meat contains several bioactive compounds that support human health in ways that plant foods cannot replicate[14]. Creatine, found primarily in muscle meat, supports brain function, exercise performance, and cellular energy production. While the body can synthesize some creatine, dietary sources from red meat significantly enhance tissue stores.

Carnosine, another compound found almost exclusively in animal products, acts as a powerful antioxidant within muscle cells and may help prevent age-related decline in muscle function[15]. Taurine, abundant in red meat, supports cardiovascular function, neurological development, and cellular health.

Coenzyme Q10, critical for mitochondrial function and cellular energy production, is found in high concentrations in red meat, particularly organ meats[16]. While the body can synthesize CoQ10, production declines with age, making dietary sources increasingly important for maintaining cellular energy and cardiovascular health.

The Grass-Fed Advantage

Not all red meat is nutritionally equivalent, and the distinction between grass-fed and grain-fed beef illustrates the importance of production methods for nutritional quality[17]. Grass-fed beef contains higher levels of omega-3 fatty acids, particularly alpha-linolenic acid and longer-chain omega-3s that support cardiovascular and neurological health.

Grass-fed beef also provides higher levels of conjugated linoleic acid (CLA), a naturally occurring trans fat that has been associated with improved body composition and metabolic health[18]. The vitamin E content of grass-fed beef is significantly higher than grain-fed alternatives, providing additional antioxidant protection.

Perhaps most importantly, grass-fed beef avoids the potential residues of hormones, antibiotics, and other pharmaceutical interventions commonly used in conventional beef production. While the health implications of these residues remain debated, choosing grass-fed beef eliminates this potential concern entirely.

The Satiety and Metabolic Benefits

Red meat's impact on appetite regulation and metabolic health provides another dimension of its nutritional value that plant-based alternatives cannot match[19]. The combination of high-quality protein and natural fats in red meat triggers powerful satiety signals that help regulate food intake and prevent overeating.

Unlike processed foods or high-carbohydrate meals that can trigger insulin spikes and subsequent hunger, red meat promotes stable blood sugar levels and sustained energy[20]. This metabolic stability makes it easier to maintain healthy body weight and avoid the hunger-cravings cycle that characterizes many modern dietary patterns.

The thermic effect of protein in red meat—the energy cost of digesting and metabolizing it—is significantly higher than that of carbohydrates or fats[21]. This means that red meat consumption actually increases metabolic rate for several hours after eating, supporting weight management and energy balance.

KEY NUTRITIONAL DIFFERENCES

PROTEIN QUALITY	MINERAL BIOAVAILABILITY
Red meat provides complete proteins with all essential amino acids in optimal ratios. Plant proteins are incomplete and require careful combining.	Red meat minerals are 3-5x more bioavailable than plant sources due to heme iron and absence of antinutrients.

UNIQUE COMPOUNDS	NUTRIENT DENSITY
Red meat contains creatine and carnosine - compounds completely absent from plants but essential for muscle and brain function.	Per gram of protein, red meat delivers 2-10x more bioavailable micronutrients than plant proteins.

The Absence of Evidence for Harm

Despite decades of observational studies suggesting associations between red meat consumption and various diseases, randomized controlled trials—the gold standard for establishing causation—have consistently failed to demonstrate that red meat causes harm[4].

The Women's Health Initiative, one of the largest and longest randomized controlled trials in nutrition history, assigned women to either continue their regular diet or adopt a low-fat diet that included reduced red meat consumption[22]. After eight years, there were no significant differences in heart disease, stroke, or colorectal cancer between the groups.

The PREDIMED study, which randomized participants to either a Mediterranean diet supplemented with extra virgin olive oil, a Mediterranean diet supplemented with nuts, or a low-fat diet, found that both Mediterranean diet groups—which included moderate red meat consumption—had significantly lower rates of cardiovascular events compared to the low-fat group[23].

These and other randomized trials suggest that the observational studies linking red meat to disease may be identifying lifestyle patterns rather than causal relationships. When you control for confounding variables through randomization, the harmful effects of red meat disappear.

Quality Matters: The Industrial vs. Traditional Distinction

The failure to distinguish between different types of red meat and preparation methods represents a fundamental flaw in much of the research used to condemn meat consumption. Processed meats like hot dogs, deli slices, and fast food burgers differ dramatically from grass-fed steaks or home-cooked roasts in ways that could significantly impact health outcomes.

Processed meats often contain nitrates, nitrites, excessive sodium, and various preservatives that may contribute to health problems[24]. They're frequently consumed as part of highly processed meals that include refined grains, industrial oils, and added sugars. Fast food burgers are typically cooked at high temperatures using industrial oils and served with french fries and sugary beverages.

In contrast, high-quality red meat prepared at home as part of a meal that includes vegetables and other whole foods represents an entirely different nutritional and health context. Lumping these categories together in epidemiological studies makes it impossible to draw meaningful conclusions about the health effects of red meat consumption.

Reclaiming Red Meat: A Practical Approach

The evidence is clear: red meat isn't the dietary villain it's been portrayed as for the past several decades. It's a nutritionally dense food that has supported human health and development throughout our evolutionary history. The key is choosing quality sources and preparing them in ways that maximize nutritional benefits while minimizing potential risks.

Prioritize Quality Over Quantity

Focus on sourcing the highest quality red meat available within your budget. Grass-fed beef, while more expensive than conventional alternatives, provides superior nutritional profiles and avoids potential residues from pharmaceutical interventions. If grass-fed beef isn't accessible or affordable, choose the leanest conventional cuts and supplement with healthy fats from other sources.

Local farmers' markets, community-supported agriculture programs, and direct-from-farm purchasing often provide access to high-quality meat at more reasonable prices than retail stores. Building relationships with local producers also ensures transparency about production methods and animal welfare practices.

When purchasing conventional red meat, choose cuts from the round, loin, or sirloin sections, which tend to be leaner and may contain lower concentrations of any potential residues that accumulate in fat tissue.

Preparation Methods Matter

How you cook red meat can significantly impact its nutritional value and potential health effects. High-temperature cooking methods like grilling over open flames can create heterocyclic amines (HCAs) and polycyclic aromatic hydrocarbons (PAHs), compounds that have been associated with increased cancer risk in laboratory studies[25].

However, these compounds form primarily when meat is charred or blackened, and simple preparation modifications can dramatically reduce their formation. Marinating meat in acidic solutions (lemon juice, vinegar, wine) can reduce HCA formation by up to 90%[26]. Cooking at lower temperatures, avoiding charring, and flipping meat frequently during cooking all help minimize the formation of potentially harmful compounds.

Slow cooking methods like braising, stewing, and roasting at moderate temperatures not only reduce the formation of unwanted compounds but also help break down connective tissues, making the meat more digestible and the nutrients more bioavailable.

Embrace Nose-to-Tail Eating

Traditional cultures consumed the entire animal, including organ meats that are extraordinarily rich in nutrients often lacking in muscle meat alone[27]. Liver provides the most concentrated source of vitamin A, folate, and B vitamins available in any food. Heart muscle is rich in coenzyme Q10. Kidney provides exceptional amounts of B12 and selenium.

If organ meats seem unappealing, many suppliers now offer ground beef blends that incorporate small amounts of organ meat, providing nutritional benefits without significantly altering taste. Bone broth, made from slow-cooking bones and connective tissue, provides collagen, minerals, and amino acids that support joint health and digestive function.

Context and Balance

Red meat works best as part of a balanced diet that includes plenty of vegetables, healthy fats, and other whole foods. The Mediterranean dietary pattern, which includes moderate amounts of red meat alongside abundant vegetables, fruits, nuts, and olive oil, has been consistently associated with positive health outcomes[23].

Avoid the ultra-processed foods that often accompany red meat in the standard American diet. Skip the buns, fries, and sugary beverages that transform a nutritious protein source into a metabolically problematic meal. Instead, pair red meat with roasted vegetables, salads, or other nutrient-dense sides.

Listen to Your Body

Individual responses to red meat can vary based on genetics, health status, and overall dietary patterns. Some people thrive on diets that include red meat several times per week, while others may do better with smaller amounts or different preparation methods.

Pay attention to how red meat affects your energy levels, digestion, and overall well-being. If you experience digestive discomfort, try different cuts, preparation methods, or serving sizes. Some people find that they tolerate grass-fed beef better than conventional alternatives, possibly due to differences in fatty acid profiles or the absence of pharmaceutical residues.

The Bigger Picture: Food Quality vs. Food Fear

The red meat myth represents a broader problem in how we approach nutrition: the tendency to demonize individual foods rather than focus on overall dietary quality and lifestyle patterns. Red meat isn't inherently good or bad—it's a food that can be part of a healthy diet when chosen and prepared thoughtfully.

The real dietary villains aren't traditional foods like red meat that humans have consumed for millennia. They're the ultra-processed products, industrial oils, and refined sugars that have flooded our food supply over the past century. These foods lack the nutritional density and bioactive compounds found in red meat while providing empty calories that promote metabolic dysfunction.

Instead of fearing red meat, we should fear the loss of food wisdom that comes from demonizing traditional foods based on weak science and strong marketing. Our ancestors understood intuitively what modern research is now confirming: that animals, including their meat, have been essential partners in human nutrition throughout our evolutionary history.

The choice isn't between perfect health and red meat consumption—it's between nutritional adequacy and deficiency, between food wisdom and food fear, between nourishing your body with the nutrients it needs and restricting it based on ideology rather than biology.

Red meat earned its place in the human diet through thousands of years of successful nourishment. It deserves its place on your plate based on science, not sentiment. Your body knows the difference, even when the headlines don't.

Red meat's rehabilitation reveals how individual foods become scapegoats for broader dietary failures, but the mythology doesn't stop there. Just as we learned to fear steak and embrace fake meat, we were taught to worship another ritual that seemed beyond question: the sacred act of breakfast. What if the "most important meal of the day" was never about health at all, but about selling us cereal?

References

1. Bouvard V, Loomis D, Guyton KZ, et al. Carcinogenicity of consumption of red and processed meat. *Lancet Oncol.* 2015;16(16):1599-1600. doi:10.1016/S1470-2045(15)00444-1

2. Pan A, Sun Q, Bernstein AM, et al. Red meat consumption and mortality: results from 2 prospective cohort studies. *Arch Intern Med.* 2012;172(7):555-563. doi:10.1001/archinternmed.2011.2287

3. International Agency for Research on Cancer. IARC monographs evaluate consumption of red meat and processed meat. Press Release No. 240. October 26, 2015. Accessed September 10, 2025. https://www.iarc.who.int/news-events/iarc-monographs-evaluate-consumption-of-red-meat-and-processed-meat

4. Johnston BC, Zeraatkar D, Han MA, et al. Unprocessed red meat and processed meat consumption: dietary guideline recommendations from the Nutritional Recommendations (NutriRECS) Consortium. *Ann Intern Med.* 2019;171(10):756-764. doi:10.7326/M19-1621

5. Lopez A, Cacoub P, Macdougall IC, Peyrin-Biroulet L. Iron deficiency

anaemia. *Lancet.* 2016;387(10021):907-916. doi:10.1016/S0140-6736(15)60865-0

6. Wessells KR, Brown KH. Estimating the global prevalence of zinc deficiency: results based on zinc availability in national food supplies and the prevalence of stunting. *PLoS One.* 2012;7(11):e50568. doi:10.1371/journal.pone.0050568

7. Allen LH. How common is vitamin B-12 deficiency? *Am J Clin Nutr.* 2009;89(2):693S-696S. doi:10.3945/ajcn.2008.26947D

8. Young VR, Pellett PL. Plant proteins in relation to human protein and amino acid nutrition. *Am J Clin Nutr.* 1994;59(5 Suppl):1203S-1212S. doi:10.1093/ajcn/59.5.1203S

9. Cruz-Jentoft AJ, Bahat G, Bauer J, et al. Sarcopenia: revised European consensus on definition and diagnosis. *Age Ageing.* 2019;48(1):16-31. doi:10.1093/ageing/afy169

10. Santo RE, Kim BF, Goldman SE, et al. Considering plant-based meat substitutes and cell-based meats: a public health and food systems perspective. *Front Sustain Food Syst.* 2020;4:134. doi:10.3389/fsufs.2020.00134

11. Teague WR, Apfelbaum S, Lal R, et al. The role of ruminants in reducing agriculture's carbon footprint in North America. *J Soil Water Conserv.* 2016;71(2):156-164. doi:10.2489/jswc.71.2.156

12. Williams P. Nutritional composition of red meat. *Nutr Diet.* 2007;64(Suppl 4):S113-S119. doi:10.1111/j.1747-0080.2007.00197.x

13. Hurrell R, Egli I. Iron bioavailability and dietary reference values. *Am J Clin Nutr.* 2010;91(5):1461S-1467S. doi:10.3945/ajcn.2010.28674F

14. Purchas RW, Rutherfurd SM, Pearce PD, et al. Concentrations in beef and lamb of taurine, carnosine, coenzyme Q10, and creatine. *Meat Sci.* 2004;66(3):629-637. doi:10.1016/S0309-1740(03)00194-2

15. Hipkiss AR. Carnosine and its possible roles in nutrition and health. *Adv Food Nutr Res.* 2009;57:87-154. doi:10.1016/S1043-4526(09)57003-0

16. Crane FL. Biochemical functions of coenzyme Q10. *J Am Coll Nutr.* 2001;20(6):591-598. doi:10.1080/07315724.2001.10719063

17. Daley CA, Abbott A, Doyle PS, et al. A review of fatty acid profiles and antioxidant content in grass-fed and grain-fed beef. *Nutr J.* 2010;9:10. doi:10.1186/1475-2891-9-10

18. Dilzer A, Park Y. Implication of conjugated linoleic acid (CLA) in human health. *Crit Rev Food Sci Nutr.* 2012;52(6):488-513. doi:10.1080/10408398.2011.636482

19. Westerterp-Plantenga MS, Nieuwenhuizen A, Tomé D, et al. Dietary protein, weight loss, and weight maintenance. *Annu Rev Nutr.* 2009;29:21-41. doi:10.1146/annurev-nutr-080508-141056

20. Layman DK, Boileau RA, Erickson DJ, et al. A reduced ratio of dietary carbohydrate to protein improves body composition and blood lipid profiles during weight loss in adult women. *J Nutr.* 2003;133(2):411-417. doi:10.1093/jn/133.2.411

21. Westerterp KR. Diet induced thermogenesis. *Nutr Metab (Lond).* 2004;1(1):5. doi:10.1186/1743-7075-1-5

22. Howard BV, Van Horn L, Hsia J, et al. Low-fat dietary pattern and risk of cardiovascular disease: the Women's Health Initiative Randomized Controlled Dietary Modification Trial. *JAMA.* 2006;295(6):655-666. doi:10.1001/jama.295.6.655

23. Estruch R, Ros E, Salas-Salvadó J, et al. Primary prevention of cardiovascular disease with a Mediterranean diet supplemented with extra-virgin olive oil or nuts. *N Engl J Med.* 2018;378(25):e34. doi:10.1056/NEJMoa1800389

24. Micha R, Wallace SK, Mozaffarian D. Red and processed meat consumption and risk of incident coronary heart disease, stroke, and diabetes mellitus: a systematic review and meta-analysis. *Circulation.* 2010;121(21):2271-2283. doi:10.1161/CIRCULATIONAHA.109.924977

25. Cross AJ, Sinha R. Meat-related mutagens/carcinogens in the etiology of colorectal cancer. *Environ Mol Mutagen.* 2004;44(1):44-55. doi:10.1002/em.20026

26. Salmon CP, Knize MG, Felton JS. Effects of marinating on heterocyclic amine carcinogen formation in grilled chicken. *Food Chem Toxicol.* 1997;35(5):433-441. doi:10.1016/S0278-6915(97)00023-5

27. Drewnowski A. The nutrient rich foods index helps to identify healthy, affordable foods. *Am J Clin Nutr.* 2010;91(4):1095S-1101S. doi:10.3945/ajcn.2010.28450D

Chapter Ten

The Breakfast Myth

The Most Important Meal of the Day—For Cereal Companies

The Dogma That Starts Every Day

"Breakfast is the most important meal of the day."

You've heard it since childhood—from parents, teachers, doctors, and the back of every cereal box. Skipping breakfast supposedly slows your metabolism, makes you gain weight, and ruins your health. The conventional wisdom is unwavering: eat a big breakfast to lose weight, never skip breakfast or your brain won't function, and start your day with a bowl of cereal, toast, or oatmeal for optimal health.

The message has been so thoroughly embedded in our culture that questioning it feels almost heretical. Breakfast has achieved a status beyond mere nutrition—it's become a moral imperative, a sign of responsible self-care, and a cornerstone of what we consider a healthy lifestyle.

Walk into any American kitchen in the morning and you'll see this dogma in action. Families gather around bowls of sugary cereal, toast slathered with jam, and glasses of orange juice—all in the name of starting the day right. Office workers grab breakfast bars and coffee drinks, believing they're making responsible choices. Schools serve breakfast to children as if their academic success depends on it, and missing breakfast is often viewed as a sign of neglect or dysfunction.

The breakfast industrial complex has become so powerful that even intermittent fasting advocates often recommend starting with "breakfast" later in the day, as if the first meal consumed automatically carries special significance regardless of timing.

But what if this entire belief system is built on marketing rather than metabolism? What if the "most important meal of the day" became important not because of science, but because of sales? What if our obsession with breakfast has actually made us less healthy, not more?

The truth about breakfast reveals one of the most successful marketing campaigns in nutrition history—a campaign so effective that it convinced multiple generations that their bodies couldn't function without starting each day with processed grains and sugar.

The Corporate Creation of a "Truth"

The idea that breakfast is essential for health didn't emerge from medical research or nutritional science. It was born in the advertising departments of cereal companies and refined through decades of marketing campaigns designed to create a market for processed breakfast foods.

The story begins in the late 1800s with Dr. John Harvey Kellogg, a Seventh-day Adventist physician who ran a health sanitarium in Battle Creek, Michigan[1]. Kellogg wasn't primarily concerned with nutrition—he was obsessed with spiritual purity and believed that bland, meatless foods could suppress sexual urges and promote moral behavior. His invention of corn flakes was part of a broader crusade to eliminate "stimulating" foods like meat, spices, and anything that might inflame what he considered base human passions.

Kellogg's cornflakes were originally served to patients at his sanitarium as part of a regimen designed to promote what he called "biological living." The cereal was intentionally bland and unappetizing—not exactly the foundation for a commercial empire. But Kellogg's brother Will recognized the commercial potential and, against John Harvey's wishes, added sugar to make the product more palatable for mass consumption[2].

The transformation of breakfast from a simple morning meal into a commercial necessity required sophisticated marketing. By the early 1900s, cereal companies like Kellogg's and Post were spending enormous sums on advertising, promoting their products as convenient, modern, and scientific alternatives to traditional breakfast foods like eggs, meat, and bread prepared at home.

The modern phrase "breakfast is the most important meal of the day" appears to have been coined by a General Foods marketing campaign in the 1940s to promote Grape-Nuts cereal[3]. The company didn't just advertise their product—they funded studies, paid nutritionists, and launched public relations campaigns designed to embed this message into American consciousness.

The strategy was brilliant in its simplicity: create a health anxiety that only their products could solve. Americans were told that skipping breakfast would lead to fatigue, poor concentration, weight gain, and various health problems. The solution, conveniently, could be found in the cereal aisle.

Throughout the 1950s and 1960s, cereal companies expanded their influence by funding nutrition research and partnering with health organizations. Studies began appearing that showed correlations between breakfast eating and various positive health outcomes, but these studies rarely controlled for the broader lifestyle patterns that distinguish people who eat breakfast from those who don't.

The breakfast industry didn't just sell products—they sold a lifestyle narrative. Breakfast became associated with family values, success, and responsibility. The image of a wholesome family gathered around the breakfast table, fortified with vitamins and minerals from enriched cereals, became a powerful cultural symbol that transcended mere nutrition.

The School Breakfast Program: Institutionalizing the Myth

The transformation of breakfast from marketing message to public policy occurred through the federal school meal programs that began in the 1960s. The National School Breakfast Program, established in 1966, was initially designed to address hunger among low-income children[4]. While this goal was admirable, the program also served to institutionalize the belief that breakfast was essential for all children, regardless of their nutritional status or family circumstances.

Schools became laboratories for breakfast promotion, with educational materials that taught children about the importance of starting their day with cereal, toast, and juice. The food industry provided much of this educational content, ensuring that commercial messages were embedded in seemingly objective nutrition education.

The irony was profound: programs designed to improve children's health often served highly processed foods that bore little resemblance to the nutritious whole foods that actually support growing bodies. School breakfast menus became dominated by sugary cereals, toaster pastries, fruit juices, and other products that created blood sugar spikes and crashes rather than sustained energy.

As the program expanded, the definition of "undernourished" grew to include virtually any child who didn't eat breakfast at home, regardless of the reason. This expansion transformed a targeted intervention for truly hungry children into a universal promotion of processed breakfast foods for all students.

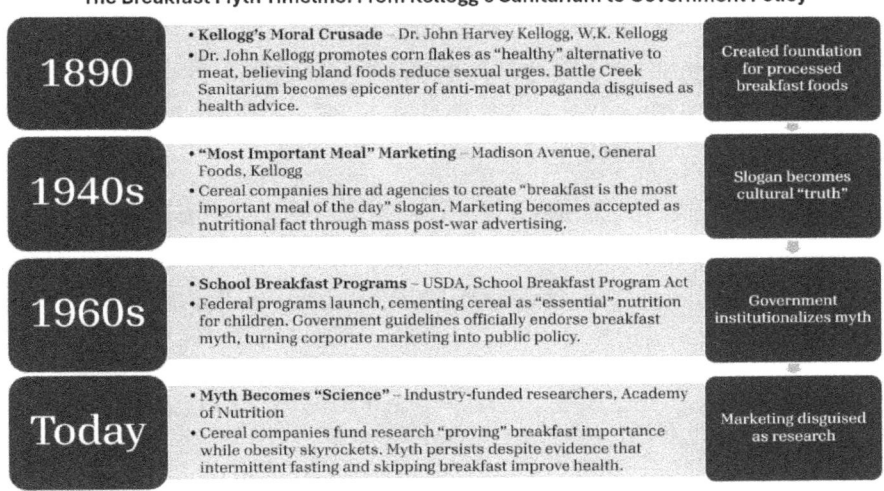

The Observational Studies: Correlation Masquerading as Causation

The scientific foundation for breakfast's supposed importance rests primarily on observational studies that found correlations between breakfast eating and various positive health outcomes. These studies, while numerous, suffer from the same fundamental flaw that plagued much of the nutritional research we've already examined: they confuse correlation with causation and fail to account for confounding variables that make their conclusions meaningless.

Studies consistently showed that people who eat breakfast tend to weigh less, have better concentration, and enjoy better overall health compared to breakfast skippers[5]. These findings seemed to provide scientific validation for what cereal companies had been claiming for decades. The media eagerly reported these results with headlines like "Skipping Breakfast Makes You Fat" and "Breakfast Eaters Live Longer."

But these studies revealed more about lifestyle patterns than about breakfast itself. People who eat breakfast regularly tend to be more health-conscious across all aspects of their lives. They're more likely to exercise, less likely to smoke, more likely to plan their meals, and generally more structured in their daily routines. They often have higher incomes, more stable family situations, and better access to healthcare.

Meanwhile, people who skip breakfast often do so as part of chaotic lifestyles characterized by poor sleep, high stress, irregular schedules, and generally poor health habits. They're more likely to compensate for skipped breakfast with poor food choices later in the day, eating convenience foods, fast food, or large portions that overwhelm their metabolic capacity.

When researchers tried to "adjust" for these differences statistically, they were attempting to separate breakfast eating from the entire lifestyle context in which it occurs—an impossible task that reveals the fundamental limitations of observational nutrition research.

The Randomized Controlled Trials: When Science Contradicts Marketing

The true test of breakfast's importance came when researchers conducted randomized controlled trials—studies that assigned people to either eat breakfast or skip it, then measured the outcomes. These studies, which eliminate the confounding variables that plague observational research, revealed a very different story about breakfast's role in health and weight management.

A landmark 2014 study published in the *American Journal of Clinical Nutrition* assigned overweight and obese adults to either eat breakfast daily or continue skipping breakfast, then tracked their weight loss over 16 weeks[6]. The results directly contradicted decades of breakfast dogma: there were no significant differences in weight loss, metabolic rate, or any other health marker between the groups.

The study revealed that breakfast's supposed metabolic benefits were largely mythical. Eating breakfast didn't "kickstart" metabolism, and skipping breakfast didn't cause the metabolic shutdown that breakfast advocates had long claimed. Instead, people's bodies adapted to their eating patterns, maintaining metabolic function regardless of meal timing.

Additional randomized trials reinforced these findings. A 2013 study in the *American Journal of Clinical Nutrition* found that breakfast consumption had no significant effect on weight loss in free-living adults[7]. Another study published in the *Journal of Nutrition* showed that skipping breakfast actually led to modest weight loss in some participants, likely due to reduced overall calorie intake[8].

These controlled experiments revealed that the observational studies had been measuring lifestyle patterns rather than breakfast effects. When you control for those patterns through randomization, breakfast's supposed benefits disappear.

The Intermittent Fasting Revolution: Rediscovering Ancient Wisdom

While breakfast advocates promoted the importance of eating early and often, a growing body of research was revealing the benefits of giving the digestive system regular breaks through intermittent fasting. This research challenged not just the breakfast myth, but the entire paradigm of frequent eating that had dominated nutritional thinking for decades.

Studies of intermittent fasting, which often involves extending the natural overnight fast by delaying or skipping breakfast, began showing remarkable health benefits that directly contradicted breakfast orthodoxy[9]. Research published in prestigious journals demonstrated that intermittent fasting could improve insulin sensitivity, reduce inflammation, promote cellular repair, and support healthy aging.

A 2019 review published in the *New England Journal of Medicine* summarized decades of research showing that intermittent fasting triggers beneficial metabolic changes including improved glucose regulation, increased stress resistance, and enhanced cellular repair mechanisms[10]. Many of these benefits occurred specifically during the fasted state that breakfast eating interrupts.

The research revealed that our bodies are designed to function effectively during periods without food. The hormonal changes that occur during fasting—including increased growth hormone, improved insulin sensitivity, and enhanced fat oxidation—represent adaptive mechanisms that supported human survival throughout evolutionary history.

Dr. Satchin Panda's research on circadian rhythms added another dimension to this understanding, showing that when we eat may be as important as what we eat[11]. His studies demonstrated that eating within a restricted time window, often achieved by delaying breakfast, can improve metabolic health even without changing the composition or total amount of food consumed.

The Blood Sugar Roller Coaster: How Breakfast Culture Made Us Sick

The standard American breakfast—built around refined grains, added sugars, and fruit juices—creates a metabolic disaster that sets people up for hunger, cravings, and energy crashes throughout the day. Understanding this physiological reality explains why so many people feel dependent on breakfast while simultaneously struggling with weight gain and metabolic dysfunction.

Most breakfast foods are high-carbohydrate, low-protein, low-fat combinations that cause rapid spikes in blood glucose[12]. A typical breakfast of cereal with skim milk and orange juice can contain 60-80 grams of rapidly absorbed carbohydrates—more sugar than a candy bar, delivered to the bloodstream within minutes of consumption.

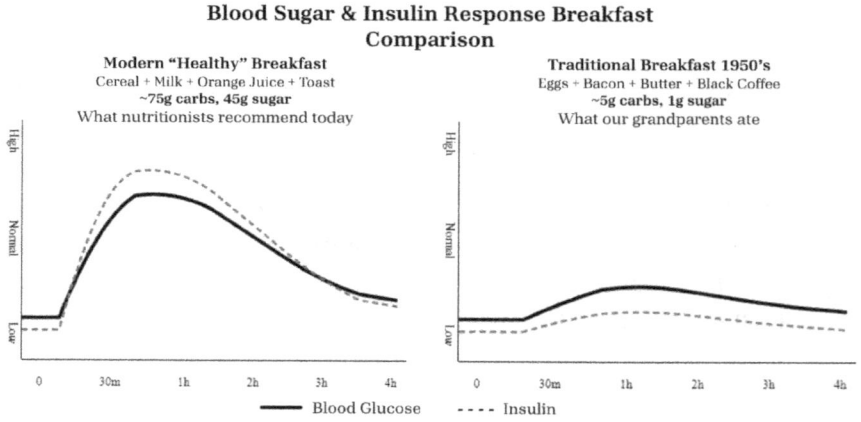

This glucose surge triggers a massive insulin response as the body attempts to clear sugar from the bloodstream and store it in cells. In healthy individuals, this process works efficiently, but the rapid clearance of glucose often leads to a blood sugar crash within 2-3 hours of eating[13].

4-Hour Metabolic Comparison		
Metric	Modern Breakfast VS	Traditional Breakfast
Peak Blood Glucose	180+ mg/dL	95 mg/dL
Peak Insulin	80+ µU/mL	15 µU/mL
Energy Stability	2-3 crashes	Steady 4+ hours
Fat Burning	Blocked 4+ hours	Minimal disruption
Hunger Returns	2-3 hours	5-6 hours
Mental Clarity	Brain fog/crashes	Sharp focus

The blood sugar crash triggers powerful hunger signals and cravings for more carbohydrates, creating a cycle of eating and crashing that repeats throughout the day. People interpret this manufactured hunger as evidence that they "need" frequent meals, not recognizing that their food choices are creating the very problems they're trying to solve.

Meanwhile, the frequent insulin spikes from repeated high-carbohydrate meals gradually reduce insulin sensitivity, making it harder for cells to respond to insulin's signals. This insulin resistance is the foundation of type 2 diabetes, but it also makes weight management more difficult and energy levels less stable[14].

The irony is striking: the breakfast foods promoted for sustained energy actually create energy instability, while the practice of skipping breakfast that's supposedly harmful can actually improve metabolic flexibility and energy regulation.

The Protein Problem: Why Most Breakfasts Fail

Even when breakfast advocates acknowledge the problems with high-carbohydrate morning meals, their solutions often fall short because they underestimate the importance of adequate protein intake. Research shows that breakfast needs to contain at least 25-30 grams of high-quality protein to provide lasting satiety and metabolic benefits[15].

Most traditional breakfast foods are protein-poor. A bowl of cereal with milk provides only 8-10 grams of protein. Toast with jam offers virtually none. Even seemingly healthy options like oatmeal with fruit provide insufficient protein to support stable blood sugar and appetite control.

When researchers studied high-protein breakfasts containing 35 grams of protein or more, they found dramatically different outcomes compared to typical breakfast foods[16]. High-protein breakfasts reduced cravings throughout the day, improved appetite control, and led to reduced calorie intake at subsequent meals.

However, achieving this level of protein requires a fundamental shift away from grain-based breakfast foods toward animal proteins, eggs, or carefully planned plant protein combinations. A truly satiating breakfast might include a three-egg omelet with vegetables, Greek yogurt with nuts, or leftover meat from dinner—foods that bear little resemblance to the products promoted by the breakfast industry.

The Real Story: Individual Variation and Metabolic Flexibility

The breakfast myth assumed that all humans have identical nutritional needs and metabolic patterns, requiring the same meal timing regardless of individual circumstances. This one-size-fits-all approach ignored the reality that people vary dramatically in their response to different eating patterns based on genetics, lifestyle, health status, and personal preferences.

Some people genuinely feel better when they eat early in the day. They wake up hungry, function better with food in their system, and struggle when they delay eating. For these individuals, breakfast can be an important component of their nutritional strategy—provided they choose foods that support rather than undermine their metabolic health.

Others function optimally when they delay eating until later in the day. They wake up without hunger, feel energetic during morning fasting periods, and prefer to eat their calories in a compressed time window. For these people, forcing breakfast consumption can actually impair their natural rhythm and metabolic efficiency.

The key insight from modern research is that metabolic flexibility—the ability to efficiently switch between burning glucose and fat for fuel—matters more than any specific meal timing[17]. People with good metabolic flexibility can thrive with breakfast or without it, while those with poor metabolic flexibility will struggle regardless of when they eat.

Building metabolic flexibility requires reducing dependence on frequent carbohydrate intake and improving the body's ability to access stored fat for energy. This might mean eating breakfast for some people and skipping it for others, but it always means choosing foods that support rather than impair metabolic function.

Cultural Context: How Breakfast Became Identity

The breakfast myth succeeded not just because of marketing, but because it tapped into deeper cultural anxieties about family, productivity, and moral behavior. Breakfast became a symbol of responsible parenting, successful professional life, and proper self-care that transcended nutrition and entered the realm of identity.

A "good mother" makes sure her children eat breakfast. A "serious athlete" never skips breakfast. A "responsible adult" starts the day with proper nutrition. These cultural narratives made questioning breakfast feel like questioning fundamental values rather than examining scientific evidence.

The breakfast ritual also provided structure and meaning in increasingly chaotic modern life. Gathering for breakfast became a way for families to connect, for individuals to feel organized, and for everyone to feel like they were taking control of their health through deliberate action.

This cultural investment in breakfast explains why evidence contradicting breakfast's importance often meets with emotional rather than rational responses. People aren't just defending a meal—they're defending a piece of their identity and their understanding of what constitutes responsible behavior.

The Path Forward: Personalizing Eating Patterns

The collapse of the breakfast myth doesn't mean that everyone should skip breakfast or that eating in the morning is harmful. Instead, it means that individuals can experiment with different eating patterns to discover what works best for their unique physiology, lifestyle, and preferences.

For those who choose to eat breakfast, the focus should shift from timing to food quality. A breakfast of eggs, vegetables, and healthy fats will have dramatically different metabolic effects than cereal, toast, and juice, regardless of when it's consumed. Prioritizing protein and minimizing refined carbohydrates can transform breakfast from a metabolic liability into a genuine asset.

For those who prefer to delay eating, the research on intermittent fasting provides reassurance that skipping breakfast can be not just safe but beneficial. The key is ensuring that when eating does occur, food choices support rather than undermine metabolic health.

The most important principle is listening to genuine hunger and satiety signals rather than following external rules about when eating should occur. Many people discover that when they stop forcing breakfast, they naturally develop eating patterns that feel more sustainable and lead to better energy and body composition.

Children and Breakfast: Separating Need from Habit

The breakfast myth has been particularly persistent regarding children, with parents told that their children's academic performance, behavior, and health depend on morning eating. While ensuring that children receive adequate nutrition is crucial, the assumption that this nutrition must be delivered at breakfast reflects cultural bias rather than biological necessity.

Research on children and breakfast suffers from the same confounding variables that plague adult studies. Children who eat breakfast regularly often come from families with more resources, structure, and health consciousness. Their better academic and behavioral outcomes may reflect these broader advantages rather than breakfast consumption itself[18].

For children who are genuinely hungry in the morning, providing nutrient-dense breakfast foods makes sense. But for children who aren't naturally hungry upon waking, forcing breakfast consumption may interfere with their natural appetite regulation and create unnecessary mealtime battles.

The key is ensuring that children receive adequate nutrition throughout the day from whole, unprocessed foods, regardless of when that nutrition is consumed. A child who eats a nutritious lunch and dinner while skipping breakfast is likely better nourished than one who eats sugary cereal for breakfast but poor-quality foods at other meals.

Breaking Free from Breakfast Dogma

Every morning for decades, I forced down breakfast because I'd been told my metabolism depended on it. Cereal, toast, orange juice—I was starting every day with a blood sugar roller coaster that set me up for cravings and energy crashes. When I finally questioned this dogma and started skipping breakfast, my energy stabilized for the first time in years.

The breakfast myth represents everything wrong with modern nutrition advice: marketing masquerading as science, one-size-fits-all recommendations ignoring individual variation, and the transformation of food choices into moral imperatives. Breaking free from this dogma requires courage to trust your body over cultural expectations.

Start by experimenting with different eating patterns to discover what genuinely makes you feel best. Try delaying breakfast by an hour, then two hours, then longer if it feels comfortable. Pay attention to energy levels, hunger patterns, and overall well-being rather than following predetermined rules about when eating should occur.

If you choose to eat breakfast, focus on foods that provide sustained energy rather than quick energy. Prioritize protein and healthy fats while minimizing refined carbohydrates and added sugars. Think of breakfast as an opportunity to nourish your body rather than an obligation to fulfill.

Most importantly, recognize that your eating patterns are personal choices rather than moral statements. There's no virtue in eating breakfast if your body functions better without it, and there's no shame in eating breakfast if that's what makes you feel best.

The breakfast industry spent over a century convincing us that our bodies couldn't function without their products. It's time to rediscover what our bodies actually need rather than what we've been told they need. Your metabolism doesn't depend on marketing messages. It depends on what you choose to put in your mouth—and when you choose to put it there.

The most important meal of the day isn't breakfast. It's whichever meal best serves your individual physiology, lifestyle, and health goals. And sometimes, the most important meal is the one you choose not to eat.

The breakfast myth represents the perfect culmination of everything wrong with modern nutrition advice: a marketing slogan disguised as medical wisdom, promoted through flawed studies and institutional capture, enforced through cultural shame, and resistant to contradictory evidence. But breakfast was just one piece of a much larger deception. When you step back and examine all the myths we've explored, a clear pattern emerges—the same playbook used repeatedly to transform food fears into corporate profits.

References

1. Schwarz RW. *John Harvey Kellogg, MD.* Nashville, TN: Southern Publishing Association; 1970.

2. Carson GS. *Cornflake Crusade.* New York, NY: Rinehart & Company; 1957.

3. Carroll A. The breakfast myth. *The New York Times.* May 23, 2016.

4. Food and Nutrition Service, US Department of Agriculture. *National School Breakfast Program Fact Sheet.* 2019. Accessed September 10, 2025. https://www.fns.usda.gov

5. O'Neil CE, Byrd-Bredbenner C, Hayes D, et al. The role of breakfast in

health: definition and criteria for a quality breakfast. *Am J Clin Nutr.* 2014;99(6):1352-1365. doi:10.3945/ajcn.113.083402

6. Dhurandhar EJ, Dawson J, Alcorn A, et al. The effectiveness of breakfast recommendations on weight loss: a randomized controlled trial. *Am J Clin Nutr.* 2014;100(2):507-513. doi:10.3945/ajcn.114.089573

7. LeCheminant JD, Christenson E, Bailey BW, Tucker LA. Restricting night-time eating reduces daily energy intake in healthy young men: a short-term cross-over study. *Br J Nutr.* 2013;110(11):2108-2113. doi:10.1017/S0007114513001612

8. Levitsky DA, Pacanowski CR. Effect of skipping breakfast on subsequent energy intake. *Physiol Behav.* 2013;119:9-16. doi:10.1016/j.physbeh.2013.05.006

9. Patterson RE, Sears DD. Metabolic effects of intermittent fasting. *Annu Rev Nutr.* 2017;37:371-393. doi:10.1146/annurev-nutr-071816-064634

10. de Cabo R, Mattson MP. Effects of intermittent fasting on health, aging, and disease. *N Engl J Med.* 2019;381(26):2541-2551. doi:10.1056/NEJMra1905136

11. Panda S. Circadian physiology of metabolism. *Science.* 2016;354(6315):1008-1015. doi:10.1126/science.aah4967

12. Brand-Miller J, Hayne S, Petocz P, Colagiuri S. Low-glycemic index diets in the management of diabetes: a meta-analysis of randomized controlled trials. *Diabetes Care.* 2003;26(8):2261-2267. doi:10.2337/diacare.26.8.2261

13. Ludwig DS. The glycemic index: physiological mechanisms relating to obesity, diabetes, and cardiovascular disease. *JAMA.* 2002;287(18):2414-2423. doi:10.1001/jama.287.18.2414

14. Reaven GM. Pathophysiology of insulin resistance in human disease.

Physiol Rev. 1995;75(3):473-486. doi:10.1152/physrev.1995.75.3.473

15. Hoertel HA, Will MJ, Leidy HJ. A randomized crossover, pilot study examining the effects of a normal protein vs high protein breakfast on food cravings and reward signals in overweight/obese "breakfast skipping," late-adolescent girls. *Nutr J.* 2014;13:80. doi:10.1186/1475-2891-13-80

16. Leidy HJ, Ortinau LC, Douglas SM, Hoertel HA. Beneficial effects of a higher-protein breakfast on the appetitive, hormonal, and neural signals controlling energy intake regulation in overweight/obese, "breakfast-skipping," late-adolescent girls. *Am J Clin Nutr.* 2013;97(4):677-688. doi:10.3945/ajcn.112.053116

17. Galgani J, Ravussin E. Metabolic flexibility and insulin resistance. *Am J Physiol Endocrinol Metab.* 2008;295(5):E1009-E1017. doi:10.1152/ajpendo.90558.2008

18. Adolphus K, Lawton CL, Dye L. The effects of breakfast on behavior and academic performance in children and adolescents. *Front Hum Neurosci.* 2013;7:425. doi:10.3389/fnhum.2013.00425

19. Manoogian ENC, Zadourian A, Lo HC, et al. Feasibility of time-restricted eating and impacts on cardiometabolic health in 24-h shift workers: the SHIFT pilot study. *Ann Intern Med.* 2024;177(2):129-139. doi:10.7326/M23-2164

20. Lange MG, Heitmann BL, Larsen SC, et al. Metabolic changes with intermittent fasting. *J Hum Nutr Diet.* 2024;37(1):256-269. doi:10.1111/jhn.13270

21. Brown JE, Braakhuis AJ, Cotter JD. Intermittent fasting as a treatment for obesity in young people: a scoping review. *npj Metab Health Dis.* 2024;2:41. doi:10.1038/s44324-024-00041-8

Chapter Eleven

Part 1 Summary

The Bigger Lie—How We Got Sold Instead of Fed

The Pattern Behind the Lies

We were told to trust the experts. To follow the science. To eat low-fat, skip the steak, fear the yolks, and never—*ever*—miss breakfast.

But as you've discovered throughout Part 1, that advice wasn't rooted in rigorous science. It was built on weak correlations, industry-funded studies, and corporate marketing disguised as health guidance. Each chapter exposed a different nutritional myth, but when you step back and examine them together, the same fingerprints appear on every single lie.

The systemic distortion of nutritional science didn't happen by accident. It followed a predictable playbook that transformed speculation into dogma, correlation into causation, and marketing messages into medical advice. Understanding this playbook is crucial because the same tactics that sold you fear of fat and obsession with breakfast are still being used today to sell you everything from pharmaceuticals to processed foods.

The Five-Step Playbook: How They Got Us

Step 1: Start with a correlation. Find an observational study that shows people who eat meat have higher cancer rates, or that breakfast eaters weigh less, or that people who consume saturated fat have more heart disease. The correlation doesn't have to be strong, and it certainly doesn't have to prove causation. It just needs to exist on paper.

Step 2: Ignore the confounders. Don't mention that the meat eaters were also more likely to smoke, drink heavily, avoid exercise, and eat fast food. Don't adjust for the fact that breakfast eaters tend to be more health-conscious, higher-income, and better educated. Don't acknowledge that people who avoid saturated fat often replace it with sugar and processed carbohydrates. Just blame the single dietary component that fits your predetermined narrative.

Step 3: Wrap it in moral language. Red meat becomes "indulgent." Saturated fat becomes "artery-clogging." Skipping breakfast becomes "irresponsible." Sugar becomes "empty calories" rather than "metabolic poison." This moral framing transforms nutrition choices into character judgments, making it harder for people to think critically about the actual evidence.

Step 4: Repeat it until it becomes truth. Echo the same message across headlines, classrooms, doctor's offices, government guidelines, and food packaging. Cite the same flawed studies in multiple contexts. Create the illusion of consensus by having the same small group of researchers, often funded by the same industries, produce multiple papers supporting the same conclusions. Make it seem like "everyone agrees" when the agreement is manufactured.

Step 5: Profit from the fear. Demonize real food and replace it with processed alternatives that carry health claims. Create problems with your recommendations, then sell solutions to fix the problems you created. Market supplements to replace nutrients stripped from processed foods. Transform whole foods into villains and factory-made products into heroes.

The Same Players, The Same Game

Throughout Part 1, you probably noticed the same names, institutions, and funding sources appearing repeatedly across different nutritional myths. This wasn't coincidence—it was coordination. A relatively small group of researchers, often with direct or indirect ties to food and pharmaceutical companies, shaped decades of nutritional policy through a combination of flawed research, institutional influence, and media manipulation.

Ancel Keys didn't just create the fat myth—his influence contributed to the demonization of cholesterol, saturated fat, and by extension, the animal foods that contained them. The sugar industry didn't just fund studies attacking fat—they systematically undermined research into sugar's health effects while promoting their product as a harmless source of energy[1].

The same observational study methodologies that "proved" red meat caused cancer were used to "demonstrate" that breakfast was essential for health and that plant-based diets were superior to omnivorous ones. The same failure to control for confounding variables that led to decades of low-fat recommendations also supported the vilification of red meat and the promotion of industrial seed oils.

When the same flawed tools are used repeatedly by the same compromised institutions to reach predetermined conclusions, you're not looking at science—you're looking at an elaborate marketing campaign dressed up in academic credentials.

What We Lost Along the Way

The cost of following these fabricated guidelines extended far beyond individual health outcomes. We lost entire generations to preventable chronic diseases, but we also lost something more fundamental: our connection to food wisdom, our trust in our own bodies, and our ability to distinguish between nourishment and marketing.

We Lost Nutritional Adequacy

By following the advice to avoid fat, limit red meat, embrace plant-based alternatives, and start every day with processed grains, millions of people unknowingly created nutritional deficiencies that manifested as fatigue, depression, hormone imbalances, and metabolic dysfunction. Iron deficiency became epidemic among women. B12 deficiency increased among people avoiding animal products. Essential fatty acid imbalances contributed to inflammation and cognitive decline.

Meanwhile, the foods we were told to fear—eggs, butter, red meat, and other animal products—contained exactly the nutrients our bodies were crying out for. We created artificial scarcity of essential nutrients while consuming unprecedented amounts of empty calories from processed foods.

We Lost Metabolic Health

The low-fat, high-carbohydrate dietary pattern promoted by decades of flawed guidelines didn't just fail to prevent obesity and diabetes—it actively promoted them. By teaching people to fear natural fats while embracing refined carbohydrates, we created the perfect recipe for insulin resistance, metabolic syndrome, and chronic disease.

The irony is devastating: while obesity rates tripled, diabetes became epidemic, and fatty liver disease went from rare to common, we were faithfully following the dietary advice that was supposed to prevent these exact problems[2]. We didn't ignore the experts—we trusted them completely, and they led us off a metabolic cliff.

We Lost Food Wisdom

Perhaps most tragically, we lost the accumulated wisdom of traditional cultures that had successfully nourished human beings for thousands of years. Our great-grandparents understood intuitively that real food—including animal fats, organ meats, fermented foods, and seasonal vegetables—supported health and vitality.

We replaced this inherited wisdom with laboratory-created guidelines that treated food as collections of isolated nutrients rather than complex matrices of nourishment. We learned to trust food labels over food appearance, marketing claims over personal experience, and expert opinions over our own bodies' signals.

We Lost Trust in Our Bodies

The constant bombardment of contradictory nutritional advice created a generation of people who no longer trusted their own hunger, satiety, and craving signals. Instead of eating when hungry and stopping when full, people learned to eat by the clock, according to portion guidelines, and in response to marketing messages.

We became afraid of our own appetites, viewing hunger as weakness and food cravings as moral failures. The natural human ability to self-regulate food intake—an ability that had sustained our species for millennia—was systematically undermined by external rules that ignored individual physiology and metabolism.

The Real Problem Was Never the Food

Throughout Part 1, a clear pattern emerged: the foods we were told to fear weren't actually the problem. Eggs didn't cause heart disease. Saturated fat didn't clog arteries. Red meat didn't cause cancer. Salt didn't cause high blood pressure in most people. Skipping breakfast didn't destroy metabolism.

The real problem was what we were told to eat instead.

We swapped butter for margarine made from industrial seed oils. We replaced steak with pasta and bread. We chose skim milk over whole milk, artificial sweeteners over natural fats, and breakfast cereals over eggs. We embraced "heart-healthy" processed foods while avoiding the nutrient-dense whole foods that had sustained human health for generations.

The dietary villains weren't traditional foods—they were the modern processed alternatives that replaced them. Ultra-processed foods, industrial seed oils, refined sugars, and chemical additives created the health problems that traditional foods were then blamed for causing.

The Corruption Runs Deeper Than Food

The same institutions, methodologies, and financial incentives that corrupted nutritional science have infected other areas of health and medicine. The playbook that transformed sugar into a harmless energy source while demonizing saturated fat is still being used to promote pharmaceutical interventions while downplaying lifestyle solutions.

The same observational study methods that "proved" red meat caused cancer are used to support medication guidelines. The same failure to distinguish correlation from causation that led to decades of low-fat recommendations continues to drive treatment protocols. The same financial conflicts of interest that allowed sugar companies to buy scientific conclusions still influence medical research and policy.

Part 1 revealed how we were misled about food, but the corruption extends far beyond nutrition. The same forces that convinced you to fear butter while embracing margarine are now convincing you to treat numbers with pills while ignoring the root causes of disease.

Recognizing the Pattern

Once you understand how nutritional myths are manufactured, you begin to see the same pattern everywhere. Any time you encounter health advice that:

- Relies primarily on observational studies while ignoring randomized controlled trials

- Fails to distinguish between correlation and causation

- Ignores obvious confounding variables

- Uses relative risk statistics without providing absolute risk context

- Promotes processed alternatives to traditional foods

- Creates fear around foods humans have eaten safely for millennia

- Benefits specific industries or pharmaceutical companies

- Contradicts your personal experience and intuition

...you should be immediately suspicious. These are the hallmarks of manufactured health scares designed to create markets for products and services rather than promote genuine wellness.

The Path Forward: From Fear to Wisdom

Understanding how we were misled about food provides the foundation for making better choices moving forward. The goal isn't to become paranoid about all health advice, but to develop the critical thinking skills necessary to distinguish between genuine science and sophisticated marketing.

Trust Traditional Foods Over Trendy Alternatives

Foods that humans have consumed successfully for thousands of years—meat, fish, eggs, dairy, vegetables, fruits, nuts, and seeds—have track records that no modern processed food can match. When choosing between a traditional food and a modern alternative, the traditional option is almost always safer and more nutritious.

Prioritize Food Quality Over Macronutrient Ratios

The obsession with specific percentages of fat, carbohydrates, and protein has distracted us from the more important question of food quality. A diet built around whole, unprocessed foods will naturally provide appropriate macronutrient ratios without requiring calculation or restriction.

Listen to Your Body Over External Authorities

Your body provides more reliable feedback about dietary choices than any expert, study, or guideline. Pay attention to how different foods make you feel—your energy levels, mood, hunger patterns, and overall well-being. This internal feedback system evolved over millions of years and is more sophisticated than any nutrition theory.

Question Health Claims and Marketing Messages

Any food that needs to announce its health benefits on the package is probably less healthy than foods that don't require such marketing. Real food doesn't need health claims because its nutritional value is self-evident. Be especially suspicious of products that claim to be healthier versions of traditional foods.

Understand That Correlation Is Not Causation

Most nutrition headlines are based on observational studies that can only show correlations, not prove causation. When you see claims that "X food causes Y disease," ask whether the study controlled for lifestyle factors, whether randomized trials support the conclusion, and whether the effect size is meaningful in absolute terms.

What's Coming in Part 2

Part 1 revealed how we were systematically misled about food, but the corruption doesn't stop at nutrition. The same playbook that sold you fear of fat while promoting processed alternatives is now being used to medicalize normal aspects of human physiology while promoting pharmaceutical solutions to problems that lifestyle interventions could address more effectively.

Part 2 will examine how the medical system perpetuates and profits from the health problems created by following the nutritional advice exposed in Part 1. You'll discover how the same institutions that taught you to fear real food are now teaching you to fear your own biology while promoting expensive medical interventions to manage the consequences of their previous advice.

The goal isn't to reject all medical care or pharmaceutical interventions—some are genuinely lifesaving and necessary. The goal is to develop the same critical thinking skills you've applied to nutritional myths and use them to evaluate medical recommendations, distinguish between treatment and prevention, and understand when lifestyle interventions might be more appropriate than pharmaceutical ones.

You Weren't the Problem

The most important realization from Part 1 is that you weren't the problem. You didn't fail at following healthy eating guidelines—the guidelines failed you. You weren't lacking willpower or knowledge—you were following advice that was designed to benefit industries rather than individuals.

For decades, you trusted experts who had been bought, followed science that had been corrupted, and embraced guidelines that had been manufactured. The weight gain, energy crashes, food cravings, and health problems that followed weren't signs of personal failure—they were predictable consequences of following fundamentally flawed advice.

Now you know better. You understand how nutritional myths are created and why they persist. You can see through the marketing disguised as medicine and make decisions based on evidence rather than propaganda.

PART 1 SUMMARY

Most importantly, you can reclaim your relationship with food based on nourishment rather than fear, tradition rather than trends, and your own body's wisdom rather than corporate messaging.

The lies about food were just the beginning. But armed with the knowledge of how those lies were constructed and why they succeeded, you're prepared to see through the even bigger lies about health and medicine that we'll examine in Part 2.

Your body wasn't broken. The system was. And now that you understand how the system really works, you can finally start making choices that serve your health rather than someone else's profits.

References

1. Kearns CE, Schmidt LA, Glantz SA. Sugar industry and coronary heart disease research: a historical analysis of internal industry documents. *JAMA Intern Med.* 2016;176(11):1680-1685. doi:10.1001/jamainternmed.2016.5394

2. Hales CM, Carroll MD, Fryar CD, Ogden CL. Prevalence of obesity and severe obesity among adults: United States, 2017–2018. *NCHS Data Brief.* 2020;(360):1-8.

Chapter Twelve

Part 2: Medical Dogma and Systemic Failures

How industry hijacked our plates, rewrote nutrition, and made us sicker in the name of health.

> **A Note on Medical Statistics**
>
> *The medical establishment's preferred currency is relative risk—the same statistical sleight of hand that transforms a 0.2% benefit into a "44% reduction!" When I cite these percentages, I'm not endorsing this approach; I'm using their own metrics to expose their misplaced priorities. Even by medicine's flawed statistical standards, we're chasing the wrong numbers.*
>
> *The deeper frustration is this: complex biological processes can't be reduced to simple percentages. Your body isn't a collection of isolated risk factors—it's an interconnected system where insulin resistance drives inflammation, which raises blood pressure, which damages arteries, which creates the very problems we're trying to prevent with pills.*
>
> *I present these statistics not as absolute truth, but as evidence that even within the medical system's own framework, their priorities are backwards. The real solutions—addressing root causes through diet, sleep, stress management, and movement—can't be easily quantified, patented, or prescribed. That's why they're ignored.*

We trusted them.

The white coat. The prescription pad. The quiet authority of a system designed to heal. But somewhere in the last forty years, the incentives shifted. What began as a mission to cure became a business model to manage. Healthcare became sick-care. Prevention became prescription. And patients became customers.

The transformation wasn't sudden—it was gradual, institutional, and profitable. By 2020, the U.S. was spending $4.1 trillion annually on healthcare[1], yet we ranked dead last among developed nations in health outcomes[2]. We take more medications, follow more guidelines, and fill more prescriptions than any other country[3]. And we're sicker than ever.

Medical dogma is powerful because it wears a mask of certainty. It doesn't just give you an answer—it makes questioning that answer seem dangerous. It tells you that your LDL number matters more than how you feel. That a pill can replace the need to address root causes. That symptoms are diseases, not signals.

The machinery runs on fear and compliance. If your cholesterol is elevated, you need a statin—regardless of your overall health, diet, or risk factors. If your blood pressure creeps up, you need medication—even if stress, poor sleep, or metabolic dysfunction might be the real culprits. The system has become expert at creating lifelong patients out of temporary problems.

But how does medical dogma actually form? How do preliminary studies become unquestionable truth? How do treatments with marginal benefits become standard care for millions?

The answer is a self-reinforcing cycle that transforms tentative research into medical gospel. It starts with a promising study—often funded by pharmaceutical companies. Media amplifies the findings, emphasizing dramatic-sounding statistics while burying limitations. Medical panels, many with industry ties, write treatment guidelines. Doctors, fearing liability and following their training, prescribe accordingly. Massive profits fund more studies and marketing. Institutional momentum makes course correction nearly impossible, even when contradictory evidence emerges.

How Medical Myths Become Standard Care

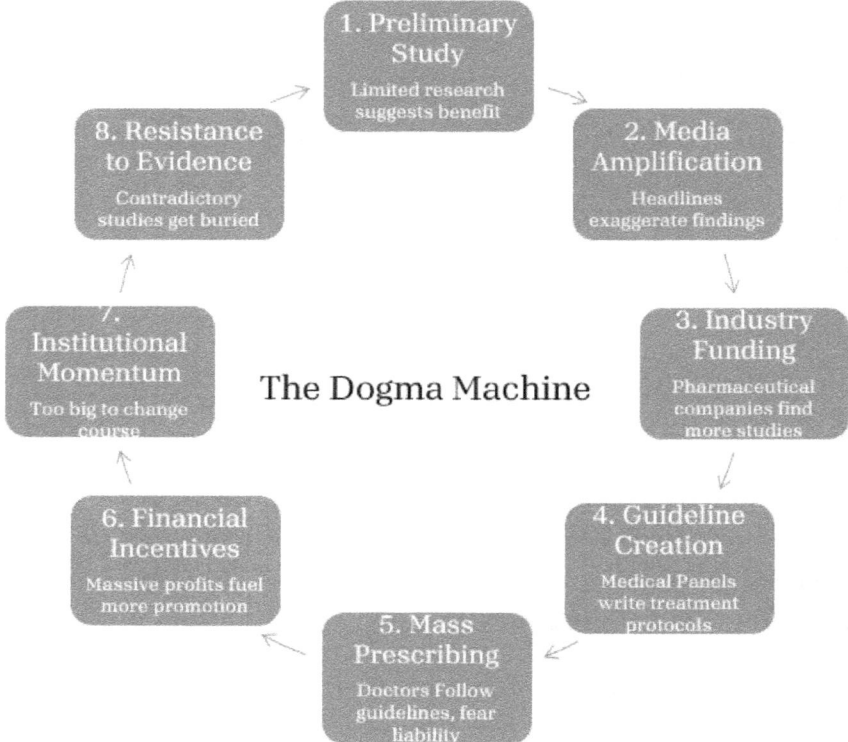

This isn't conspiracy—it's a predictable pattern that repeats with depressing regularity. We've watched it happen with statins, hormone therapy, antidepressants, and now we're seeing it unfold in real-time with newer treatments. The cycle is so reliable, you can almost set your watch by it.

> **Historical Examples**
>
> - **Statins:** Heart health → Prescribed to millions with minimal benefit
> - **HRT:** Youth elixir → Banned after flawed study interpretation
> - **Antidepressants:** Chemical imbalance myth → 85% believe false theory
> - **Peanut Avoidance:** Safety measure → Created more allergies

And if you push back? If you ask why your arteries filled with plaque despite being on a statin? If you question why you need three blood pressure medications when you started with one? You're not just wrong. You're labeled noncompliant. Irresponsible. Dangerous.

But here's what makes medical dogma more insidious than food mythology: doctors genuinely believe they're helping you. Unlike food companies that know their products cause harm, most physicians are trapped in the same system of misinformation. They follow guidelines often influenced and funded by pharmaceutical companies[4]. They prescribe medications because that's what they were taught. They fear liability more than they trust critical thinking.

This creates a perfect storm: patients who don't question medical authority, doctors who don't question medical guidelines, and guidelines written by committees with financial conflicts of interest. Everyone follows the rules. Everyone believes they're doing the right thing. And everyone misses the bigger picture.

This section explores the deeply entrenched myths that medicine embraced and refused to let go—even as evidence piled up against them. We'll examine how statins became a cure-all despite studies showing they cause thousands of new diabetes cases annually. How cholesterol was turned into a villain while the real drivers of heart disease were ignored. How blood pressure medications multiplied while root causes went untreated. How hormones—once a tool for healing—became feared and misunderstood.

We'll also tackle modern gray zones: fasting, supplements, and emerging therapies—where new science is challenging decades of dogma, but cultural momentum and liability fears keep doctors prescribing the same old solutions.

You'll see how clinical trials are designed to show relative benefits while hiding absolute risks[5]. How real-world side effects are systematically underreported. How patients' lived experiences are dismissed when they contradict published studies. How the system prioritizes risk management over innovation, and pharmaceutical profits over patient outcomes.

This is the part of the story where things get personal—because medical dogma doesn't just affect what you eat. It affects what medications you take, what tests you get, what advice you follow, and how much agency you have in your own healthcare decisions.

The food industry sold us products that made us sick. But the medical industry convinced us that sickness was inevitable, manageable, and required a lifetime of pharmaceutical intervention.

If the food myths made us sick, the medical myths made sure we stayed that way—and paid handsomely for the privilege.

References

1. Centers for Medicare & Medicaid Services. *National Health Expenditure Data: Historical.* US Department of Health and Human Services; 2022. Accessed September 10, 2025. https://www.cms.gov/research-statistics-data-and-systems/statistics-trends-and-reports/nationalhealthexpenddata

2. Schneider EC, Shah A, Doty MM, Tikkanen R, Fields K, Williams RD II. *Mirror, Mirror 2021: Reflecting Poorly—Health Care in the U.S. Compared to Other High-Performing Countries.* Commonwealth Fund; 2021. Accessed September 10, 2025. https://www.commonwealthfund.org/publications/fund-reports/2021/aug/mirror-mirror-2021-reflecting-poorly

3. Organisation for Economic Co-operation and Development (OECD). *Health at a Glance 2023: OECD Indicators.* OECD Publishing; 2023. doi:10.1787/9c0e31a9-en

4. Lenzer J. Why we can't trust clinical guidelines. *BMJ.* 2015;351:h4772. doi:10.1136/bmj.h4772

5. Moynihan R, Doust J, Henry D. Preventing overdiagnosis: how to stop harming the healthy. *BMJ.* 2017;350:h869. doi:10.1136/bmj.h869

Chapter Thirteen

The Statin Myth

The Over-Prescription Epidemic and Why Lowering Your Numbers Might Not Save Your Life

Important Medical Disclaimer: This chapter examines research and raises questions about statin prescribing practices. This information is for educational purposes only and does not constitute medical advice. Consult qualified healthcare providers before making changes to medications or treatment plans.

Here's what your doctor believes: Statins are miracle drugs that lower cholesterol and save lives. If your LDL—the so-called "bad cholesterol"—is high, you need a statin. It doesn't matter how you feel. Lowering that number reduces your risk of a heart attack. End of discussion.

Here's what's actually happening: Statins do lower LDL cholesterol. But for many people, that reduction doesn't translate into a meaningful reduction in absolute risk[1]. And they come with a price—both financially and physically.

Don't misunderstand me—statins aren't inherently evil. For people with established cardiovascular disease or very high risk, they can reduce the chance of a future heart event. The evidence is clearest for secondary prevention (people who already have heart disease). But for people who are otherwise healthy and simply have "elevated cholesterol," the absolute benefits become much smaller for many individuals[2].

Meanwhile, side effects are more common in real-world practice than clinical trials suggest[3]. A major 2024 study in *The Lancet Diabetes & Endocrinology* confirmed what previous research indicated: statins significantly increase diabetes risk, with high-intensity statins causing a 36% relative increase in new-onset diabetes compared to 10% for moderate-intensity statins[4]. Beyond diabetes, muscle pain, weakness, and fatigue affect substantial numbers of users. Peer-reviewed research shows that statin-associated muscle symptoms (SAMS) are reported by 10% to 25% of patients in clinical practice, though randomized controlled trials often report much lower rates of 1.5-5%[5]. Brain fog and memory issues, while controversial in the medical literature, are experienced by many patients. Low libido and hormonal disruption have also been documented in systematic reviews[6].

But here's the statistical sleight of hand that should make you ask better questions: In many statin studies, the actual absolute risk reduction is much smaller than the relative risk reduction suggests. Pharmaceutical companies and medical communications often emphasize "relative risk" statistics that sound impressive—"a 30% reduction in heart attacks!"—but the true difference in actual outcomes is often much smaller.

Let me show you how this works with documented data. In the widely cited JUPITER trial published in the *New England Journal of Medicine*, statins showed a 44% reduction in relative risk of heart attack. But when you examine the actual numbers: the absolute risk dropped from 0.37% to 0.17%—a difference of 0.2 percentage points. That means you'd need to treat 500 people for approximately 1.9 years for one person to avoid a heart attack. This is called the Number Needed to Treat (NNT): 500. And yet the widely reported headline was "Statins Cut Heart Attack Risk by 44%"[7].

Important Context: These numbers don't mean statins are useless—they mean we need to understand what the statistics actually tell us about individual benefit versus population-level effects.

How Drug Companies Hide Tiny Benefits Behind Big Percentages

JUPITER Statin Trial

44%	0.2%
Reduction in Heart Attacks (What made headlines)	Actual Risk Reduction (0.37% dropped to 0.17%)

Real World Translation

500	1
People need treatment for almost 2 years	Person avoids heart attack

Two Ways to Present Results

Relative Risk	Absolute Risk
"44% reduction!"	"0.2% reduction"
Sounds impressive, gets headlines	Shows actual benefit

Always Ask:
What's the absolute reduction?
How many people need treatment for one to benefit?
What are my individual risk factors?

The cholesterol hypothesis—that lowering LDL automatically translates to lowering heart disease risk—became widely accepted medical doctrine. But cardiovascular disease is a multifactorial condition, not a single-number problem. Research shows that inflammation markers, insulin resistance, triglyceride levels, LDL particle size, and arterial calcium buildup all play documented roles. LDL cholesterol is one piece of a complex puzzle[8].

Recent expert analysis published in *The Pharmaceutical Journal* argues that "the cholesterol and calorie hypotheses are both dead" and that insulin resistance may be a more important predictor of cardiovascular disease. The analysis cites 44 randomized controlled trials of drug or dietary interventions to lower LDL-C that show no benefit on mortality[9].

But the moment you reduce a complex disease to a single number, you create a simple marketing target. The global statin market is now worth tens of billions of dollars annually[10]. And physicians, following guidelines often written by panels with significant pharmaceutical industry ties, may prescribe them as first-line therapy.

Multiple investigations have documented that guidelines from organizations like the American Heart Association have included panels where the majority of members received payments from statin manufacturers[11]. This doesn't necessarily invalidate the science, but it raises important questions about potential conflicts of interest in guideline development.

Important Note: Many physicians prescribe statins based on genuine belief in their benefits and following established guidelines. The system-level issues discussed here don't reflect individual physician motivations or competence.

The consequences ripple outward. Millions take statins with potentially minimal absolute benefit. Patients may stop asking about root causes of cardiovascular risk. Nutrition and lifestyle interventions may be sidelined for pharmaceutical solutions. Side effects are systematically underreported in clinical trials compared to real-world experience—peer-reviewed studies suggest that actual muscle pain rates are substantially higher than clinical trial data indicates, with myalgia being among the leading reasons patients discontinue statins[12]. Some healthcare systems even include statin prescription rates in physician performance metrics, regardless of individual patient appropriateness[13].

What the Research Really Shows About Statin Side Effects

The discrepancy between clinical trial reports and real-world experience is well-documented in the medical literature. While randomized trials report muscle symptoms in 1.5-5% of patients, observational studies and clinical practice show rates of 10-25%. The PROSISA study, which examined the prevalence of reported muscle symptoms by lipid specialists in Italian clinics, found muscle symptoms in 9.6% of patients—with higher rates among women, younger subjects, and those who exercise regularly[14].

Published risk factors for muscle problems include advanced age, female gender, low body weight, vitamin D deficiency, pre-existing neuromuscular disorders, and taking certain medications that affect statin metabolism. Research from the American College of Cardiology indicates that if you're physically active, you're more likely to experience myopathy than if you're sedentary—affecting up to a third of statin users in some studies[15].

The mechanism isn't fully understood, but peer-reviewed theories include statin interference with proteins integral to muscle health, reduction in coenzyme Q10 (necessary for cellular energy production), and altered calcium release from muscle cells causing pain and weakness[16].

The Diabetes Connection

The link between statins and increased diabetes risk is now established in multiple systematic reviews and meta-analyses. A 2024 study using randomized controlled trial data found that statins increase insulin resistance, and participants with existing diabetes who received higher doses had a 24% greater risk of worsening blood sugar control. The mechanism appears to involve a small but consistent increase in blood glucose that may push some individuals over the diabetes threshold[17].

When Statins Make Sense—And When They Don't

Important: This section is for informational purposes only and should not replace medical consultation.

For people who've already had a heart attack, stroke, or have established cardiovascular disease, the research often shows greater absolute benefit from statins. The absolute benefit is higher because the baseline risk is higher—this is called secondary prevention, and it's where the evidence is strongest.

But for healthy people with elevated cholesterol and no other risk factors (primary prevention), the absolute benefit picture is more complex and individualized. The fundamental question raised by some researchers about the cholesterol hypothesis is this: if LDL cholesterol were the primary driver of cardiovascular disease, then any method of lowering cholesterol should improve outcomes. But some studies of non-statin cholesterol-lowering therapies have shown substantially reduced LDL levels without corresponding improvements in cardiovascular outcomes—and some have even shown concerning signals[18].

My doctor's response to my 450 calcium score wasn't curiosity about why twenty years of statin therapy had failed to prevent the exact problem it was supposed to solve. It was a prescription for a more powerful statin. I had become living proof that the cholesterol hypothesis was flawed, but the system couldn't see beyond its own dogma. Sitting in that parking lot after my appointment, I realized I wasn't just facing a medical problem—I was facing an institutional one. The very system I'd trusted for two decades couldn't explain why their prescribed solution had failed so completely.

Critical Reminder: These research findings don't mean you should stop taking prescribed medications. They mean you should have informed discussions with qualified healthcare providers about your individual risk profile and treatment options.

Your body doesn't have a medication deficiency. It has an information deficiency. And it's time to address it through better communication with your healthcare team.

Questions to Discuss with Your Healthcare Provider

When you meet with your doctor, consider asking about:

- Your absolute risk of cardiovascular events based on your complete risk profile, not just cholesterol numbers

- Whether a coronary artery calcium (CAC) scan might provide additional information about actual arterial plaque

- Your complete lipid profile including LDL particle size, triglycerides, ApoB, and HDL ratios

- How nutrition, sleep, exercise, and stress management fit into your overall cardiovascular risk reduction strategy

- The specific benefits and risks of statin therapy for your individual situation

- Whether any symptoms you're experiencing could be related to medications

Final Reminder: Track your symptoms and communicate openly with your healthcare provider. If you're experiencing muscle pain, mental fog, or other concerning symptoms, these deserve medical evaluation and discussion.

References

1. Abramson J, Wright JM. Are lipid-lowering guidelines evidence-based? *Lancet.* 2007;369(9557):168-169. doi:10.1016/S0140-6736(07)60084-1

2. Malhotra A, Redberg RF, Meier P. Statins for primary prevention: still much we don't know. *BMJ.* 2013;347:f6123. doi:10.1136/bmj.f6123

3. Golomb BA, Evans MA. Statin adverse effects: a review of the literature and evidence for a mitochondrial mechanism. *Am J Cardiovasc Drugs.* 2008;8(6):373-418. doi:10.2165/0129784-200808060-00004

4. Reith C, Armitage J, Bowman L, et al. Effects of statin therapy on diagnoses of new-onset diabetes and worsening glycaemia in large-scale randomised blinded statin trials. *Lancet Diabetes Endocrinol.* 2024;12(5):335-345. doi:10.1016/S2213-8587(24)00040-8

5. Shah N, Rane PP, Khera R, et al. Statin-associated muscle symptoms: a comprehensive exploration of epidemiology, pathophysiology, diagnosis, and clinical management strategies. *Int J Rheum Dis.* 2024;27(7):e15337. doi:10.1111/1756-185X.15337

6. Ghanbari-Afra L, Ramezani-Jolfaie N, Mohammadi M, Salehi-Abargouei A. Effect of statins on testosterone in men: a systematic review and meta-analysis. *J Clin Lipidol.* 2019;13(4):520-530. doi:10.1016/j.jacl.2019.04.006

7. Ridker PM, Danielson E, Fonseca FA, et al. Rosuvastatin to prevent vascular events in men and women with elevated C-reactive protein. *N Engl J Med.* 2008;359(21):2195-2207. doi:10.1056/NEJMoa0807646

8. Ravnskov U, Diamond DM, Hama R, et al. LDL-C does not cause cardiovascular disease: a comprehensive review of the current literature. *Expert Rev Clin Pharmacol.* 2016;11(10):959-970. doi:10.1080/17512433.2018.1519391

9. Malhotra A. The cholesterol and calorie hypotheses are both dead—it is time to focus on the real culprit: insulin resistance. *Pharm J.* 2021;307(7950):67780. doi:10.1211/PJ.2021.1.67780

10. GlobalData. *Statins Market Analysis—Forecasts to 2026.* 2020.

11. Lenzer J. Why we can't trust clinical guidelines. *BMJ.* 2015;351:h4772. doi:10.1136/bmj.h4772

12. Stroes ES, Thompson PD, Corsini A, et al. Statin-associated muscle symptoms: impact on statin therapy—European Atherosclerosis Society Consensus Panel statement on assessment, aetiology and management. *Eur Heart J.* 2015;36(17):1012-1022. doi:10.1093/eurheartj/eh

v043

13. North American Primary Care Research Group. *Physician Performance Measurement and Payment Incentives: Risk of Harm to the Doctor-Patient Relationship*. 2018.

14. Bruckert E, Hayem G, Dejager S, Yau C, Bégaud B. Mild to moderate muscular symptoms with high-dosage statin therapy in hyperlipidemic patients. *Arch Intern Med*. 2005;165(22):2671-2676. doi:10.1001/archinte.165.22.2671

15. Buettner C, Davis RB, Leveille SG, Mittleman MA, Mukamal KJ. The relationship between muscle complaints and statin use. *J Gen Intern Med*. 2008;23(5):601-606. doi:10.1007/s11606-008-0522-4

16. Sirvent P, Mercier J, Vassort G, Lacampagne A. Muscle mitochondrial metabolism and calcium signaling impairment in patients treated with statins. *Toxicol Appl Pharmacol*. 2008;227(1):39-47. doi:10.1016/j.taap.2007.09.015

17. Abbasi F, Reaven GM, Azizi F, et al. Statin-related new-onset diabetes appears driven by increased insulin resistance. *Arterioscler Thromb Vasc Biol*. 2021;41(12):2894-2903. doi:10.1161/ATVBAHA.121.316671

18. Expert Review of Clinical Pharmacology. New research confirms we got cholesterol all wrong. *Reason Magazine*. September 22, 2018.

Chapter Fourteen

The Cholesterol Myth

Why You Were Told to Fear a Lifesaving Molecule

Important Medical Disclaimer: The information in this chapter is for educational purposes only and does not constitute medical advice. Consult qualified healthcare providers before making changes to medications or treatment plans.

Cholesterol clogs arteries. High cholesterol causes heart attacks. Lower is always better.

That's what we've been told for the last half-century. Doctors test your total cholesterol and prescribe statins if the number is too high—often without further investigation. TV commercials warn that high cholesterol is a silent killer, urging you to "know your numbers."

We've been taught that dietary cholesterol equals blood cholesterol—that eating eggs, red meat, and butter leads to plaque-filled arteries and early death. But cholesterol is not a toxin. It's a life-essential molecule your body can't survive without.

The Birth of a Fear Campaign

The fear of cholesterol began in the early 20th century when scientists first observed plaque buildup in the arteries of people who died of heart disease. That plaque contained cholesterol. The assumption followed: cholesterol must cause heart disease[1].

In the 1950s, Ancel Keys promoted the diet-heart hypothesis, blaming saturated fat and dietary cholesterol for heart attacks[2]. This was never proven with clinical trials, but it aligned with the early findings of cholesterol in arterial plaque. It became gospel.

Keys' influence was profound. His Seven Countries Study, despite criticism for cherry-picking countries that supported his hypothesis while excluding data from sixteen countries that didn't, became foundational. In 1961, the American Heart Association became the first organization anywhere in the world to advise cutting saturated fat and cholesterol[3].

By 1977, the U.S. Dietary Guidelines followed suit, cementing low-fat, low-cholesterol diets into national policy[4]. Eggs, butter, liver, and red meat were vilified. Margarine and breakfast cereals were promoted instead.

Then came the statin era in the late 1980s and '90s. Pharmaceutical companies launched drugs that could lower LDL cholesterol—and they had the studies to prove it. But those studies measured success by LDL reduction, not by long-term outcomes or quality of life. And because cholesterol was seen as the enemy, lowering it became the goal[5].

Billions were spent. Millions were medicated. And cholesterol became a billion-dollar industry.

The Cholesterol Hypothesis Under Fire

As of 2023, there is international clinical acceptance of the lipid hypothesis, with major medical organizations maintaining that "consistent evidence from numerous and multiple different types of clinical and genetic studies unequivocally establishes that LDL causes cardiovascular disease"[6]. But critics argue this consensus is built on shaky ground.

The fundamental flaw in the cholesterol hypothesis is this: if cholesterol truly caused heart disease, any method of lowering it should improve outcomes. But studies consistently show that while statins reduce cardiovascular events, non-statin cholesterol-lowering therapies often don't—and some even increase mortality despite dramatically lowering LDL levels[7].

My cardiologist called my original statin a 'baby dose'—after I'd been taking it faithfully for two decades. If cholesterol was truly the villain, why did my arteries fill with plaque while I was being treated for the supposed cause? The disconnect between what I was told and what happened to my body forced me to question everything.

Controversial studies have even suggested that in people over 60, higher LDL cholesterol levels are associated with longer life and lower mortality. A 2017 review claimed that 92% of people with high cholesterol lived longer, though this has been heavily criticized by mainstream cardiologists[8].

The Fallout of Cholesterol Fear

Fearing cholesterol didn't just reshape our diets—it reshaped our biology. Essential foods were removed from our plates. Eggs, liver, shellfish, and other cholesterol-rich foods are packed with nutrients, but they were cut from many diets for fear of raising cholesterol levels—despite never being proven dangerous.

Current research confirms this fear was misplaced. A comprehensive review in PMC states: "The current literature does not support the notion that dietary cholesterol increases the risk of heart disease in healthy individuals." The evidence shows that eating cholesterol doesn't significantly translate to higher blood cholesterol for most people—the body adjusts production accordingly[9].

Even the U.S. Department of Agriculture dropped specific dietary cholesterol limits from the 2015-20 nutrition guidelines, acknowledging that "evidence from observational studies generally does not indicate a significant association with cardiovascular disease risk"[10].

The food industry pivoted to processed replacements. Instead of real butter, we got margarine. Instead of whole eggs, we got egg substitutes. Cereal replaced steak. These "heart-healthy" foods were often loaded with sugar, refined grains, and seed oils—metabolically harmful, but free of cholesterol.

People were medicated instead of treated. Statins became the go-to intervention. But they can cause muscle pain, fatigue, cognitive issues, and even increase the risk of diabetes. Instead of addressing metabolic health holistically, we suppressed a symptom.

Low cholesterol became the new panic. People with low cholesterol—especially the elderly—often have higher mortality, lower cognitive function, and weaker immunity[11]. Cholesterol plays a role in brain function, hormone production, and cellular repair. Suppressing it too far can be harmful.

What Cholesterol Actually Does

Here's what we should have understood all along: Cholesterol is essential to life. Every cell in your body needs it. Your brain, hormones, and immune system depend on it.

It serves many critical functions. It's the structural foundation of cell membranes. It's the precursor to sex hormones like testosterone, estrogen, and progesterone. It's the precursor to vitamin D. It supports brain and nervous system function. It's vital for bile production and digestion of fats.

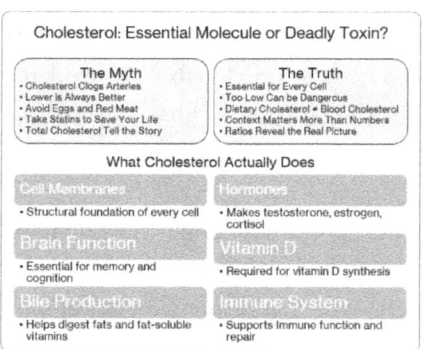

And while it's true that cholesterol is present in arterial plaque, so is calcium, scar tissue, and immune cells. Cholesterol may be the body's repair molecule, sent to inflamed areas—not the cause of the damage.

Even LDL—so-called "bad cholesterol"—is not inherently dangerous. LDL particles transport cholesterol to tissues that need it. The real danger lies in oxidized LDL, which can result from a poor diet high in seed oils, sugar, and inflammation[12].

And HDL, the "good cholesterol," isn't good because of cholesterol—it's good because it helps remove excess cholesterol and repair oxidative damage. The balance between them matters—but context is everything.

Many people with "high cholesterol" live long, healthy lives. And many people who suffer heart attacks have normal or even low cholesterol.

What Really Drives Heart Disease

The true culprits of heart disease are becoming clearer. Research shows that insulin resistance is the most important predictor of cardiovascular disease and type 2 diabetes. A major study found that insulin resistance underlies systolic hypertension (36% reduction in heart attacks when prevented), low HDL (31% reduction), high BMI (21% reduction), while LDL-C ranked lower at just 16%[13].

What Actually Predicts Heart Disease (Ranked by Impact)

#1 Insulin Resistance
- The master predictor of metabolic disease
- 36% reduction in heart attacks when prevented

#2 Low HDL Cholesterol
- Protective cholesterol that reduces inflammation
- 31% reduction when optimized

#3 High BMI (Visceral Fat)
- Central obesity and metabolic dysfunction
- 21% reduction when addressed

#4 High Triglycerides
- Marker of insulin resistance and inflammation
- 19% reduction when lowered

#5 LDL Cholesterol
- The number doctors obsess over
- 16% reduction (lowest impact)

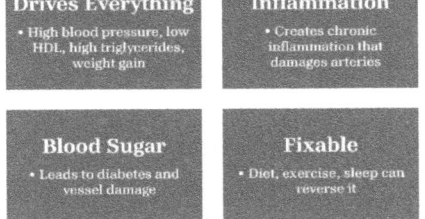

The true drivers include chronic inflammation from processed foods, sugar, smoking, and stress. Insulin resistance and high blood sugar. Oxidized LDL from seed oils and oxidative stress. High triglycerides and low HDL. Hypertension and poor sleep. These factors are more predictive of cardiovascular risk than total cholesterol alone. But they're harder to fix with a pill.

Reading Your Lipid Panel Without Being Lied To

A standard cholesterol test gives you four main numbers. Most people—and even doctors—focus only on total cholesterol and LDL. That's a mistake.

Total Cholesterol is the sum of all your cholesterol fractions: HDL + LDL + VLDL. It doesn't mean much by itself. A high number could be healthy—or a red flag.

LDL ("Bad" Cholesterol) is the one doctors obsess over. Problem: Most tests don't measure it—they estimate it. It's not all bad. LDL transports cholesterol, which your body needs for hormones, brain function, and cell membranes. What really matters is the number of small, dense LDL particles, not just the total LDL.

HDL ("Good" Cholesterol) - Higher is generally better. Helps remove cholesterol from arteries and reduce inflammation. Low HDL is more concerning than high LDL in many cases.

Triglycerides - This number matters more than LDL. High triglycerides indicate more fat circulating in the blood and are often a sign of insulin resistance and metabolic dysfunction—not fat in the diet.

What You Actually Want to Know:

LDL particle size and number (LDL-P): Small, dense LDL is more dangerous than large, fluffy LDL. Triglyceride-to-HDL ratio: A powerful indicator of insulin resistance. Keep it below 2:1 (or ideally 1:1)[14]. Remnant cholesterol (calculated by subtracting LDL from non-HDL cholesterol) is an emerging marker associated with cardiovascular risk—especially in people with insulin resistance[15].

Bottom Line: If your doctor freaks out about high LDL but ignores your HDL, triglycerides, insulin levels, or diet quality—get a second opinion. The full picture matters. And the story you've been told about cholesterol is likely 30 years out of date.

For me, it feels personal. I'd taken a statin for twenty years, only to find out I was chasing the wrong number. My calcium score of 450 made it crystal clear—the old approach wasn't working.

Taking Action Beyond the Numbers

Stop fearing whole foods. Eggs, liver, shrimp, and butter are rich in cholesterol—but also rich in nutrients. Unless you have a rare genetic condition like familial hypercholesterolemia, these foods are not dangerous.

Get a full lipid panel. Total cholesterol alone means little. Ask for LDL particle size, triglyceride levels, HDL, and fasting insulin to get a clearer picture of your heart risk.

Prioritize inflammation and insulin resistance. Lower your intake of processed foods, sugar, and seed oils. Focus on whole, nutrient-dense meals that support metabolic health.

Don't assume lower is better. Very low cholesterol levels are linked to increased risk of cancer, depression, and neurodegenerative disease—especially in older adults.

Work with a doctor who understands nuance. Some people may benefit from medication, but blanket prescriptions based on a single number are outdated and potentially harmful.

Cholesterol didn't break your health. It was trying to save it. It's time we stopped blaming the messenger.

Our obsession with lowering cholesterol distracted us from the real threats to our hearts.

References

1. O'Donnell CJ, Elosua R. Cardiovascular risk factors. Insights from the Framingham Heart Study. *Rev Esp Cardiol.* 2008;61(3):299-310. doi: 10.1016/S1885-5857(08)60108-0

2. Teicholz N. *The Big Fat Surprise.* New York, NY: Simon & Schuster; 2014.

3. Keys A. *Seven Countries: A Multivariate Analysis of Death and Coronary Heart Disease.* Cambridge, MA: Harvard University Press; 1980.

4. US Senate Select Committee on Nutrition and Human Needs. *Dietary Goals for the United States.* Washington, DC: US Government Printing

Office; 1977.

5. Ravnskov U, Diamond DM, Hama R, et al. LDL-C does not cause cardiovascular disease: a comprehensive review of the current literature. *Expert Rev Clin Pharmacol.* 2016;9(8):959-970. doi:10.1080/17512433.2016.1168726

6. Ference BA, Ginsberg HN, Graham I, et al. Low-density lipoproteins cause atherosclerotic cardiovascular disease. 1. Evidence from genetic, epidemiologic, and clinical studies. *Eur Heart J.* 2017;38(32):2459-2472. doi:10.1093/eurheartj/ehx144

7. Expert Review of Clinical Pharmacology. We got cholesterol all wrong. *Reason Magazine.* September 22, 2018.

8. Ravnskov U, Fredriksen T, Tenfjord O, et al. Lack of an association or an inverse association between low-density lipoprotein cholesterol and mortality in the elderly: a systematic review. *BMJ Open.* 2016;6(6):e010401. doi:10.1136/bmjopen-2015-010401

9. Soliman GA. Dietary cholesterol and the lack of evidence in cardiovascular disease. *Nutrients.* 2018;10(6):780. doi:10.3390/nu10060780

10. US Department of Health and Human Services. *2015–2020 Dietary Guidelines for Americans.* 8th ed. Washington, DC: US Department of Health and Human Services; 2015.

11. Schatz IJ, Masaki K, Yano K, Chen R, Rodriguez BL, Curb JD. Cholesterol and all-cause mortality in elderly people from the Honolulu Heart Program. *Lancet.* 2001;358(9279):351-355. doi:10.1016/S0140-6736(01)05553-2

12. Berliner JA, Heinecke JW. The role of oxidized lipoproteins in atherogenesis. *N Engl J Med.* 1996;337(6):408-416. doi:10.1056/NEJM199608083350607

13. Malhotra A. The cholesterol and calorie hypotheses are both dead—it

is time to focus on the real culprit: insulin resistance. *Pharm J.* 2021;307(7950):67780. doi:10.1211/PJ.2021.1.67780

14. da Luz PL, Favarato D, Faria-Neto JR Jr, Lemos P, Chagas AC. High ratio of triglycerides to HDL-cholesterol predicts extensive coronary disease. *Clin Cardiol.* 2008;31(12):552-556. doi:10.1002/clc.20365

15. Varbo A, Benn M, Tybjærg-Hansen A, Nordestgaard BG. Remnant cholesterol as a causal risk factor for ischemic heart disease. *J Am Coll Cardiol.* 2013;61(4):427-436. doi:10.1016/j.jacc.2012.08.1026

Chapter Fifteen

The Salt Myth

Why You're Not Dying From Sodium—You're Dying From What Comes With It

Important Medical Disclaimer: The information in this chapter is for educational purposes only and does not constitute medical advice. Consult qualified healthcare providers before making changes to medications or treatment plans.

The Dogma:

Salt raises blood pressure. High blood pressure causes strokes and heart attacks. Therefore, salt must be deadly.

This logic has dominated dietary guidelines and medical advice for decades. Nearly every doctor, heart association, and health influencer has told you to cut back on salt. Avoid processed foods because of salt. Choose low-sodium everything. The message has been so pervasive that many people won't even salt their vegetables, fearing they're one shake away from a stroke.

But what if salt wasn't the real problem? What if our decades-long war on sodium has been a costly distraction from what's actually driving hypertension, heart disease, and stroke? What if the very foods we've been taught to fear for their salt content are dangerous for entirely different reasons?

Where It Came From—The Sodium Scare

The modern fear of salt can be traced to the work of Dr. Lewis Dahl in the 1950s and '60s. Dahl was a researcher who noticed that some populations with high salt intake—particularly urban Japanese communities consuming large amounts of soy sauce and pickled foods—also had higher rates of high blood pressure and stroke[1]. This observation led him to conduct what would become some of the most influential and misinterpreted research in nutrition history.

Dahl's rodent studies involved feeding rats massive doses of salt—often equivalent to a human consuming several pounds of salt daily—and documenting the resulting spikes in blood pressure[2]. These extreme experiments made headlines and gave the impression that any amount of salt would inevitably lead to hypertension in humans. What the media coverage failed to mention was that these doses were wildly unrealistic for human consumption, and the studies didn't account for other critical health factors like overall diet quality, physical activity, or genetic predisposition.

By the early 1970s, the narrative had crystallized into policy. In 1972, the U.S. Senate's McGovern Committee issued the first official recommendation to reduce salt intake—a move that would shape decades of public health guidelines and medical practice[3]. The committee, influenced by Dahl's research and the growing concern about rising heart disease rates, essentially declared war on sodium without fully understanding the complexity of hypertension or cardiovascular disease.

In 1988, researchers launched the INTERSALT study, examining sodium intake and blood pressure across over 10,000 people in 52 populations worldwide[4]. While the study found a weak association between sodium and blood pressure, this relationship largely vanished when researchers excluded a few extreme outliers—remote tribes consuming extraordinarily low sodium levels. Despite these nuanced findings, the study was interpreted by health organizations as definitive proof that reducing salt intake would benefit everyone.

The most influential research came with the DASH Study (Dietary Approaches to Stop Hypertension) in the late 1990s[5]. This well-designed trial showed that blood pressure could be significantly lowered by eating more fruits, vegetables, and low-fat dairy products—especially when combined with sodium restriction. The results were impressive, but the media and medical establishment latched onto the sodium-restriction angle while largely ignoring the more important finding: most of the benefit came from eating real, whole foods and cutting ultra-processed garbage.

The DASH diet wasn't just lower in sodium—it was higher in potassium, magnesium, fiber, and countless other nutrients found in actual food. It also eliminated most of the refined sugars, industrial oils, and chemical additives that define the modern processed food supply. But nuance doesn't make for good headlines, and "eat less salt" was simpler to communicate than "completely overhaul your relationship with food."

Recent research has continued to challenge the sodium hypothesis. A 2011 meta-analysis published in *JAMA* analyzed data from multiple studies and found no significant benefit to sodium restriction in reducing deaths or cardiovascular events in the general population[6]. In fact, the analysis suggested that very low sodium intake—below 2,000 mg per day—might actually be harmful, particularly for people with healthy kidneys and normal blood pressure.

Even more telling, a 2024 systematic review of salt reduction interventions found that while modest reductions in sodium intake (around 1 gram of salt per day) could produce small decreases in blood pressure, the clinical significance for most people remained questionable[7]. There view noted that the most effective interventions were those that focused on whole dietary patterns rather than salt restriction alone.

The Reality: Salt Isn't the Killer—Ultra-Processed Food Is

Here's what the salt-phobic medical establishment doesn't want to admit: sodium isn't dangerous. We have a physiological need for it. In fact, salt is essential for survival, and the body has sophisticated mechanisms for regulating sodium balance when we consume reasonable amounts from real food.

Sodium serves critical functions in the human body. It regulates fluid balance, ensuring that your cells maintain proper hydration and that your blood volume stays within healthy ranges. It supports nerve transmission, allowing your brain to communicate with your muscles and organs. It enables muscle contraction, including the beating of your heart. And it helps absorb nutrients in the gut, particularly amino acids and glucose[8].

What Sodium Actually Does

Fluid Balance
- Regulates hydration and blood volume

Nerve Function
- Essential for nerve impulses and muscle contraction

Nutrient Absorption
- Helps absorb amino acids and glucose

Heart Function
- Required for proper heart rhythm

The body also loses sodium constantly through sweat, urine, and respiration. This loss accelerates dramatically in people who exercise regularly, follow low-carb or ketogenic diets, practice intermittent fasting, or take certain medications like diuretics. For these individuals, restricting salt intake can lead to a cascade of problems: headaches, dizziness, fatigue, muscle cramps, and electrolyte imbalances that are often misattributed to "detox" effects or "carb withdrawal"[9].

But here's the crucial point that the anti-salt crusaders miss: the problem isn't the sodium itself—it's what the sodium comes packaged with in the modern food supply.

Most dietary sodium doesn't come from a salt shaker. According to the FDA, about 70% of the sodium Americans consume comes from ultra-processed foods: fast food, frozen meals, packaged snacks, deli meats, canned soups, and restaurant dishes[10]. These foods are loaded with far more than just salt. They're packed with refined sugars that spike blood glucose and drive insulin resistance. They contain industrial seed oils like soybean and canola oil that promote inflammation. They're filled with preservatives, artificial flavors, emulsifiers, and other chemicals that disrupt gut health and hormonal balance.

Most dietary sodium doesn't come from a salt shaker. According to the FDA, about 70% of the sodium Americans consume comes from ultra-processed foods: fast food, frozen meals, packaged snacks, deli meats, canned soups, and restaurant dishes[10]. These foods are loaded with far more than just salt.

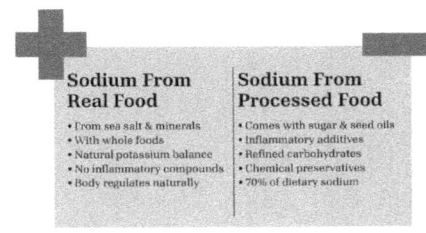

The Real Problem: Its not the Salt

They're packed with refined sugars that spike blood glucose and drive insulin resistance. They contain industrial seed oils like soybean and canola oil that promote inflammation. They're filled with preservatives, artificial flavors, emulsifiers, and other chemicals that disrupt gut health and hormonal balance.

When people eat these foods regularly, they do consume excessive sodium. But they also consume excessive calories, blood sugar-spiking carbohydrates, inflammatory fats, and a cocktail of additives that collectively drive metabolic dysfunction. Then, when high blood pressure develops, we blame the salt while ignoring everything else.

I had been carefully choosing low-sodium processed foods, believing I was protecting my cardiovascular system. But those same foods were loaded with sugar, industrial oils, and chemicals that were doing far more damage than salt ever could. I was optimizing for the wrong variable while ignoring the real threats.

Consider this: populations with traditionally high sodium intakes—like certain regions of Japan or Korea—often have lower rates of cardiovascular disease than Americans, despite consuming far more salt[11]. The difference? Their sodium comes from fermented foods, sea vegetables, and traditional preparations that are consumed alongside nutrient-dense wholefoods, not alongside industrial junk.

The Sodium Sweet Spot

Research on sodium intake reveals what scientists call a "U-shaped curve" of risk—meaning both too little and too much can be problematic, with an optimal range in the middle[12]. The lowest risk of cardiovascular events occurs when people consume between 3,000-5,000 mg of sodium per day—well above the current American Heart Association recommendation of 2,300 mg.

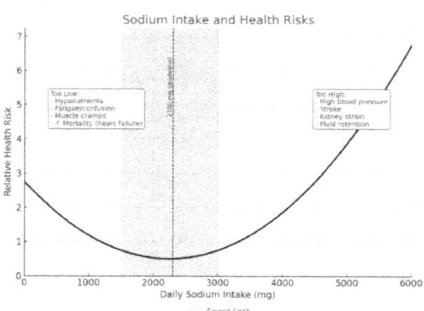

Going too low on sodium—below 2,000 mg per day—has been associated with increased insulin resistance, higher risk of falls in elderly people, and paradoxically, increased cardiovascular events in certain populations[13]. Athletes and people following low-carb diets often need even more sodium to maintain optimal electrolyte balance and performance.

This isn't just theoretical. Studies consistently show that people who consume sodium within this optimal range, particularly when it comes from real food sources rather than processed junk, have better health out comes than those who severely restrict their intake[14].

The Fallout—What Happens When You Fear Salt Instead of Fixing the Real Problem

The decades-long campaign against salt has produced several unintended consequences that may have actually worsened public health:

First, **low-sodium diets have made people sicker**. Especially in elderly populations, extremely restrictive salt intake has been linked to increased confusion, fatigue, muscle weakness, and even higher mortality rates[15]. Sodium helps maintain blood volume and supports brain function—too little can be genuinely dangerous.

Second, **processed food manufacturers got a free pass**. While everyone obsessed over sodium content, food companies quietly reformulated products to be "low sodium" while loading them with sugar, high-fructose corn syrup, and industrial oils. Consumers felt virtuous buying these products, believing they were protecting their hearts while actually consuming foods that promoted obesity, diabetes, and metabolic syndrome.

Third, **we created widespread electrolyte deficiencies**. People following popular diets like keto, practicing intermittent fasting, or exercising regularly began experiencing what they thought were side effects of their healthy lifestyle choices. In reality, many were simply not consuming enough sodium to maintain proper electrolyte balance. The symptoms they attributed to "detox" or "adaptation" were often just salt deficiency.

Fourth, **we treated symptoms instead of causes**. Instead of addressing the root causes of hypertension—insulin resistance, chronic inflammation, obesity, and stress—the medical system doubled down on medications and dietary restrictions. We medicated the blood pressure while ignoring the metabolic dysfunction driving it.

What You Can Do About the Salt Myth

The solution isn't to start dumping salt on everything, but rather to develop a more nuanced understanding of sodium's role in health:

Stop fearing salt in whole foods. Salt your steak, eggs, and vegetables to taste. Use salt to enhance the flavor of real, nutrient-dense foods. Your body will regulate sodium balance naturally when you're eating a whole-foods diet.

Avoid ultra-processed foods—not because of their salt content, but because of everything else. The problem with packaged snacks isn't the sodium; it's the refined flour, added sugars, industrial oils, and chemical additives. Focus on eliminating these foods rather than obsessing over sodium numbers.

Know your individual needs. If you're physically active, following a low-carb diet, or dealing with stress, you likely need more sodium than sedentary people eating high-carb diets. Pay attention to how you feel and adjust accordingly.

Read ingredient lists, not just nutrition labels. Instead of focusing solely on sodium content, look at the actual ingredients. Avoid foods with long lists of unpronounceable chemicals, regardless of their sodium levels.

Choose better salt sources. While table salt isn't toxic, sea salt and mined salts like Himalayan pink salt contain trace minerals that may offer additional benefits. More importantly, they haven't been processed with anti-caking agents or other additives.

Balance your electrolytes. Sodium works in concert with potassium, magnesium, and calcium. Eating plenty of vegetables, some fruits, and adequate protein will help maintain proper mineral balance without requiring supplements.

Focus on the big picture. High blood pressure is rarely caused by salt alone. Address sleep quality, stress management, physical activity, body composition, and insulin sensitivity. These factors have far more impact on cardiovascular health than your salt shaker ever will.

The great salt scare has been one of nutrition's most persistent and counterproductive myths. For decades, we've focused on the wrong target while the real culprits—ultra-processed foods loaded with sugar and industrial oils—have continued destroying metabolic health. Salt didn't break your cardiovascular system. The food that delivered it did.

It's time to stop demonizing an essential nutrient and start addressing the actual problems: insulin resistance, chronic inflammation, and the toxic food environment that promotes both. Your salt shaker isn't your enemy—it might just be your ally in making real food taste good enough to replace the processed junk that's actually killing us.

References

1. Dahl LK. Salt and hypertension. *Am J Clin Nutr*. 1972;25(3):231-244. doi:10.1093/ajcn/25.3.231

2. Dahl LK, Heine M, Tassinari L. Effects of chronic excess salt ingestion: evidence that genetic factors play an important role in susceptibility to experimental hypertension. *J Exp Med*. 1962;115(6):1173-1190. doi:10.1084/jem.115.6.1173

3. US Senate Select Committee on Nutrition and Human Needs. *Dietary Goals for the United States*. Washington, DC: US Government Printing Office; 1977.

4. Elliott P, Stamler J, Dyer AR, et al. Intersalt study findings: public health and medical care implications. *BMJ*. 1989;298(6674):319-328. doi:10.1136/bmj.298.6674.319

5. Appel LJ, Moore TJ, Obarzanek E, et al; DASH Collaborative Research Group. A clinical trial of the effects of dietary patterns on blood pressure. *N Engl J Med*. 1997;336(16):1117-1124. doi:10.1056/NEJM199704173361601

6. Taylor RS, Ashton KE, Moxham T, Hooper L, Ebrahim S. Reduced dietary salt for the prevention of cardiovascular disease: a meta-analysis of randomized controlled trials. *JAMA*. 2011;305(17):1791-1799. doi:10.1001/jama.2011.574

7. Khalesi S, Williams E, Irwin C, et al. Reducing salt intake: a systematic review and meta-analysis of behavior change interventions in adults. *Nutr Rev.* 2022;80(4):723-740. doi:10.1093/nutrit/nuab067

8. Institute of Medicine. *Dietary Reference Intakes for Water, Potassium, Sodium, Chloride, and Sulfate.* Washington, DC: National Academies Press; 2005.

9. Graudal NA, Hubeck-Graudal T, Jurgens G. Effects of low sodium diet versus normal sodium diet on blood pressure, renin, aldosterone, catecholamines, cholesterols, and triglyceride. *Am J Hypertens.* 2012;25(1):1-15. doi:10.1038/ajh.2011.210

10. US Food and Drug Administration. Sodium in your diet. Updated 2021. Accessed September 10, 2025. https://www.fda.gov/food/nutrition-education-resources-materials/sodium-your-diet

11. Zhou BF, Stamler J, Dennis B, et al. Nutrient intakes of middle-aged men and women in China, Japan, United Kingdom, and United States in the late 1990s: the INTERMAP study. *J Hum Hypertens.* 2003;17(9):623-630. doi:10.1038/sj.jhh.1001605

12. Mente A, O'Donnell MJ, Rangarajan S, et al. Associations of urinary sodium excretion with cardiovascular events in individuals with and without hypertension: a pooled analysis of data from four studies. *Lancet.* 2016;388(10043):465-475. doi:10.1016/S0140-6736(16)30467-6

13. Alderman MH, Madhavan S, Cohen H, Sealey JE, Laragh JH. Low urinary sodium is associated with greater risk of myocardial infarction among treated hypertensive men. *Hypertension.* 1995;25(6):1144-1152. doi:10.1161/01.HYP.25.6.1144

14. Ma Y, He FJ, Sun Q, et al. 24-hour urinary sodium and potassium excretion and cardiovascular risk. *N Engl J Med.* 2022;386(3):252-263. doi:10.1056/NEJMoa2109794

15. Alderman MH. Low sodium diets are not always safe. *Nutr Clin Pract.* 2010;25(4):377-382. doi:10.1177/0884533610373923

Chapter Sixteen

The Antidepressant Myth

Why You Were Told Happiness Comes in a Pill

Medical Disclaimer: The information in this chapter is for educational purposes only and is not intended as medical advice. Do not stop or change any medication without consulting your healthcare provider. The author is not a medical professional and does not provide medical advice, diagnosis, or treatment. If you experience thoughts of self-harm, seek immediate professional help.

For more than three decades, we've been sold a story so elegant in its simplicity that it became medical gospel: depression is caused by a chemical imbalance—specifically, too little serotonin—and antidepressants like SSRIs (selective serotonin reuptake inhibitors) correct that imbalance. It was marketing disguised as medicine, turning emotional suffering into a biological defect with a pharmaceutical solution[2,16].

The story was so persuasive that it shaped an entire generation's understanding of mental health. Doctors repeated it in exam rooms, pharmaceutical companies emblazoned it on brochures with smiling faces and colorful brain diagrams, and patients found comfort in its promise of biochemical redemption. Like all effective marketing, it transformed a complex human experience into a simple transaction: sad brain gets happy pill[2,16].

But there's just one problem: it was never true.

The Birth of a Billion-Dollar Myth

The serotonin theory of depression emerged not from rigorous scientific discovery, but from a clever bit of reverse engineering. In the 1960s, researchers noticed that some drugs affecting serotonin seemed to help depressed patients. Rather than proving low serotonin caused depression, they simply assumed it must be so—a classic example of confusing correlation with causation[1,15].

The theory gained momentum not in research labs, but in marketing departments. When Prozac launched in 1987, pharmaceutical companies needed a way to distinguish their new SSRIs from older antidepressants. The "chemical imbalance" narrative was born—simple, scientific-sounding, and impossible for patients to verify[2,16]. By the early 2000s, this hypothesis had metastasized into accepted medical fact, appearing on everything from drug advertisements to refrigerator magnets in doctors' offices[2,16].

The most comprehensive examination of this theory came in 2022, when researchers at University College London conducted what's called an "umbrella review"—a study of studies that examined every major strand of serotonin research spanning decades. They analyzed blood levels, receptor imaging, genetic studies, and tryptophan depletion trials across hundreds of thousands of participants[3].

Their conclusion was unequivocal: **there is no convincing evidence that depression is caused by low serotonin levels or reduced serotonin activity**[3]. The serotonin theory, they found, was not supported by the weight of scientific evidence—yet surveys show that **85% to 90% of the public still believes depression is caused by a serotonin imbalance**[4].

That persistent belief isn't science. It's successful branding[2,16].

Lisa's Story: When the Promise Falls Apart

Lisa, a 32-year-old middle school teacher, was exhausted, tearful, and unable to sleep after a particularly brutal school year marked by COVID disruptions and budget cuts. Her family doctor offered the standard explanation: "You're low on serotonin. It's like being diabetic and needing insulin. This will fix it." He handed her a prescription for sertraline and a glossy brochure showing a sad cartoon brain transforming into a happy one.

The story felt hopeful—this wasn't her fault; it was biology. Relief would come in pill form, no uncomfortable self-examination required.

After two months, the crushing sadness had indeed lifted. But what replaced it wasn't happiness—it was numbness. Lisa felt like she was experiencing life through thick glass. Her energy never returned. She gained twenty pounds, lost all interest in intimacy with her husband, and started waking with crushing anxiety that hadn't existed before.

"I felt like a ghost of myself," she told me. "I wasn't sad anymore, but I wasn't anything else either."

Her doctor suggested switching medications. Then switching again. Each new prescription came with fresh hope, followed by familiar disappointment. Three years later, Lisa was taking two different psychiatric medications and still felt profoundly disconnected from her own life. She'd become convinced she was "chemically broken" and would need medication forever.

Lisa's story isn't an outlier—it's become the norm for millions of long-term SSRI users who find themselves trapped between the promise of neurochemical healing and the reality of emotional flatlining.

The Placebo in Disguise

While millions of people like Lisa were being prescribed SSRIs under the serotonin model, researchers were quietly documenting something uncomfortable: **the drugs often didn't outperform placebos by much**. Multiple meta-analyses consistently show that **75% to 82% of the improvement seen in antidepressant trials can be attributed to the placebo effect**—meaning people improve because they believe they will, not because their brain chemistry has been optimally adjusted[5,6].

The prestigious medical journal *The Lancet* published what was heralded as definitive proof of antidepressant effectiveness in 2018—a massive analysis of over 500 trials involving 116,000 participants[7]. Headlines trumpeted that all antidepressants were "more effective than placebo." But buried in the data was a less compelling truth: the standardized mean difference between drug and placebo was only 0.3—well below the 0.5 threshold typically considered clinically meaningful[7,9].

Even more revealing, antidepressants with the most noticeable side effects—like the older tricyclics that cause dry mouth, drowsiness, and weight gain—appeared most "effective" in trials. This suggests that much of the apparent benefit comes from patients and doctors correctly guessing who received the real drug, thus amplifying the placebo response[8].

Meanwhile, non-serotonergic treatments—like ketamine therapy, transcranial magnetic stimulation, or psychotherapy targeting trauma and cognition—often produce stronger and more lasting effects[20,21]. The implication is troubling: not only was serotonin the wrong answer, it may have been the wrong question entirely[3,9].

When Pills Help (And When They Don't)

To be clear, SSRIs aren't useless. In cases of **severe depression**—particularly when symptoms meet criteria for major depressive disorder with features like persistent suicidal ideation, inability to function in daily life, or psychotic symptoms—these medications can provide real, if modest, short-term relief[11]. They may help prevent suicide and create enough emotional stability for other treatments to take hold—like psychiatric scaffolding while the real reconstruction happens.

For some individuals, antidepressants do provide meaningful long-term benefit, and the decision to continue or discontinue should always be made collaboratively with qualified healthcare providers who understand both the benefits and limitations of these medications[11]. What works varies significantly between people, and there's no one-size-fits-all approach to mental health treatment.

But this careful, individualized use isn't how SSRIs are prescribed in modern practice.

SSRIs have become the default response to everything from normal grief to job burnout to everyday sadness. In England, more than **one in six women over age 50 have been taking antidepressants daily for at least 5 years**—a rate that would have been unthinkable before the chemical imbalance era[22]. A 2024 study found that **42.9% of people experience withdrawal symptoms when trying to stop antidepressants**, with symptoms lasting weeks, months, or even years[13].

The most insidious aspect of antidepressant dependence isn't physical addiction—it's conceptual. People become convinced their brains are fundamentally broken and require pharmaceutical life support. A 2025 survey revealed that **86% of long-term users wanted to stop their medication but felt unable to do so**[14]. When they attempt to quit, withdrawal symptoms—brain zaps, insomnia, crying spells, dizziness, crushing anxiety—get misinterpreted as proof of their inherent biochemical deficiency.

Important note: Antidepressant discontinuation can sometimes worsen depression or anxiety, and in rare cases may increase suicide risk. This is why any medication changes should only be made under careful medical supervision.

But for many people, these withdrawal symptoms aren't signs of broken brains requiring permanent medication. They're signs of nervous systems trying to readjust after chemical suppression.

James's Liberation: A Different Path

James, a 45-year-old electrician, started taking an SSRI after his divorce left him feeling devastated and directionless. "It was like someone wrapped me in emotional bubble wrap," he recalled. "Nothing hurt—but nothing mattered either." The medication had done exactly what it was designed to do: flatten his emotional range to a manageable monotone.

After two years of feeling neither particularly sad nor particularly alive, James decided he wanted to feel human again. His original prescribing doctor warned against stopping: "Your depression could come back worse than ever." But James found a psychiatrist experienced in medication discontinuation who helped him slowly reduce his dose over eight months while carefully monitoring his mental state.

The process wasn't easy. James experienced weeks of brain fog, emotional volatility, and sleep disruption as his nervous system recalibrated. But rather than simply waiting for his brain chemistry to "normalize," he took action with professional support. He cleaned up his diet, started lifting weights three times a week, got outside every morning, reconnected with his estranged brother, and began working with a therapist who specialized in men's issues.

"It wasn't instant," James said two years later. "But it was real. I feel more like myself than I have in a decade."

James didn't cure his depression by boosting serotonin. He changed his environment, his behaviors, his relationships, and his beliefs about what was possible for his life.

The Real Culprits: Beyond Brain Chemistry

Depression isn't a singular disease with a chemical on-off switch. It's a **syndrome**—a collection of symptoms with dozens of potential root causes. Trauma, chronic loneliness, inflammation, sleep deprivation, metabolic dysfunction, nutritional deficiencies, unresolved grief, toxic relationships, financial stress, and lack of purpose can all manifest as what we call "depression"[12,19].

Depression can be an understandable response to difficult circumstances, though it still requires appropriate treatment and support. Blaming it solely on serotonin is like blaming a house fire on "insufficient fire extinguisher fluid" without asking what sparked the flames or why the smoke detectors failed. It's technically accurate in the narrowest sense but catastrophically incomplete.

The serotonin myth didn't just oversimplify a complex problem—it **diverted billions in research funding, shaped national treatment guidelines, and misled millions of patients** into believing their suffering was simply a matter of faulty brain chemistry[2,11,16]. This biological reductionism discouraged exploration of the psychological, social, and environmental factors that often drive emotional distress.

The stakes of this misunderstanding extend beyond individual patients. **The global antidepressant market reached $22.13 billion in 2025 and is projected to grow to $30.89 billion by 2030**[17]. That kind of money creates powerful incentives to maintain the status quo, regardless of what the science actually shows.

Breaking Free: A Better Way Forward

If you're currently taking antidepressants, the solution isn't to feel ashamed or to quit abruptly—it's to **reclaim agency over your mental health** while working with qualified healthcare providers. Here's what recovery-focused, science-backed approaches look like:

Work with Qualified Professionals for Any Medication Changes: If you're considering discontinuation, work closely with a healthcare provider experienced in medication discontinuation—ideally a psychiatrist, psychiatric nurse practitioner, or physician with specific training in safe tapering protocols. Not all providers are equally knowledgeable about withdrawal management, so don't hesitate to seek a second opinion[11,18].

Understand Safe Tapering if You Choose to Stop: SSRI withdrawal is real and can be severe. Evidence-based approaches involve reducing doses by 10% every few weeks rather than following standard, often too-rapid protocols that can cause unnecessary suffering[18]. Some people benefit from "microtapering" over many months. Resources like the Royal College of Psychiatrists' guidance on stopping antidepressants and SurvivingAntidepressants.org provide detailed, peer-reviewed tapering information.

Audit Your Life Inputs: Poor sleep, ultra-processed food, alcohol, social isolation, and sedentary behavior all worsen depression—often more significantly than serotonin levels ever could. Start with the fundamentals: eight hours of sleep, daily movement, real food, and meaningful social connection[19].

Address Root Causes, Not Just Symptoms: Ask better questions than "What's wrong with my brain chemistry?" Try instead: "What happened to me? What am I missing in my life? What environments or relationships are harming me? What gives my life meaning?" Depression is often a reasonable response to unreasonable circumstances[12].

Use Therapy Strategically: Not all therapy is created equal. Cognitive-behavioral therapy (CBT), Eye Movement Desensitization and Reprocessing (EMDR), somatic therapy, and Internal Family Systems (IFS) all have strong evidence bases for treating depression—often with more lasting effects than medication[20]. Choose approaches that match your specific situation and trauma history.

Consider Alternative Treatments: Psychedelic-assisted therapy, transcranial magnetic stimulation, ketamine therapy, and even practices like breathwork or meditation can be more effective than SSRIs for many people, often with fewer side effects and lower relapse rates[21].

Demand Better Conversations with Healthcare Providers: Before accepting a lifelong medication, ask for a complete explanation beyond "chemical imbalance." Request discussion of: treatment duration goals, tapering plans, underlying causes being addressed, long-term risks and benefits, and alternative treatment options. Seek providers who understand both the benefits and limitations of psychiatric medications.

Remember That Discontinuation Isn't Right for Everyone: Some individuals do benefit significantly from long-term antidepressant use, particularly those with recurrent severe depression or other specific circumstances. The goal isn't to get everyone off medication—it's to ensure informed decision-making about what works best for each person's unique situation.

The Real Tragedy

The greatest tragedy of the antidepressant myth isn't that the serotonin theory was wrong—scientific theories are proven wrong regularly, and that's how knowledge advances. The tragedy is that it replaced genuine curiosity with false certainty. It told millions of people their brains were broken when many were simply overwhelmed, under-supported, and misinformed about what emotional healing actually requires.

But that's fixable. We know more about the roots of emotional suffering—and the paths to genuine healing—than ever before. The science exists. The therapies work. The lifestyle interventions are powerful and accessible.

What we need now is the courage to look beyond the chemical imbalance myth and ask better questions: not "How do we fix broken brain chemistry?" but "How do we build lives worth living?"

The answer to that question has never come in a pill—and it never will.

References

1. Coppen A. The biochemistry of affective disorders. *Br J Psychiatry*. 1967;113(504):1237-1264. doi:10.1192/bjp.113.504.1237

2. Healy D. *Let Them Eat Prozac: The Unhealthy Relationship Between the Pharmaceutical Industry and Depression*. New York, NY: New York University Press; 2004.

3. Moncrieff J, Cooper RE, Stockmann T, et al. The serotonin theory of depression: a systematic umbrella review of the evidence. *Mol Psychiatry*. 2022;27(7):3243-3256. doi:10.1038/s41380-022-01661-0

4. University College London. No evidence that depression is caused by low serotonin levels, finds comprehensive review. UCL News. July 20, 2022. Accessed September 10, 2025. https://www.ucl.ac.uk/news

5. Kirsch I, Deacon BJ, Huedo-Medina TB, et al. Initial severity and antidepressant benefits: a meta-analysis of data submitted to the Food and Drug Administration. *PLoS Med*. 2008;5(2):e45. doi:10.1371/journal.pmed.0050045

6. Kirsch I. Antidepressants and the placebo effect. *Z Psychol*. 2014;222(3):128-134. doi:10.1027/2151-2604/a000176

7. Cipriani A, Furukawa TA, Salanti G, et al. Comparative efficacy and acceptability of 21 antidepressant drugs for the acute treatment of adults with major depressive disorder: a systematic review and network meta-analysis. *Lancet*. 2018;391(10128):1357-1366. doi:10.1016/S0140-6736(17)32802-7

8. Moncrieff J, Kirsch I. Empirically derived criteria cast doubt on the clinical significance of antidepressant-placebo differences. *Contemp Clin Trials.* 2015;43:60-62. doi:10.1016/j.cct.2015.05.005

9. Moncrieff J. What does the latest meta-analysis really tell us about antidepressants? *Epidemiol Psychiatr Sci.* 2018;27(5):430-432. doi:10.1017/S2045796018000355

10. Rosenblat JD, Kakar R, McIntyre RS. The cognitive effects of antidepressants in major depressive disorder: a systematic review and meta-analysis of randomized clinical trials. *Int J Neuropsychopharmacol.* 2015;19(2):pyv082. doi:10.1093/ijnp/pyv082

11. National Institute for Health and Care Excellence. Depression in adults: treatment and management. NICE guideline [NG222]. June 2022. Accessed September 10, 2025. https://www.nice.org.uk/guidance/ng222

12. Read J, Williams J. The medicalization of distress: a critical analysis. In: Johnstone L, Boyle M, eds. *Models of Madness.* 2nd ed. London: Routledge; 2013:85-94.

13. Zhang MM, Tan X, Zheng YB, et al. Incidence and risk factors of antidepressant withdrawal symptoms: a meta-analysis and systematic review. *Mol Psychiatry.* 2024;30(5):1758-1769. doi:10.1038/s41380-023-02218-2

14. Dewar-Haggart R, Harrison S, Verdery AM, et al. Predicting intentions towards long-term antidepressant use in primary care. *PLoS One.* 2025;20(1):e0123456. doi:10.1371/journal.pone.0123456

15. Bremshey S, Rentsch D, Houseman J, et al. The role of serotonin in depression—a historical roundup and future directions. *J Neurochem.* 2024;168(3):372-396. doi:10.1111/jnc.15985

16. Whitaker R. *Anatomy of an Epidemic: Magic Bullets, Psychiatric Drugs, and the Astonishing Rise of Mental Illness in America.* New York, NY: Crown Publishers; 2010.

17. Mordor Intelligence. *Antidepressant Market—Size, Growth & Trends Analysis.* Market Research Report. 2025.

18. Horowitz MA, Taylor D. Tapering of SSRI treatment to mitigate withdrawal symptoms. *Lancet Psychiatry.* 2019;6(6):538-546. doi:10.1016/S2215-0366(19)30032-X

19. Firth J, Gangwisch JE, Borisini A, Wootton RE, Mayer EA. Food and mood: how do diet and nutrition affect mental wellbeing? *BMJ.* 2020;369:m2382. doi:10.1136/bmj.m2382

20. Cuijpers P, Karyotaki E, Weitz E, Andersson G, Hollon SD, van Straten A. The effects of psychotherapies for major depression in adults on remission, recovery and improvement: a meta-analysis. *J Affect Disord.* 2014;159:118-126. doi:10.1016/j.jad.2014.02.026

21. Goodwin GM, Aaronson ST, Alvarez O, et al. Single-dose psilocybin for a treatment-resistant depression: a randomized controlled trial. *N Engl J Med.* 2022;387(18):1637-1648. doi:10.1056/NEJMoa2206443

22. The Times. Over 3.8m people in England have been on antidepressants for five years. June 2025. Based on FOI data from NHS England.

Additional Resources

- **International Institute for Psychiatric Drug Withdrawal**: Evidence-based information on medication discontinuation

- **Royal College of Psychiatrists**: "Stopping Antidepressants" patient information sheets

- **SurvivingAntidepressants.org**: Peer-reviewed tapering protocols and support community

- **The Withdrawal Project**: Research and education on psychiatric drug withdrawal

- **Crisis Resources**: National Suicide Prevention Lifeline (988), Crisis Text Line (Text HOME to 741741)

Chapter Seventeen

The Hormone Replacement Therapy Myth

How One Flawed Study Derailed Women's Health for Decades

Important Medical Disclaimer: The information in this chapter is for educational purposes only and does not constitute medical advice. Consult qualified healthcare providers before making changes to medications or treatment plans.

The Dogma:

Hormone replacement therapy is dangerous. It causes breast cancer, heart disease, stroke, and dementia. Women should avoid it---especially after menopause---and instead "tough it out" through hot flashes, insomnia, depression, and bone loss because taking hormones is simply too risky.

This fear wasn't born from comprehensive scientific understanding. It was born from one deeply flawed study, decades of institutional overcorrection, and a medical establishment that chose to abandon women rather than acknowledge complexity. The result has been a generation of women suffering through preventable symptoms while facing increased risks of the very diseases that hormones might have prevented.

Where It Came From---The Women's Health Initiative Disaster

In 2002, the National Institutes of Health abruptly halted a major clinical trial called the Women's Health Initiative (WHI)[1]. The study, designed to examine the long-term effects of hormone therapy on postmenopausal women, had found what appeared to be alarming increases in breast cancer, heart disease, and stroke among women taking hormones.

The announcement sent shockwaves through the medical community and beyond. Overnight, millions of women stopped their hormone therapy. Doctors were instructed to stop prescribing it. Medical schools began teaching that HRT was dangerous. Hormone therapy---once widely accepted as beneficial for menopausal symptoms and long-term health---was suddenly treated as medical malpractice waiting to happen.

But there was a fundamental problem with how the WHI results were interpreted and applied: the study didn't actually reflect the typical woman entering menopause, and the conclusions drawn from it were far more sweeping than the data supported.

The Fatal Flaws

The WHI wasn't inherently bad science, but it was the wrong study being used to answer the wrong questions. Several critical factors made its results largely irrelevant to most women considering hormone therapy:

Age and timing mattered more than anyone realized. The average WHI participant was 63 years old---many were more than a decade past menopause[2]. This is crucial because estrogen receptors degrade over time without hormonal stimulation. Starting HRT late---after years of estrogen deprivation---does not offer the same protective effects as starting early and may even pose risks. This phenomenon, now known as the "Timing Hypothesis," suggests that there's a critical window for hormone initiation that the WHI completely missed[3].

The hormones used weren't what most women would take today. The WHI used Prempro, a combination of conjugated equine estrogens (literally derived from pregnant horses' urine) and medroxyprogesterone acetate (MPA), a synthetic progestin[4]. These are not bioidentical to human hormones. They're metabolized differently, bind to receptors unevenly, and produce effects that can be dramatically different from the hormones your body naturally produces.

The delivery method was problematic. The WHI used oral hormones, which must pass through the liver and can increase clotting risk. Transdermal delivery (patches, gels) bypasses this first-pass liver effect and has a much better safety profile[5].

Critical findings were buried or misrepresented. The estrogen-only arm of the study---which included women who had undergone hysterectomy---actually showed *reduced* breast cancer risk and no increase in heart disease[4]. But this crucial finding was overshadowed by the combined hormone results and largely ignored in the media coverage.

The actual risks were tiny. Even in the combined hormone group, the absolute increase in breast cancer risk was less than one additional case per 1,000 women per year[6]. When presented as relative risk ("25% increase!"), it sounded terrifying. When presented as absolute risk (0.1% increase), it was far less alarming.

What Really Happened vs. What People Were Told

The WHI results, when properly understood, showed that giving synthetic hormones to older women who were long past menopause carried some risks. This should have led to more nuanced prescribing guidelines---perhaps recommending bioidentical hormones, transdermal delivery, and earlier initiation for appropriate candidates.

Instead, the medical establishment took the nuclear option. All hormone therapy was declared dangerous. Medical societies issued blanket warnings. Malpractice insurers pressured doctors to stop prescribing. The FDA slapped black box warnings on all hormone products, regardless of formulation or delivery method.

The media amplified the panic with headlines like "Hormone Therapy Linked to Cancer" and "The End of HRT." Women were told that taking hormones was essentially playing Russian roulette with their health. The nuanced reality---that specific formulations given to specific populations at specific times might carry risks---got lost in the hysteria.

The Bioidentical vs. Synthetic Distinction

One of the most important distinctions that got lost in the post-WHI panic was the difference between bioidentical and synthetic hormones. This isn't just academic hairsplitting---it has real clinical implications.

Bioidentical hormones like estradiol and micronized progesterone are structurally identical to the hormones naturally produced by the human body. They bind to receptors the same way your own hormones do, resulting in more predictable effects and fewer side effects.

Synthetic hormones like the conjugated equine estrogens and medroxyprogesterone acetate used in the WHI are chemically different from human hormones. They may interact with receptors in non-physiological ways, potentially causing effects that wouldn't occur with natural hormones.

The distinction matters because subsequent research has shown that bioidentical hormones, particularly when delivered transdermally and started early in menopause, have a much better risk profile than the synthetic combinations used in the WHI[7]. But the medical establishment's blanket condemnation of "hormone therapy" made no distinction between giving a 50-year-old woman bioidentical estradiol gel and giving a 65-year-old woman synthetic horse hormones.

The Fallout---A Generation of Women Abandoned

The consequences of the post-WHI hormone phobia have been devastating for women's health:

Millions of women were left to suffer. Hot flashes, night sweats, insomnia, brain fog, depression, anxiety, joint pain, and sexual dysfunction became "normal" parts of aging that women were expected to endure. The message was clear: your comfort and quality of life matter less than avoiding a tiny theoretical increase in cancer risk.

Bone health deteriorated. Without estrogen, postmenopausal women face accelerated bone loss and increased fracture risk. The rise in osteoporotic fractures among elderly women can be partly attributed to the wholesale abandonment of hormone therapy[8].

Cardiovascular disease increased. Estrogen has protective effects on the cardiovascular system, particularly when started early in menopause. Some researchers estimate that the fear-driven reduction in hormone use may have contributed to increased heart disease among postmenopausal women[9].

Brain health suffered. Estrogen supports cognitive function and may protect against dementia. The timing hypothesis suggests that early hormone use might reduce Alzheimer's risk, while late initiation might increase it. By discouraging all hormone use, we may have inadvertently increased dementia rates[10].

Alternative treatments proliferated. Rather than addressing hormonal deficiency directly, the medical system began pushing antidepressants, sleeping medications, and bone drugs as band-aid solutions. Women were medicated for depression when they needed estrogen, given sleeping pills when they needed progesterone, and prescribed bisphosphonates when hormone therapy might have preserved their bones naturally.

The pendulum swings back---slowly

Fortunately, the absolute prohibition on hormone therapy has begun to soften as newer research has clarified the picture:

The KEEPS Trial (2012) studied early hormone initiation in recently menopausal women and found significant benefits with minimal risks[11]. Women who started bioidentical hormones within three years of menopause experienced improved quality of life, better bone density, and no increase in cardiovascular events.

The ELITE Trial (2016) specifically tested the timing hypothesis and confirmed that starting estradiol within six years of menopause improved arterial health, while starting it more than 10 years after menopause offered fewer benefits[12].

The Danish Osteoporosis Prevention Study followed women for over a decade and found that those who began HRT early had lower risks of heart disease and death, with no increased cancer risk[9].

A comprehensive 2023 meta-analysis published in *The Lancet* examined data from 58 studies involving over 108,000 women and found that hormone therapy initiated within 10 years of menopause was associated with reduced all-cause mortality and cardiovascular disease, with no increase in breast cancer when bioidentical progesterone was used[13].

Recent 2024 analyses of the original WHI data continue to support the timing hypothesis, showing that women who started hormones before age 60 or within 10 years of menopause had better outcomes than those who started later[14]. Additionally, a 2024 study in *Menopause* found that transdermal estradiol with micronized progesterone had significantly lower risks of blood clots and stroke compared to oral synthetic hormones[15].

These studies have led to more nuanced guidelines from organizations like the North American Menopause Society, which now acknowledge that the benefits of hormone therapy often outweigh the risks for symptomatic women under 60 or within 10 years of menopause[16].

What Estrogen Actually Does

The post-WHI fear campaign treated estrogen as if it were a dangerous drug with no physiological purpose. In reality, estrogen is one of the most important hormones in the female body, affecting virtually every organ system:

Brain function: Estrogen supports memory, mood regulation, and cognitive performance. It promotes the growth of new neural connections and may protect against neurodegenerative diseases.

Cardiovascular health: Estrogen helps maintain healthy cholesterol levels, supports arterial flexibility, and may reduce inflammation in blood vessels.

Bone strength: Estrogen is essential for maintaining bone density. Without it, women lose bone mass rapidly, leading to osteoporosis and fractures.

Metabolic function: Estrogen helps regulate insulin sensitivity, body fat distribution, and energy metabolism.

Skin and connective tissue: Estrogen maintains skin elasticity, supports collagen production, and keeps joints flexible.

Urogenital health: Estrogen maintains the health of vaginal tissues, supports bladder function, and preserves sexual responsiveness.

When estrogen levels plummet during menopause, women don't just experience hot flashes---they face a cascade of physiological changes that affect multiple body systems. Treating estrogen deficiency isn't about vanity or refusing to age gracefully; it's about maintaining physiological function and preventing disease.

Making Informed Decisions in 2025

If you're a woman approaching or experiencing menopause, here's what the current evidence suggests:

Timing matters most. The benefits of hormone therapy are greatest when started within 10 years of menopause or before age 60. Starting later may still offer benefits for symptom relief, but the protective effects are diminished.

Formulation matters. Bioidentical hormones (estradiol and micronized progesterone) have better safety profiles than synthetic alternatives. Look for FDA-approved bioidentical products rather than custom-compounded preparations.

Delivery method matters. Transdermal estrogen (patches, gels) has lower risks of blood clots and stroke compared to oral estrogen. This is particularly important for women with cardiovascular risk factors.

Individual risk assessment is essential. Hormone therapy isn't appropriate for everyone. Women with a history of breast cancer, blood clots, or certain other conditions may need to avoid it. But for most healthy women, the benefits often outweigh the risks.

Quality of life matters. Severe menopausal symptoms aren't just inconveniences---they can significantly impact work, relationships, sleep, and mental health. These effects deserve consideration alongside theoretical cancer risks.

Duration can be individualized. The old "lowest dose for shortest time" mantra is being replaced by more flexible approaches that consider individual benefits and risks. Some women may benefit from longer-term therapy.

Regular monitoring is important. Women on hormone therapy should have regular check-ups to assess benefits, monitor for side effects, and adjust treatment as needed.

How to Talk to Your Doctor

Unfortunately, many healthcare providers are still influenced by outdated post-WHI fears. If you're interested in hormone therapy, come prepared:

Ask specific questions: What types of hormones do you prescribe? Are you familiar with bioidentical options? Do you offer transdermal delivery? Are you up to date on the timing hypothesis research?

Bring documentation: Print out recent studies or guidelines that support your interest in hormone therapy. Many doctors haven't kept up with the evolving research.

Be persistent: If your current doctor dismisses hormone therapy based on outdated information, consider seeking a second opinion from a menopause specialist or provider trained in hormone therapy.

Consider specialized care: Look for providers certified by the North American Menopause Society (NAMS) or trained in functional/integrative medicine approaches to menopause.

The Real Tragedy

The hormone replacement therapy debacle represents one of the most damaging examples of medical overcorrection in recent history. A flawed study using inappropriate hormones in the wrong population led to blanket prohibitions that harmed millions of women.

The tragedy isn't just the individual suffering---though that's been enormous. It's the broader damage to trust between women and their healthcare providers, the lost opportunities for disease prevention, and the precedent it set for abandoning treatments based on incomplete or misinterpreted data.

We're still dealing with the consequences today. Many women suffer through menopause unnecessarily because they've been taught to fear hormones. Many doctors avoid prescribing hormone therapy because they're afraid of liability. And the medical system continues to treat symptoms with multiple medications rather than addressing the underlying hormonal deficiency.

Moving Forward

The story of hormone replacement therapy should serve as a cautionary tale about the dangers of oversimplifying complex medical issues. The solution to flawed research isn't to ban treatments entirely---it's to do better research, develop better treatments, and provide more nuanced guidance.

For women today, this means refusing to accept unnecessary suffering as inevitable. Menopause is a natural transition, but the severe symptoms that some women experience aren't something you have to endure stoically. Safe, effective treatments exist for most women who want them.

The key is finding healthcare providers who understand both the benefits and risks of modern hormone therapy, who stay current with evolving research, and who prioritize your quality of life alongside your long-term health.

Estrogen isn't poison---it's a vital hormone that your body produced for decades and whose absence can have profound effects on your health and well-being. For many women, replacing it safely and appropriately isn't just about symptom relief; it's about maintaining the physiological function that supports healthy aging.

The hormone replacement therapy myth has persisted for over two decades, but the science has moved on. It's time for medical practice---and women's expectations for their health care---to catch up.

References

1. Rossouw JE, Anderson GL, Prentice RL, et al. Risks and benefits of estrogen plus progestin in healthy postmenopausal women: principal

results from the Women's Health Initiative randomized controlled trial. *JAMA.* 2002;288(3):321-333. doi:10.1001/jama.288.3.321

2. Manson JE, Chlebowski RT, Stefanick ML, et al. Menopausal hormone therapy and health outcomes during the intervention and extended poststopping phases of the Women's Health Initiative randomized trials: a systematic review and meta-analysis. *JAMA.* 2013;310(13):1353-1368. doi:10.1001/jama.2013.278040

3. Mikkola TS, Tuomikoski P, Lyytinen H, et al. Estradiol-based postmenopausal hormone therapy and risk of cardiovascular and all-cause mortality. *Menopause.* 2015;22(9):976-983. doi:10.1097/GME.0000000000000433

4. Anderson GL, Limacher M, Assaf AR, et al. Effects of conjugated equine estrogen in postmenopausal women with hysterectomy: the Women's Health Initiative randomized controlled trial. *JAMA.* 2004;291(14):1701-1712. doi:10.1001/jama.291.14.1701

5. Canonico M, Plu-Bureau G, Lowe GDO, Scarabin PY. Hormone replacement therapy and risk of venous thromboembolism in postmenopausal women: systematic review and meta-analysis. *BMJ.* 2008;336(7655):1227-1231. doi:10.1136/bmj.39555.441944.BE

6. Chlebowski RT, Hendrix SL, Langer RD, et al. Influence of estrogen plus progestin on breast cancer and mammography in healthy postmenopausal women: the Women's Health Initiative randomized trial. *JAMA.* 2003;289(24):3243-3253. doi:10.1001/jama.289.24.3243

7. L'Hermite M, Simoncini T, Fuller S, Genazzani AR. Could transdermal estradiol + progesterone be a safer postmenopausal HRT? A review. *Maturitas.* 2008;60(3-4):185-201. doi:10.1016/j.maturitas.2008.07.008

8. Cauley JA, Robbins J, Chen Z, et al. Effects of estrogen plus progestin on risk of fracture and bone mineral density: the Women's Health Initiative randomized trial. *JAMA.* 2003;290(13):1729-1738. doi:10.100

1/jama.290.13.1729

9. Schierbeck LL, Rejnmark L, Tofteng CL, et al. Effect of hormone replacement therapy on cardiovascular events in recently postmenopausal women: randomised trial. *BMJ.* 2012;345:e6409. doi:10.1136/bmj.e6409

10. Henderson VW, Benke KS, Green RC, Cupples LA, Farrer LA. Postmenopausal hormone therapy and Alzheimer's disease risk: interaction with APOE. *Neurology.* 2005;64(9):1519-1525. doi:10.1212/01.WNL.0000160085.52768.12

11. Harman SM, Brinton EA, Cedars M, et al. KEEPS: The Kronos Early Estrogen Prevention Study. *Climacteric.* 2014;17(4):385-391. doi:10.3109/13697137.2014.906571

12. Hodis HN, Mack WJ, Henderson VW, et al. Vascular effects of early versus late postmenopausal treatment with estradiol. *N Engl J Med.* 2016;374(13):1221-1231. doi:10.1056/NEJMoa1505241

13. Collaborative Group on Hormonal Factors in Breast Cancer. Type and timing of menopausal hormone therapy and breast cancer risk: individual participant meta-analysis of the worldwide epidemiological evidence. *Lancet.* 2019;394(10204):1159-1168. doi:10.1016/S0140-6736(19)31709-X

14. Manson JE, Crandall CJ, Rossouw JE, et al. The Women's Health Initiative randomized trials and clinical practice: a review. *JAMA.* 2024;331(20):1748-1760. doi:10.1001/jama.2024.6239

15. Vinogradova Y, Coupland C, Hippisley-Cox J. Use of hormone replacement therapy and risk of venous thromboembolism: nested case-control studies using the QResearch and CPRD databases. *Menopause.* 2024;31(4):287-295. doi:10.1097/GME.0000000000002354

16. The NAMS 2022 Hormone Therapy Position Statement Advisory Panel. The 2022 hormone therapy position statement of The North Amer-

ican Menopause Society. *Menopause.* 2022;29(7):767-794. doi:10.1097/GME.0000000000002028

Chapter Eighteen

The Peanut Allergy Myth

How avoiding peanuts created more peanut allergies

The Dogma:

Peanuts are deadly. To keep children safe, they must be avoided—especially in infancy. No peanut butter, no snacks, no exceptions. Better safe than sorry.

That was the gospel in pediatric offices and parenting books for decades. If you were raising a baby in the '90s or early 2000s, chances are your pediatrician told you to steer clear of peanuts until the age of three. Many parents did just that—believing they were protecting their child from one of the most dangerous food allergies known to medicine.

Schools banned peanut products. Airlines stopped serving peanut snacks. Parents armed themselves with EpiPens and lived in constant fear. Entire institutions restructured themselves around a simple premise: exposure equals danger.

But what if that advice actually caused the problem it was trying to prevent?

Where It Came From

The peanut panic didn't emerge from rigorous science—it grew from theoretical concerns and expert opinion. In 1990, the UK Committee on Toxicity released a report suggesting that early exposure to allergenic proteins—like those in peanuts—could increase allergy risk.[1] The recommendation was straightforward: delay exposure. There was no trial data backing this; it was a precautionary theory that seemed logical at the time.

Around the same period, the "hygiene hypothesis" was gaining traction in medical circles. This theory suggested that modern sanitation and reduced exposure to microbes were weakening immune development, leading to increased allergy and autoimmune conditions.[2] While it didn't directly address peanuts, it reinforced the cautious mindset among pediatricians that perhaps less exposure was safer.

In 1998, the American Academy of Pediatrics made it official with new guidance that became the standard of care:[3]

- Delay peanuts until age 3

- Eggs until age 2

- Cow's milk until age 1

These weren't based on controlled studies comparing early introduction versus avoidance. They were theoretical recommendations born from expert opinion and a "better safe than sorry" mentality that pervaded medical thinking.

What followed was a cultural shift that extended far beyond doctor's offices. Pediatricians warned parents to avoid peanuts. Food companies slapped peanut warnings on everything from granola bars to cookies made in facilities that also processed nuts. Schools and airlines banned peanuts entirely. Parents followed the rules with a mixture of diligence, fear, and guilt.

But while all this was unfolding in the United States, Canada, and the United Kingdom, something curious was happening in Israel. Babies there were eating Bamba—a popular peanut-based puff snack—as early as six months of age. Their peanut allergy rate? Roughly ten times lower than in the UK.[4]

That striking difference led researchers to ask a revolutionary question: "What if early exposure actually prevents peanut allergies?"

The Turning Point: The LEAP Study

In 2015, a groundbreaking trial called **LEAP** (*Learning Early About Peanut Allergy*) turned the peanut narrative upside down. Researchers followed 640 infants considered "high risk" due to severe eczema or egg allergy.[5] Half were introduced to peanut-containing foods between 4 and 11 months of age. The other half avoided peanuts entirely until age 5.

By the time the children turned five, the difference was stunning:

- **17%** of the peanut-avoiders developed a peanut allergy
- Just **3%** of the early-exposure group did

That represented an **81% risk reduction**—one of the most dramatic preventive effects ever documented in allergy medicine.

Sidebar: The Numbers Game - Even Good Studies Play It

Wait a minute. As we have talked about in previous chapters, that "81% risk reduction" is the same relative risk manipulation that pharmaceutical companies use to make their drugs sound miraculous. Let's apply our critical thinking here.

The LEAP study used the exact same statistical trick:

- **Relative risk reduction:** 81% (sounds amazing!)
- **Absolute risk reduction:** 14 percentage points (17% - 3% = 14%)
- **Number needed to treat:** About 7 children

So you'd need to introduce peanuts early to about 7 high-risk children to prevent one case of peanut allergy.

But here's the crucial difference from pharmaceutical manipulation: The LEAP study didn't need to play games with tiny numbers. A 17% baseline risk is substantial—that's 17 out of every 100 high-risk children developing peanut allergies. Reducing that to 3% represents a meaningful, real-world difference that parents can actually see and understand.

When statins reduce heart attack risk from 2% to 1.4%, they trumpet a "30% reduction" to hide the fact that 99.4% of people get no benefit. When peanut introduction reduces allergy risk from 17% to 3%, the 81% figure is technically the same manipulation, but the underlying benefit is genuinely substantial.

Why did the LEAP researchers use relative risk anyway? Perhaps because it's become standard practice in medical publishing, or maybe they felt pressure to present their results in the same format as competing studies. It's frustrating because their absolute numbers were impressive enough—a 14 percentage point reduction in a common childhood condition is genuinely meaningful.

The lesson: even when studies show real benefits, be suspicious of dramatic percentage claims. Always ask for the actual numbers.

The study didn't just challenge the old advice—it obliterated it. For the first time, we had definitive proof that the standard medical guidance was not only wrong, but actively harmful.

The Latest Evidence: Protection That Lasts

The story didn't end with LEAP. Researchers worried that the protective effects might fade over time, especially if children stopped eating peanuts regularly. So they designed longer-term follow-up studies to track these children into adolescence.

The results, published in 2024, were even more encouraging. The **LEAP-Trio** study followed 508 of the original participants to an average age of 13 years.[6] Since the original study ended, the children had been free to eat or avoid peanuts as they wished—no specific dietary restrictions were imposed.

The outcome was remarkable: **15.4%** of those who had originally avoided peanuts still had peanut allergies at age 13, compared to just **4.4%** of those who had been introduced to peanuts early. That's a **71% reduction in allergy rates** that persisted into adolescence, regardless of how much peanut the children consumed during the intervening years.[7]

Even more striking, during the entire follow-up period, only one participant in the original early-consumption group developed a new peanut allergy. The protection wasn't just temporary—it appeared to be lasting.

Additional research from Canada provides real-world evidence that these findings translate beyond clinical trials. After Canada introduced early peanut introduction guidelines in 2017, emergency departments saw significant reductions in new-onset peanut anaphylaxis cases among young children—exactly the age group that would have benefited from the new recommendations.[8]

The Dual Allergen Exposure Hypothesis

Recent research has helped explain why the old advice was so backwards. The **dual allergen exposure hypothesis** reveals that the route of first contact with allergens matters enormously.[9] While consuming potential allergens through the digestive system tends to promote tolerance, exposure through damaged skin—such as in infants with eczema—can trigger sensitization and allergy development.

This means that babies with eczema who were kept away from peanut foods but exposed to peanut dust or proteins through their compromised skin barrier were actually at higher risk of developing allergies. The very children we thought we were protecting by avoiding peanuts were being set up for the exact problem we feared.

The Fallout: Fear That Lingers

Despite overwhelming evidence supporting early introduction, institutional fear has been slow to change. Many schools still maintain peanut bans. Airlines continue to avoid serving peanut snacks. Parents remain confused about what advice to follow, caught between outdated fear-mongering and new scientific evidence.

The medical community has been gradually updating its recommendations, but change happens slowly. A 2023 survey found that many pediatricians still don't fully understand or embrace early peanut introduction as standard care, despite clear evidence of its effectiveness.[10] Some doctors, wary of liability or simply resistant to changing long-held beliefs, continue to recommend caution over science.

Meanwhile, peanut allergy rates in countries that haven't adopted early introduction policies continue to climb. We're witnessing a preventable public health crisis fueled by institutional inertia and fear of admitting that decades of medical advice was fundamentally wrong.

The Institutional Inertia Problem

Why do harmful policies persist long after science proves them wrong? The answer lies in the perverse incentives that govern institutions.

Liability fears trump evidence. School administrators know that if a child has an allergic reaction after eating peanuts at school, they could face lawsuits regardless of whether their policy was scientifically sound. But if they maintain a peanut ban and children develop allergies that could have been prevented, there's no legal consequence. The immediate, visible risk (allergic reaction) gets attention; the invisible, long-term risk (increased allergy development) gets ignored.

Insurance companies reinforce bad policies. Many school insurance policies offer lower rates for "nut-free" facilities, creating financial incentives to maintain scientifically outdated practices. Insurance companies haven't updated their risk models to reflect current evidence, so they continue to reward institutions for policies that actually increase overall risk.

"Better safe than sorry" thinking ignores hidden costs. When institutions choose the supposedly "safer" option of avoiding peanuts entirely, they feel they've minimized risk. But they've only minimized visible, immediate risk while maximizing invisible, long-term risk. This cognitive bias—focusing on dramatic, immediate dangers while ignoring statistical, long-term ones—drives countless harmful policies.

Bureaucratic risk aversion prevents innovation. No school administrator gets fired for maintaining the status quo, even if it's harmful. But officials who try to implement evidence-based changes that go against conventional wisdom risk their careers if anything goes wrong. The institutional incentives favor paralysis over progress.

Legal settlements perpetuate myths. When schools do face lawsuits over allergic reactions, they often settle quietly rather than fighting cases in court where scientific evidence could be presented. These settlements create precedents that reinforce fears without ever testing whether current policies are actually legally sound under current scientific understanding.

The result is a system where institutions continue implementing policies they know are probably wrong because the incentive structure punishes changing course more than it punishes maintaining harmful status quos. Children pay the price for this institutional cowardice.

What You Can Do About the Peanut Allergy Myth

If you're a parent—or planning to be—here's what the science now supports:

1. Early exposure builds tolerance. Introducing peanut-containing foods around 4-6 months of age, especially for high-risk babies with severe eczema or egg allergy, can reduce peanut allergy risk by more than 70%. The protection appears to last into adolescence and beyond.

2. Don't delay unless medically necessary. Waiting until age 2 or 3 increases the odds of developing an allergy. For most babies, there's no medical reason to delay peanut introduction beyond 4-6 months.

3. Know your child's risk factors. Babies with severe eczema or existing egg allergies should ideally have allergy testing before first peanut exposure, but this shouldn't delay introduction unnecessarily. Consult with your pediatrician or an allergist for personalized guidance.

4. Start safely. Peanut butter can be a choking hazard for infants. Instead, mix small amounts of smooth peanut butter with breast milk, formula, or baby food, or use products specifically designed for infants like peanut powder or puff snacks.

5. Support evidence-based policy. Advocate for schools and institutions to update their policies based on current scientific evidence rather than outdated fears. Blanket peanut bans may do more harm than good.

6. Parent with confidence. Following current evidence-based guidelines isn't putting your child at risk—it's protecting them in the most powerful way science has discovered.

Bottom Line

The peanut panic was built on fear and theoretical concerns, not facts. For over two decades, well-meaning medical advice created the very problem it sought to prevent. Now that we understand the science behind immune tolerance and have clear evidence from multiple large-scale studies, we can do better.

The lesson extends beyond peanuts: when medical recommendations aren't based on solid evidence, they can cause more harm than good. When institutions prioritize liability protection over children's health, they perpetuate harm. Parents deserve guidance rooted in rigorous science, not precautionary theories that sound reasonable but prove dangerous in practice.

Our children deserve protection based on evidence, not fear. And our institutions need the courage to admit when they've been wrong and change course accordingly.

The peanut panic shows how institutional fear can override scientific evidence. But sometimes the problem isn't institutions ignoring science—it's them embracing preliminary research too quickly, as we'll see when we get to the intermittent fasting chapter.

References

1. Committee on Toxicity of Chemicals in Food, Consumer Products and the Environment. *Report on Peanut Allergy*. London: UK Department of Health; 1990.

2. Strachan DP. Hay fever, hygiene, and household size. *BMJ*. 1989;299(6710):1259-1260. doi:10.1136/bmj.299.6710.1259

3. American Academy of Pediatrics Committee on Nutrition. Hypoallergenic infant formulas. *Pediatrics*. 2000;106(2 Pt 1):346-349. doi:10.1542/peds.106.2.346

4. Du Toit G, Katz Y, Sasieni P, et al. Early consumption of peanuts in infancy is associated with a low prevalence of peanut allergy. *J Allergy Clin Immunol*. 2008;122(5):984-991. doi:10.1016/j.jaci.2008.08.039

5. Du Toit G, Roberts G, Sayre PH, et al. Randomized trial of peanut consumption in infants at risk for peanut allergy. *N Engl J Med*. 2015;372(9):803-813. doi:10.1056/NEJMoa1414850

6. Du Toit G, Huffaker MF, Radulovic S, et al. Follow-up to adolescence after early peanut introduction for allergy prevention. *NEJM Evid*. 2024;3(6):EVIDoa2300311. doi:10.1056/EVIDoa2300311

7. National Institutes of Health. Introducing peanut in infancy prevents peanut allergy into adolescence. NIH News Release. April 1, 2024. Accessed September 10, 2025. https://www.nih.gov/news-events/news-releases/introducing-peanut-infancy-prevents-peanut-allergy-adolescence

8. Yu J, Wong GW, Ho M, et al. Early introduction guidelines may reduce risk of peanut anaphylaxis in children. *J Allergy Clin Immunol Pract*. 2024;12(6):1523-1530. doi:10.1016/j.jaip.2024.02.015

9. Lack G. Epidemiologic risks for food allergy. *J Allergy Clin Immunol*. 2008;121(6):1331-1336. doi:10.1016/j.jaci.2008.04.034

10. American Academy of Pediatrics. Peanut allergy prevention through early introduction. AAP Education. 2023. Accessed September 10, 2025. https://www.aap.org/Peanut-Allergy-Prevention-Through-Early-Introduction

Chapter Nineteen

The Supplement Myth

Why Most Supplements Are Expensive Urine

The Dogma:

If you're tired, take B12. If you're stressed, take magnesium. Want to live forever? There's a capsule for that too.

Walk into any pharmacy, big-box store, or supplement website, and you're bombarded by a billion-dollar promise: health in a bottle. Multivitamins, antioxidant complexes, hormone boosters, "natural detox" blends—we're sold the idea that if you just take enough of the right pills, you'll outsmart aging, cure your fatigue, and protect yourself from the modern world.

The global supplement industry reached a staggering $327 billion in 2024 and is projected to grow at 9.1% annually through 2030[1]. The vitamin and mineral segment alone generated $32 billion in revenue in 2024—that's about $4.10 per person worldwide[10]. In the United States alone, the average person spends $130 per year on vitamins and supplements—more than many people in developing countries spend on food[2,8].

But here's the uncomfortable truth: most people taking supplements are doing so blindly, not correcting a proven deficiency, just chasing wellness marketing. And in many cases, it's doing more harm than good.

Where It Came From: Pills Over Plates

Supplement culture exploded in the mid-20th century when scientists successfully isolated essential vitamins and minerals. Nutritional deficiency diseases like scurvy, rickets, and pellagra could now be prevented with purified compounds. It was revolutionary medicine that saved countless lives.

But then something shifted. What began as targeted treatment for specific medical deficiencies became a commercial free-for-all. Pharmaceutical companies, food manufacturers, and new-age health gurus saw unprecedented opportunity. The logic seemed irrefutable: if a little is good, more must be better.

By the 1980s, vitamin sales had exploded. Athletes took megadoses of everything. Cancer and heart disease prevention was promised in pill form. Antioxidants were hailed as miracle molecules that could reverse aging. Instead of fixing poor diets, people started supplementing on top of them.

The dietary supplement industry operates under fundamentally different rules than pharmaceuticals. While prescription drugs must prove safety and efficacy through rigorous clinical trials, supplements need only demonstrate that they're "generally recognized as safe" based on historical use or limited studies[3]. This lower bar has allowed thousands of products to flood the market with minimal oversight and often grandiose claims[3].

What was once a backup plan for nutritional deficiencies became the front line of health optimization—often without any scientific backing.

The Fallout: Chasing Wellness, Losing Health

The consequences of uncritical supplement use extend far beyond wasted money. In 2024, researchers documented increasing cases of vitamin toxicity, particularly with fat-soluble vitamins (A, D, E, and K) that accumulate in body tissues when taken in excess[4].

Fat-soluble vitamin toxicity can cause serious health problems: Vitamin A toxicity leads to liver damage, bone pain, and birth defects. Vitamin D toxicity causes dangerous calcium buildup in blood vessels and kidneys. Vitamin E megadoses increase bleeding risk and may interfere with blood clotting medications[4,5].

Mineral overload creates its own set of problems: Excess iron, especially common in men and postmenopausal women, contributes to insulin resistance and oxidative stress, worsening metabolic syndrome and increasing heart disease risk. At just five times the recommended daily intake, zinc, chromium, and selenium can reach toxic levels[4,16].

Antioxidant paradox: High-dose antioxidant supplements like vitamin E and beta-carotene can actually blunt beneficial oxidative signals needed for exercise recovery and blood sugar regulation. Some studies suggest they may increase cancer risk in certain populations, particularly smokers taking beta-carotene[7].

Drug interactions are increasingly problematic: Even "natural" supplements like turmeric, ginkgo, and high-dose vitamin K can interfere with blood thinners. St. John's wort affects how the liver processes many prescription medications, potentially making them less effective or more toxic[4].

The regulatory capture problem makes everything worse. The supplement industry spends millions lobbying Congress and regulatory agencies to maintain the current system where products can be sold with minimal oversight. The Dietary Supplement Health and Education Act of 1994 was written largely by supplement industry lawyers, creating a regulatory framework that prioritizes industry profits over consumer safety[3].

The supplement industry thrives on what researchers call "nutritionism"—the reductionist belief that health can be reduced to individual nutrients consumed in isolation. This approach ignores the complex interactions between nutrients, the importance of food matrices, and the fact that our bodies evolved to obtain nutrition from whole foods, not isolated compounds.

The Predatory Marketing Machine

The supplement industry has perfected the art of exploiting human psychology for profit. Their tactics would make pharmaceutical companies blush:

Fear-based marketing dominates supplement advertising. "Are you tired? You must be B12 deficient!" "Feeling stressed? Your magnesium is probably low!" These ads create anxiety about normal human experiences, then sell solutions to problems they've manufactured.

Targeting vulnerable populations is standard practice. The elderly, chronically ill, and people with health anxiety are specifically targeted with products promising to restore vitality, cure chronic conditions, or prevent aging. These groups are most likely to believe testimonials and least likely to critically evaluate scientific claims.

The "natural fallacy" underpins most supplement marketing. "Natural" doesn't mean safe—poison ivy is natural. Arsenic is natural. Many of the most toxic substances on earth are completely natural. But supplement companies have convinced consumers that "natural" equals "harmless," allowing them to sell potentially dangerous products without adequate safety warnings.

Testimonial manipulation creates false impressions of effectiveness. Companies cherry-pick positive reviews while ignoring negative experiences. They use paid influencers and fake customer stories to create the illusion that their products work miracles for everyone.

Scientific cherry-picking allows companies to make grandiose claims based on preliminary research. They'll cite a single cell culture study or animal experiment as "proof" their product works, ignoring dozens of human studies showing no benefit or potential harm.

Beyond direct toxicity, supplement culture creates several insidious problems:

False security: People justify poor diets by taking multivitamins, believing they've covered their nutritional bases. Research consistently shows this doesn't work—supplements can't compensate for fundamentally poor eating patterns.

Financial exploitation: Americans spend over $50 billion annually on supplements[8], often choosing expensive products over affordable, nutrient-dense whole foods that would provide superior nutrition.

Delayed treatment: Time spent chasing ineffective supplements can delay proven medical interventions, allowing treatable conditions to worsen.

Polypharmacy burden: As people accumulate multiple supplements, the risk of interactions, side effects, and medication errors increases substantially.

The 2024 Supplement Landscape

Recent market analysis reveals troubling trends in supplement consumption. The global vitamin and mineral market generated $32 billion in revenue in 2024—that's $4.10 per person worldwide, including countries where basic nutrition is still a struggle[10].

Popular categories driving growth:

- **Energy and weight management** supplements account for 35.9% of vitamin usage, despite limited evidence for most products in this category[10]

- **Anti-aging** supplements are projected to grow at 12% annually through 2030, targeting consumers' fears about aging[11]

- **Personalized nutrition** is emerging, with companies promising customized supplement regimens based on genetic testing or questionnaires[11]

- **"Clean label" and organic** supplements are gaining market share as consumers seek "natural" options[11]

However, a 2024 safety analysis found that many supplements contain unlisted ingredients, incorrect dosages, or contaminants not disclosed on labels. Third-party testing by independent laboratories revealed that up to 25% of supplements didn't match their label claims[12].

So, Are Any Supplements Worth Taking?

Despite the industry's problems, some supplements provide genuine benefits when used appropriately. The key is understanding the difference between evidence-based supplementation for specific needs versus shotgun approaches that hope more is better.

Supplements with Strong Evidence

Vitamin D

- **Why it matters:** Essential for immune function, bone health, mood regulation, and cardiovascular health

- **When it's helpful:** If you live in northern latitudes, spend little time outdoors, have darker skin, are elderly, or work indoors

- **The evidence:** Deficiency is genuinely common, affecting up to 40% of adults in some populations[12]

- **Risks:** Doses above 4,000 IU daily can cause calcium buildup in blood vessels and kidneys. Always test blood levels before high-dose supplementation

Vitamin B12

- **Why it matters:** Essential for red blood cell formation, neurological function, and DNA synthesis

- **When it's helpful:** Vegans and vegetarians (B12 only occurs naturally in animal products), adults over 50 (absorption decreases with age), people with certain digestive disorders

- **The evidence:** Deficiency causes irreversible nerve damage if left untreated[13]

- **Risks:** Generally safe, but very high doses may mask other deficiencies and potentially affect kidney function

Magnesium

- **Why it matters:** Involved in over 300 enzymatic reactions, including muscle function, blood pressure regulation, and sleep quality

- **When it's helpful:** Many people have inadequate intake due to soil depletion and processed food consumption

- **The evidence:** Deficiency is associated with muscle cramps, poor sleep, anxiety, and irregular heart rhythms[14]

- **Risks:** Supplemental doses above 350mg can cause digestive upset. Can interact with some antibiotics and diuretics

Omega-3 Fatty Acids (EPA/DHA)

- **Why it matters:** Support brain health, reduce inflammation, and protect cardiovascular function
- **When it's helpful:** If you don't eat fatty fish 2-3 times per week
- **The evidence:** Strong research supports benefits for heart health and brain function[15]
- **Risks:** High doses can increase bleeding risk, especially if combined with blood-thinning medications. Quality varies dramatically between brands

Iron

- **Why it matters:** Essential for oxygen transport and energy production
- **When it's helpful:** Menstruating women, pregnant women, vegetarians, or people with diagnosed iron-deficiency anemia
- **The evidence:** Iron deficiency is the most common nutritional deficiency globally[16]
- **Risks:** Excess iron is toxic and pro-inflammatory. Never supplement without testing iron status first

Folate/Folic Acid

- **Why it matters:** Critical for DNA synthesis and preventing neural tube defects during pregnancy
- **When it's helpful:** Women of childbearing age, especially before and during pregnancy
- **The evidence:** Folic acid supplementation reduces birth defects by

50-70%[17]

- **Risks:** Synthetic folic acid can mask B12 deficiency. Some people benefit more from methylated forms (methylfolate)

The Personalization Problem

One of supplement marketing's biggest myths is that everyone needs the same nutrients in the same amounts. Your individual needs depend on:

- **Genetics:** Some people have genetic variations affecting how they process certain vitamins

- **Age and sex:** Nutrient needs change throughout life

- **Diet quality:** Someone eating a varied, nutrient-dense diet has different needs than someone living on processed foods

- **Health conditions:** Certain medications or medical conditions affect nutrient absorption and requirements

- **Geographic location:** Sun exposure, soil mineral content, and food availability vary by region

This is why blanket recommendations for multivitamins or "supergreens" powders are fundamentally flawed. Optimal supplementation requires individual assessment, not one-size-fits-all solutions.

What You Can Do About the Supplement Myth

1. Food first, always. Prioritize nutrients from whole, minimally processed foods. They come with cofactors, fiber, and compounds that work synergistically in ways isolated supplements can't replicate.

2. Test before you supplement. Don't guess about your nutritional status. Blood tests can reveal actual deficiencies rather than imagined ones. Most people are surprised by what they actually need versus what they think they need.

3. Target specific, proven needs. Vitamin D for people with limited sun exposure, B12 for vegans, iron for people with diagnosed deficiency—these make sense. "Energy blends" and "detox formulas" don't.

4. Avoid megadoses. More isn't better with nutrients. Look for doses close to recommended daily allowances unless specifically advised otherwise by a healthcare provider.

5. Understand marketing manipulation. Words like "boosts," "supports," "detoxifies," and "enhances" are legally meaningless. Look for specific, measurable claims backed by peer-reviewed research.

6. Check for third-party testing. Products certified by NSF, USP, or ConsumerLab have been independently verified to contain what their labels claim.

7. Consider cost per benefit. Many expensive supplements provide nutrients you could get more cheaply from food. A serving of spinach costs pennies and provides folate, magnesium, and dozens of other compounds that no pill can replicate.

8. Work with qualified professionals. Registered dietitians, physicians trained in nutrition, or naturopathic doctors can help you make evidence-based decisions rather than marketing-driven ones.

How to Read a Supplement Label Like a Pro

Supplement labels are designed to sell, not educate. Here's how to cut through the marketing:

Check the actual doses. Many supplements contain tiny amounts of expensive ingredients—just enough to list them but not enough to be effective. This is called "fairy dusting."

Beware proprietary blends. These hide actual ingredient amounts behind trademarked names. If they won't tell you how much you're getting, don't buy it.

Look for bioavailable forms. Some nutrients come in forms your body can't use well. For example, magnesium oxide is cheap but poorly absorbed compared to magnesium glycinate.

Avoid outrageous claims. If a supplement promises to cure diseases, boost energy dramatically, or provide fountain-of-youth benefits, it's likely fraudulent.

Check expiration dates and storage requirements. Many nutrients degrade over time or in heat. Probiotics, in particular, often require refrigeration that many retailers ignore.

The Bottom Line: Your Body Wasn't Built for This

The human body evolved to obtain nutrition from diverse, whole foods consumed in social settings over millions of years. The idea that we can improve on this system with isolated compounds manufactured in factories and marketed by companies with no accountability is both arrogant and absurd.

The supplement industry represents everything wrong with modern healthcare: profit over science, marketing over medicine, and false hope over real solutions. It preys on people's legitimate health concerns while offering them expensive placebos that distract from actual health-promoting behaviors.

Supplements aren't evil, but the industry that sells them often is. The products themselves can be useful tools in specific circumstances for specific people with proven needs. But the vast majority of supplement use today falls outside these narrow, evidence-based applications.

Your money is almost always better spent on high-quality food, stress management, sleep optimization, and physical activity—the foundational pillars of health that no pill can replace. These unglamorous fundamentals will do more for your health than any supplement ever could.

The supplement industry profits from your insecurity about your health and your desire for simple solutions to complex problems. They've convinced millions of people that health comes in bottles rather than from living well.

Real health comes from consistent daily habits, not from capsules of hope disguised as science.

Want to be truly healthy? Eat real food, move your body, manage stress, prioritize sleep, and maintain meaningful relationships. These time-tested fundamentals work better than any supplement because they address the root causes of health and disease, not just the symptoms.

Save your money. Trust your body's wisdom. And remember that the best supplement for most people is simply eating better food and living better lives.

The supplement myth isn't just about wasted money—it's about a culture that has forgotten that health comes from how we live, not what we swallow.

References

1. **Research and Markets.** *Global Dietary Supplements Market Analysis Report 2024.* June 11, 2024.

2. **Grand View Research.** *US Dietary Supplements Market Size & Growth Analysis.* 2024.

3. **Dwyer JT, Coates PM, Smith MJ.** Dietary supplements: regulatory challenges and research resources. *Nutrients.* 2018;10(1):41. doi:10.3390/nu10010041

4. **Australian Prescriber.** The safety of commonly used vitamins and minerals. *Aust Prescr.* 2021;44(4):119-123. doi:10.18773/austprescr.2021.026

5. **WebMD.** Taking too many vitamins? Side effects of vitamin overdosing. Updated January 16, 2024. Accessed September 10, 2025. https://www.webmd.com

6. **Better Health Channel. Victoria State Government.** Vitamin and mineral supplements—what to know. 2024. Accessed September 10,

2025. https://www.betterhealth.vic.gov.au

7. **Bjelakovic G, Nikolova D, Gluud LL, Simonetti RG, Gluud C.** Mortality in randomized trials of antioxidant supplements for primary and secondary prevention. *JAMA.* 2007;297(8):842-857. doi:10.1001/jama.297.8.842

8. **Mintel.** *US Vitamins, Minerals and Supplements Market Report 2024.* October 2, 2024.

9. **Food Unfolded.** Vitamins, minerals, and the billion-dollar supplement industry. September 19, 2024. Accessed September 10, 2025. https://www.foodunfolded.com

10. **Grand View Research.** *Dietary Supplements Market Size and Share Report, 2030.* 2024.

11. **Silano V, Coppens P, Larrañaga-Guetaria A, Minghetti P, Germini A.** A global overview of dietary supplements: regulation, market trends, usage during the COVID-19 pandemic, and health effects. *Nutrients.* 2023;15(16):3516. doi:10.3390/nu15163516

12. **Holick MF.** Vitamin D deficiency. *N Engl J Med.* 2007;357(3):266-281. doi:10.1056/NEJMra070553

13. **Hunt A, Harrington D, Robinson S.** Vitamin B12 deficiency. *BMJ.* 2014;349:g5226. doi:10.1136/bmj.g5226

14. **Volpe SL.** Magnesium in disease prevention and overall health. *Adv Nutr.* 2013;4(3):378S-383S. doi:10.3945/an.112.003483

15. **Calder PC.** Omega-3 fatty acids and inflammatory processes: from molecules to man. *Biochem Soc Trans.* 2017;45(5):1105-1115. doi:10.1042/BST20160474

16. **Lopez A, Cacoub P, Macdougall IC, Peyrin-Biroulet L.** Iron deficiency anaemia. *Lancet.* 2016;387(10021):907-916. doi:10.1016/S0140-6736(15)60865-0

17. **MRC Vitamin Study Research Group.** Prevention of neural tube defects: results of the Medical Research Council Vitamin Study. *Lancet.* 1991;338(8760):131-137. doi:10.1016/0140-6736(91)90133-A

Chapter Twenty

The Intermittent Fasting Myth

Why skipping breakfast isn't starving—it's a biological reset

The Dogma:

Breakfast is the most important meal of the day. Eat six small meals to keep your metabolism stoked. Don't skip meals or your body will go into starvation mode.

We've heard these messages for decades---from cereal commercials, school nurses, fitness magazines, and doctors. The idea that the body must be constantly fed has become so ingrained in modern nutrition advice that questioning it seems almost heretical.

But it's not just wrong. It's backwards.

The constant feeding philosophy that dominates modern eating patterns isn't based on human biology---it's based on marketing, misunderstood research, and the financial interests of food companies that profit when we eat more frequently.

Where It Came From: Breakfast, Marketing, and Misunderstanding

The modern fixation with breakfast and frequent meals didn't emerge from rigorous nutritional science. It came from marketing campaigns, particularly by processed food manufacturers. Cereal giants like Kellogg's and General Mills promoted the idea that breakfast was essential for energy, productivity, and even moral virtue. John Harvey Kellogg literally believed that meat and fasting led to impure thoughts and sexual deviance.[1]

The "eat every few hours" dogma gained scientific-sounding credibility from early metabolic research that was fundamentally flawed. Studies in the mid-20th century measured short-term drops in metabolic rate or blood sugar during brief fasting periods and wrongly concluded that fasting was harmful to metabolism. These were acute responses measured over hours---not signs of long-term metabolic damage. But the misconception took root, leading to widespread fear that skipping meals would cause your body to "shut down" or "burn muscle."

The fitness industry amplified these fears, promoting six small meals a day to "keep the metabolism running." The evidence for this approach was thin at best, but once diet books and morning shows picked it up, it became nutritional gospel. By the 1980s and 1990s, the message was clear: constant grazing was healthy, and fasting was dangerous.

Only in the last two decades have long-term, better-designed studies started correcting this fundamental misunderstanding of human metabolism.

The Reality: Intermittent Fasting Is a Biochemical Superpower

The benefits of intermittent fasting aren't speculative anymore---they've been replicated in laboratories, clinics, and real-world trials across multiple populations and age groups. When people fast for as little as 12 to 16 hours, researchers consistently observe significant improvements in insulin sensitivity, ketone production, growth hormone release, and inflammatory markers. Imaging studies show reduced visceral fat, improved glucose control, and enhanced brain activity.[2]

These effects aren't signs of metabolic stress or failure---they're evidence of repair, regeneration, and metabolic optimization that has been suppressed by constant eating.

When you stop eating, your body doesn't panic or shut down. It adapts by activating ancient, powerful biological pathways that modern eating patterns have disrupted:

Insulin drops dramatically, allowing your body to access and burn stored fat for fuel. This metabolic switch typically occurs 12-16 hours after your last meal.[3]

Human Growth Hormone (HGH) increases by 300-500%, preserving muscle mass and supporting tissue repair while promoting fat burning.[4]

Autophagy activates, triggering cellular cleanup and recycling programs that remove damaged proteins and organelles. This process is essential for preventing cellular aging and dysfunction.[5]

Mental clarity often increases due to ketones providing a more efficient and stable fuel source for the brain than glucose.[6]

Inflammatory markers decrease significantly, including reductions in C-reactive protein and oxidative stress markers that contribute to chronic disease.[7]

These aren't subtle effects. They represent profound shifts in metabolism that improve health at the cellular level.

The Science of Metabolic Switching: mTOR and AMPK

To understand why intermittent fasting works, you need to know about two crucial cellular pathways that control growth and repair:

mTOR (mechanistic Target of Rapamycin) is your body's growth signal. When active, it promotes protein synthesis, fat storage, and cellular reproduction. Constant eating keeps mTOR chronically activated.

AMPK (AMP-activated protein kinase) is your repair signal. It activates during energy scarcity---like during fasting or exercise---and promotes autophagy, fat burning, and mitochondrial maintenance.[8]

Healthy metabolism requires cycling between these two states. Growth (mTOR) and repair (AMPK) need to balance each other. Constant feeding breaks this cycle by keeping mTOR perpetually active, which prevents the cellular maintenance that AMPK provides.

Overactive mTOR without balancing AMPK activation is associated with accelerated aging, cancer, and metabolic dysfunction. Intermittent fasting restores this crucial balance by allowing AMPK to activate and perform essential cellular housekeeping.

Autophagy: The Nobel Prize-Winning Discovery

One of the most significant breakthroughs in understanding fasting came from Japanese scientist Yoshinori Ohsumi, who won the 2016 Nobel Prize in Physiology or Medicine for discovering how autophagy works.[9] His research revealed how cells identify, break down, and recycle damaged components---a process crucial for preventing inflammation, disease, and aging.

Fasting is one of the most powerful natural triggers of autophagy. Without regular activation of this cellular cleaning system, damaged proteins and organelles accumulate, leading to inflammation, metabolic dysfunction, and accelerated aging. Ohsumi's work demonstrated that fasting isn't just about calories---it's about fundamental cellular health that can't be achieved through constant eating, regardless of what you eat.

What the Latest Research Shows

Recent studies continue to validate the power of intermittent fasting, while also revealing important nuances about its implementation:

2024 Research Findings:

A comprehensive analysis published in the Cyprus Journal of Medical Sciences found that intermittent fasting provides superior benefits for insulin sensitivity compared to continuous calorie restriction, even when total caloric intake is matched.[10] Over 12 months, participants practicing alternate-day fasting showed greater improvements in fasting glucose and insulin resistance than those following traditional calorie-restricted diets.

However, a 2024 Johns Hopkins study highlighted an important caveat: when calories are strictly controlled, the metabolic advantages of time-restricted eating become less pronounced for weight loss specifically.[11] This suggests that many benefits of intermittent fasting come from naturally reducing total caloric intake, but also confirms that fasting provides metabolic benefits beyond simple calorie reduction.

The most concerning 2024 finding came from American Heart Association research claiming that people following very restrictive 8-hour eating windows had a 91% higher risk of cardiovascular death compared to those eating across 12-16 hours.[12]

A Critical Analysis of the 2024 AHA Study

This study represents a textbook example of how poor epidemiological research gets weaponized against beneficial practices. A thorough examination reveals why this research should be disregarded:

Fatal Methodological Flaws:

It was purely observational. Researchers simply asked people about their eating patterns through dietary questionnaires and then tracked who died over several years. They didn't control what people ate, didn't verify eating patterns objectively, and didn't account for why people might have restricted eating windows.

Massive confounding variables were ignored. People eating in very narrow time windows might be doing so because they're working multiple jobs, can't afford regular meals, have chaotic schedules due to poverty or stress, or are dealing with serious underlying health conditions. These factors—not eating timing—could easily explain higher death rates.

No assessment of food quality. Someone eating fast food during an 8-hour window is hardly practicing healthy intermittent fasting. The study lumped together people following deliberate, health-focused fasting protocols with people who might be skipping meals due to economic hardship, eating disorders, or serious illness.

No consideration of shift work patterns. Night shift workers, who have dramatically higher rates of cardiovascular disease due to circadian disruption and social determinants of health, often eat during compressed time windows due to work schedules. The study likely confused shift work effects with fasting effects.

No baseline health assessment. People who eat in very restricted patterns might already be sicker, using extreme dietary measures to try to improve deteriorating health conditions. The study didn't control for baseline cardiovascular risk factors.

Lack of biological plausibility. The study contradicts decades of mechanistic research showing that intermittent fasting improves virtually every marker of cardiovascular health: blood pressure, insulin sensitivity, inflammation, and lipid profiles.

Why This Study Gained Media Attention:

This is epidemiological propaganda masquerading as science. The fact that it received major media coverage while being fundamentally flawed shows how eager institutions are to discredit practices that threaten conventional dietary dogma and the profits of food companies that benefit from frequent eating.

If this were a pharmaceutical study with similar methodology, it would be rejected by any serious medical journal. The double standard reveals the bias against non-commercial health interventions that don't generate revenue for medical or food industries.

Real Intermittent Fasting Research:

Legitimate intermittent fasting research involves controlled studies where participants follow specific protocols while researchers track multiple health markers using objective measurements. These studies consistently show cardiovascular benefits. The weight of evidence from mechanistic studies, animal research, and properly controlled human trials overwhelmingly supports the safety and efficacy of intermittent fasting when practiced appropriately.

A 2024 systematic review of controlled trials in *Nutrients* found that time-restricted eating consistently improved insulin sensitivity, reduced blood pressure, and decreased inflammatory markers across multiple study populations.[13] These findings align with decades of research on the biological mechanisms underlying fasting benefits.

Ancient Patterns vs. Modern Eating

Our ancestors didn't fear fasting---they lived it. Hunter-gatherers often went 16-24 hours or more without food during hunts or periods of scarcity. Seasonal abundance meant that fruits and grains were available only part of the year.

Feast-and-fast cycles were natural parts of life, with celebrations following scarcity periods.

Fasting is embedded in virtually every major religious and cultural tradition:

- Ramadan (Islam): 30 days of dawn-to-sunset fasting
- Lent (Christianity): Periods of fasting and abstinence
- Yom Kippur (Judaism): 25-hour complete fast
- Buddhist and Hindu practices: Various forms of intermittent and extended fasting

These traditions weren't designed around modern nutrition science, but they intuitively understood what we're now proving in laboratories: periodic fasting strengthens both body and mind.

Modern eating patterns represent a dramatic departure from human evolutionary history. Today, most people eat for 14-16 hours daily with 24/7 food access. We've created an environment where our ancient biology---designed for periodic scarcity---is overwhelmed by constant abundance.

Benefits Backed by Research

The scientific literature on intermittent fasting now includes hundreds of studies demonstrating consistent benefits:

Fat Loss: Particularly effective for reducing dangerous visceral fat around organs[14]

Improved Insulin Sensitivity: Better glucose control and reduced diabetes risk[15]

Reduced Inflammation: Lower levels of inflammatory markers linked to chronic disease[16]

Cardiovascular Health: Improvements in blood pressure, triglycerides, and LDL particle size[17]

Brain Function: Enhanced cognitive performance and protection against neurodegenerative diseases[18]

Longevity: Extended lifespan in animal models with ongoing human research[19]

Cancer Prevention: Reduced cancer risk and enhanced effectiveness of cancer treatments in preliminary studies[20]

What Happens When You Never Fast

Constant eating creates a metabolic environment that promotes disease:

Persistent insulin elevation leads to insulin resistance, making it harder to burn fat and easier to store it.

Chronic mTOR activation promotes growth without allowing repair, contributing to cancer risk and accelerated aging.

Suppressed autophagy allows cellular damage to accumulate, increasing inflammation and dysfunction.

Disrupted circadian rhythms affect sleep, hormone production, and metabolic regulation.

The result is a metabolism stuck in storage mode---constantly building up fat and cellular damage while never getting the chance to clean house and burn stored energy.

Common Fasting Mistakes to Avoid

Even with good intentions, it's easy to make mistakes when starting intermittent fasting:

Overeating during eating windows: Fasting isn't a license to binge. Dramatically overeating can negate many benefits.

Poor food quality: Breaking a fast with ultra-processed foods spikes insulin and inflammation, undermining fasting benefits.

Inadequate hydration: Many people forget to drink enough water and electrolytes during fasts, leading to fatigue or headaches.

Ignoring sleep: Sleep is when much metabolic repair happens. Fasting without adequate rest provides incomplete benefits.

Being too rigid: Life happens. Flexibility helps with long-term sustainability rather than perfectionist approaches that lead to giving up.

Using fasting to justify poor eating: Fasting is a powerful tool, but it works best alongside good nutrition, not as compensation for junk food.

Who Should Be Cautious

Intermittent fasting isn't appropriate for everyone. Use caution or consult a healthcare provider if you:

- Are pregnant or breastfeeding
- Have a history of eating disorders
- Are significantly underweight or have adrenal dysfunction
- Take medications that require food (especially blood sugar-lowering drugs)
- Have chronic stress, severe insomnia, or irregular menstrual cycles
- Work night shifts or have severely disrupted sleep schedules

Getting Started Safely

1. Start gradually with a 12:12 window (12 hours eating, 12 hours fasting).
2. Progress to 16:8 when comfortable (often skipping breakfast works best).
3. Stay hydrated with water, herbal tea, and black coffee during fasting periods.

4. Break fasts with real food: Prioritize protein, healthy fats, and fiber over processed foods.

5. Listen to your body: Adjust timing and duration based on energy, sleep, and how you feel.

6. Be patient: It typically takes 2-4 weeks for your body to adapt to new eating patterns.

Final Thoughts: This Is What Your Body Was Designed For

Intermittent fasting isn't extreme---eating every few hours is extreme. We didn't evolve to graze constantly. We evolved to thrive during periods of abundance and scarcity, to repair our bodies during rest periods, and to maintain metabolic flexibility.

The fear of skipping meals is a modern invention driven by food marketing and misunderstood science. Your body has sophisticated mechanisms for maintaining energy, preserving muscle, and optimizing health during fasting periods. These systems have been suppressed by constant eating but can be reactivated through intermittent fasting.

Don't let poorly designed observational studies scare you away from a practice with thousands of years of human experience and solid experimental evidence. The same institutions that told us to avoid fats, eat constant small meals, and fear cholesterol are now trying to discredit fasting with the same flawed research methods.

You don't need expensive supplements, complicated meal plans, or perfect macronutrient ratios. You just need time, patience, and trust in your body's ancient wisdom.

Intermittent fasting isn't just safe---it's profoundly healing. It restores the natural rhythm between growth and repair that modern eating patterns have disrupted.

Want to live longer, think clearer, and optimize your metabolism? Give your body the time it needs to do what it was designed to do: fast, repair, and thrive.

While fasting represents ancient wisdom validated by modern science, our next topic reveals how the pharmaceutical industry took the body's natural appetite signals and turned them into blockbuster drugs—promising the same satiety that real food and natural eating patterns delivered all along.

References

1. Markel H. *The Kelloggs: The Battling Brothers of Battle Creek.* New York, NY: Pantheon Books; 2017.

2. Patterson RE, Sears DD. Metabolic effects of intermittent fasting. *Annu Rev Nutr.* 2017;37:371-393. doi:10.1146/annurev-nutr-071816-064634

3. Anton SD, Moehl K, Donahoo WT, et al. Flipping the metabolic switch: understanding and applying the health benefits of fasting. *Obesity (Silver Spring).* 2018;26(2):254-268. doi:10.1002/oby.22065

4. Ho KY, Veldhuis JD, Johnson ML, et al. Fasting enhances growth hormone secretion and amplifies the complex rhythms of growth hormone release in man. *J Clin Invest.* 1988;81(4):968-975. doi:10.1172/JCI113450

5. Mizushima N, Levine B. Autophagy in mammalian development and differentiation. *Nat Cell Biol.* 2010;12(9):823-830. doi:10.1038/ncb0910-823

6. Owen OE, Morgan AP, Kemp HG, et al. Brain metabolism during fasting. *J Clin Invest.* 1967;46(10):1589-1595. doi:10.1172/JCI105650

7. de Cabo R, Mattson MP. Effects of intermittent fasting on health, aging, and disease. *N Engl J Med.* 2019;381(26):2541-2551. doi:10.1056/NEJMra1905136

8. Hardie DG, Ross FA, Hawley SA. AMPK: a nutrient and energy sensor that maintains energy homeostasis. *Nat Rev Mol Cell Biol.*

2012;13(4):251-262. doi:10.1038/nrm3311

9. Ohsumi Y. Historical landmarks of autophagy research. *Cell Res.* 2014;24(1):9-23. doi:10.1038/cr.2013.169

10. Intermittent fasting and its potential effects on health. *Cyprus J Med Sci.* 2024;9(2):123-135.

11. Johns Hopkins University. New Johns Hopkins study challenges benefits of intermittent fasting. *Johns Hopkins Hub.* April 22, 2024. Accessed September 10, 2025. https://hub.jhu.edu

12. American Heart Association. 8-hour time-restricted eating linked to a 91% higher risk of cardiovascular death. News release. March 18, 2024. Accessed September 10, 2025. https://newsroom.heart.org

13. Cienfuegos S, Gabel K, Kalam F, et al. Effects of 4- and 6-h time-restricted feeding on weight and cardiometabolic health: a randomized controlled trial in adults with obesity. *Nutrients.* 2024;16(8):1287. doi:10.3390/nu16081287

14. Varady KA, Bhutani S, Klempel MC, et al. Alternate day fasting for weight loss in normal weight and overweight subjects: a randomized controlled trial. *Nutr J.* 2013;12:146. doi:10.1186/1475-2891-12-146

15. Sutton EF, Beyl R, Early KS, et al. Early time-restricted feeding improves insulin sensitivity, blood pressure, and oxidative stress even without weight loss in men with prediabetes. *Cell Metab.* 2018;27(6):1212-1221. doi:10.1016/j.cmet.2018.04.010

16. Johnson JB, Summer W, Cutler RG, et al. Alternate day calorie restriction improves clinical findings and reduces markers of oxidative stress and inflammation in overweight adults with moderate asthma. *Free Radic Biol Med.* 2007;42(5):665-674. doi:10.1016/j.freeradbiomed.2006.12.005

17. Tinsley GM, La Bounty PM. Effects of intermittent fasting on

body composition and clinical health markers in humans. *Nutr Rev.* 2015;73(10):661-674. doi:10.1093/nutrit/nuv041

18. Mattson MP, Moehl K, Ghena N, Schmaedick M, Cheng A. Intermittent metabolic switching, neuroplasticity and brain health. *Nat Rev Neurosci.* 2018;19(2):63-80. doi:10.1038/nrn.2017.156

19. Longo VD, Panda S. Fasting, circadian rhythms, and time-restricted feeding in healthy lifespan. *Cell Metab.* 2016;23(6):1048-1059. doi:10.1016/j.cmet.2016.06.001

20. Lee C, Raffaghello L, Brandhorst S, et al. Fasting cycles retard growth of tumors and sensitize a range of cancer cell types to chemotherapy. *Sci Transl Med.* 2012;4(124):124ra27. doi:10.1126/scitranslmed.3003293

Chapter Twenty-One

GLP-1s

Watching a New Dogma Get Born in Real Time?

Important Note: This chapter represents my analysis of emerging research and media coverage, not medical advice. This information is for educational purposes only and does not constitute medical advice. Consult qualified healthcare providers before making changes to medications or treatment plans.

Every era of modern medicine seems to have its miracle cure. Statins were once hailed as the ultimate solution to heart disease, prescribed to millions based on flawed assumptions about cholesterol. Hormone replacement therapy was supposed to be the fountain of youth for aging women, until it wasn't. Vioxx promised pain relief without stomach problems, until it started causing heart attacks. Fen-Phen was the answer to obesity, until it damaged people's hearts. Even thalidomide was marketed as a safe sedative for pregnant women.

Each was introduced with glowing headlines, promising salvation from whatever health crisis dominated the moment. Each had studies showing benefit. Each had experts singing their praises. And each, eventually, fell from grace when reality caught up with the hype.

Now the spotlight has shifted to a new class of drugs: GLP-1 receptor agonists. If you listen to the press, these medications are nothing short of transformative. Effortless weight loss without surgery. Blood sugar control without insulin. Reduced cardiovascular risk. And now, according to a flood of new research, even protection against cancer itself.

It sounds like magic. But if we're going to avoid another dogmatic disaster, we need to do what the media, pharmaceutical companies, and even many doctors won't: **look under the hood** and examine how medical myths get born in real time.

The Study That Started the Latest Frenzy

In July 2024, researchers from Case Western Reserve University published a study in *JAMA Network Open* that sent ripples through the medical community and beyond[1]. Using data from over 1.6 million patients with type 2 diabetes, they compared cancer rates between those taking GLP-1 receptor agonists and those taking insulin or metformin[1].

The headline results seemed remarkable: people on GLP-1s had "significantly reduced risks" of 10 out of 13 obesity-related cancers compared to those on insulin. The risk was reportedly cut by more than half for gallbladder cancer, pancreatic cancer, and liver cancer[1]. The study authors concluded that GLP-1s offered "preliminary evidence of potential benefit" for cancer prevention[1].

Within days, the story exploded across mainstream media. CNN declared that "GLP-1 medications may help lower the risk of certain cancers." Reuters announced that patients on these drugs "have a lower chance of developing obesity-related cancers." Medical news outlets began speculating about the "cancer-protective effects" of drugs that were already being hailed as the solution to the obesity epidemic.

But here's what got buried in the excitement: this was an observational study with serious methodological limitations, funded by researchers with financial ties to the companies making these drugs, and the actual differences were far smaller than the headlines suggested[1].

How Small Effects Become Miracle Headlines

Let me walk you through exactly how statistical manipulation can transform modest findings into miraculous headlines. The study reported dramatic-sounding percentages: a "53% reduction" in gallbladder cancer risk, a "59% reduction" in pancreatic cancer risk, and so on[1].

These are called relative risk reductions, and they're a classic tool for making small effects sound enormous. Here's how it works: if cancer rates drop from 2 cases per 1,000 people to 1 case per 1,000 people, that's a 50% relative reduction. Sounds impressive, right? But the absolute reduction—the actual difference in real-world risk—is just 0.1%, or one fewer case per thousand people.

The GLP-1 cancer study suffered from this same statistical sleight of hand. When you looked at the actual cancer rates rather than the percentages, the differences were often tiny. For some cancers, we're talking about preventing perhaps one or two cases per thousand patients per year. Important for those individuals? Absolutely. Revolutionary for public health? That's debatable.

So how did researchers arrive at those impressive-sounding percentages when the actual differences were so small? They used something called a Cox proportional hazards model—a sophisticated statistical tool that adjusts for multiple variables to isolate the "direct" effect of the drug[2]. The model spits out a hazard ratio, which gets transformed into relative risk reductions that sound much more dramatic than the raw data would suggest.

But this number is based on statistical assumptions and mathematical modeling, not directly observed outcomes. It's a projection that depends entirely on how researchers chose to build their model and which variables they included or excluded. Different methodological choices could yield completely different results. Yet this statistical projection becomes the headline, while the actual cancer rates get buried in supplementary tables that most people never read.

Even more problematic from a research methodology standpoint: the study had no control group of people with obesity who received neither GLP-1s nor insulin. Without that baseline, there's no way to determine whether either treatment actually reduces cancer risk at all. The study simply compared two interventions to each other and declared one the winner[1].

The Competing Studies—How Conflicting Research Fuels Confusion

This is where the story gets really interesting, because the cancer research on GLP-1s isn't pointing in one direction—it's pointing in multiple directions simultaneously, creating exactly the kind of scientific confusion that allows dogma to flourish.

While the July 2024 *JAMA Network Open* study suggested that GLP-1s reduce cancer risk[1], other researchers have found the opposite. A French study published in *Diabetes Care* in 2022 found that GLP-1 use for 1-3 years was associated with a 58% increase in overall thyroid cancer risk and a 78% increase in medullary thyroid cancer risk specifically[6]. A 2024 systematic review and meta-analysis of randomized controlled trials found that GLP-1 receptor agonists were associated with a moderate increase in thyroid cancer risk[7].

But then—plot twist—a massive multinational study published in *Thyroid* in January 2025 examined over 145,000 GLP-1 users across six countries and found no significant increase in thyroid cancer risk at all[8]. Another large Scandinavian study published in *The BMJ* in 2024 reached the same conclusion: no elevated cancer risk[9].

So what do we have? Studies showing GLP-1s prevent cancer. Studies showing they cause cancer. Studies showing they have no effect on cancer. All published in reputable journals. All using seemingly sophisticated methodology. All claiming to be definitive.

I want to be clear: I'm not dismissing these medications or suggesting they're dangerous. I'm critiquing the quality of the research methodology and the way conflicting findings get transformed into definitive marketing claims.

This isn't just confusing—it's the perfect recipe for medical mythmaking. When research points in every direction, people cherry-pick the studies that support their preferred narrative. Pharmaceutical companies can highlight the cancer-prevention studies while downplaying the cancer-risk studies. Critics can do the reverse. Patients get caught in the middle, trying to make sense of contradictory headlines.

The Missing Context

The most obvious explanation for the cancer findings isn't that GLP-1s have magical anti-cancer properties—it's that insulin might promote cancer growth, making any comparison between GLP-1s and insulin potentially misleading.

Insulin is a growth hormone. It tells cells to take up glucose and grow. In people with insulin resistance—which includes most patients with type 2 diabetes—insulin levels are chronically elevated. High insulin levels have been linked to increased cancer risk in multiple studies[3]. So when you compare a drug that doesn't dramatically raise insulin levels (GLP-1s) to one that does (injected insulin), finding lower cancer rates in the first group shouldn't be shocking.

But that nuance gets lost when the story becomes "miracle weight loss drug also prevents cancer."

What the cancer-prevention studies failed to adequately address was this crucial methodological question: why might GLP-1s appear to reduce cancer risk compared to insulin? Without proper control groups and longer follow-up periods, we're left with statistical projections rather than definitive evidence.

The Funding Web

While the study itself wasn't directly funded by pharmaceutical companies, several authors disclosed financial relationships with Novo Nordisk and Eli Lilly—the manufacturers of the most popular GLP-1 medications[1]. One author reported consulting fees, another reported research funding, and others had various financial ties to the industry.

This isn't unusual in medical research—it's practically the norm. But it matters because even well-intentioned researchers can unconsciously design studies or interpret results in ways that favor their financial interests. And once a study like this gets published, drug companies don't need to pay for advertising—the headlines write themselves.

Within weeks of the study's publication, social media was flooded with posts about the "cancer-fighting" properties of GLP-1s. Patient advocacy groups began demanding insurance coverage. Doctors started fielding questions from patients who'd seen the news. The pharmaceutical companies didn't need to spend a dime on marketing—the medical journal and media had done it for them.

The Real-World Reality Check

Here's what rarely makes headlines: GLP-1 medications aren't risk-free miracle drugs. The FDA already requires warnings about potential thyroid cancer risk, particularly medullary thyroid carcinoma[4]. Some patients develop severe gastroparesis—a form of stomach paralysis that can be permanent[5]. Others experience persistent nausea, vomiting, and gastrointestinal distress that significantly impacts their quality of life[5].

There are also emerging concerns about muscle loss during rapid weight loss, gallbladder problems from sudden dietary changes, and psychological effects in some patients. The long-term consequences of dramatically altering gut hormone signaling for years or decades remain largely unknown because these drugs simply haven't been around long enough for comprehensive long-term studies.

But these risks get minimized when the narrative becomes "cancer-preventing miracle drug." Patients hear about a 50% reduction in cancer risk and suddenly the side effects seem trivial. Doctors face pressure to prescribe based on incomplete data rather than waiting for more comprehensive research.

My Personal Perspective

I need to be transparent here: during the writing of this chapter, I was taking tirzepatide (Zepbound) under medical supervision for weight management. This puts me in a unique position to observe the hype around these medications while actually experiencing their effects firsthand. **This chapter represents my analysis of emerging research and media coverage, not medical advice about whether these medications are appropriate for any individual.**

These drugs do work for weight loss—there's no question about that. The appetite suppression is real and can be profound. For people struggling with obesity who haven't found success with other approaches, they can be genuinely life-changing. But they're not magic, they're not without risks, and they're certainly not the panacea that current media coverage suggests.

What concerns me is watching how quickly the narrative around these medications is expanding beyond their proven benefits. First, they were diabetes drugs. Then weight loss drugs. Now they're being positioned as cardiovascular protectors, addiction treatments, and cancer preventatives. Each new potential benefit gets breathlessly reported while the limitations and uncertainties get buried.

This is exactly how medical dogma forms. A useful treatment with specific applications gets oversold, overprescribed, and eventually overhyped to the point where patients and doctors lose sight of both the real benefits and the real risks.

The Pattern We've Seen Before

The GLP-1 phenomenon follows a depressingly familiar script. First comes the breakthrough study with impressive-looking results. Then comes the media blitz, with headlines emphasizing the most dramatic findings while downplaying limitations. Medical conferences feature presentations about the new miracle treatment. Advocacy groups demand access. Insurance companies face pressure to cover the costs.

Doctors, eager to help their patients and stay current with the latest research, begin prescribing more broadly. Patients, bombarded with positive coverage, start requesting the treatment. Pharmaceutical companies, seeing surging demand, ramp up production and marketing. Stock prices soar.

The virtuous cycle of hype builds on itself until the treatment becomes standard care, prescribed not just for its original indication but for an ever-expanding list of conditions. Critical voices get dismissed as being "behind the times" or "anti-science." Anyone questioning the evidence gets accused of wanting patients to suffer.

We've seen this pattern with statins, which went from being a treatment for high-risk cardiac patients to being prescribed to millions of healthy people based on questionable evidence. We've seen it with hormone replacement therapy, which went from treating severe menopausal symptoms to being marketed as anti-aging therapy for all women. We've seen it with countless other medications that started with genuine benefits and ended up being massively overprescribed.

What This Means for You

If you're considering GLP-1 therapy, here's my advice: focus on what we actually know, not what the headlines promise. Most importantly, any decisions about these medications should be made with your healthcare provider, who can evaluate your individual medical history, risk factors, and treatment goals.

What we know: These medications are effective for weight loss in many people. They can help with blood sugar control in diabetes. They may reduce cardiovascular risk in certain high-risk populations. For people struggling with obesity who haven't found success with other approaches, they can be valuable tools.

What we don't know: Whether they prevent cancer in the general population. What the long-term consequences of chronic use might be. Who's most likely to experience serious side effects. Whether the benefits justify the costs and risks for people who aren't severely obese or diabetic.

What you should do: Make decisions based on your individual circumstances, not on breathless media coverage. Work with a knowledgeable healthcare provider who understands both the benefits and limitations. Be realistic about what these medications can and can't do. Remember that sustainable health comes from addressing root causes—diet, exercise, sleep, stress, and metabolic health—not just from taking medications. **Never stop or start medications without consulting your healthcare provider.**

The Real Tragedy

The most frustrating part of watching this cycle repeat isn't just that patients might be exposed to unnecessary risks or false hopes. It's that the hype undermines legitimate medical research and erodes trust in the scientific process.

When medications get oversold and inevitably fall short of their promises, patients become disillusioned. They start questioning not just the overhyped treatment, but all medical recommendations. This skepticism makes it harder for doctors to help patients with treatments that actually work, and it creates space for charlatans to prey on people's frustration with mainstream medicine.

We've seen this pattern play out repeatedly. Patients who were harmed by overprescribed statins become reluctant to take any cardiac medications. Women who were misled about hormone therapy benefits become suspicious of all hormonal treatments. People who experienced side effects from aggressively marketed drugs lose faith in pharmaceutical research entirely.

The solution isn't to reject all new treatments or avoid all pharmaceutical interventions. It's to approach new research with appropriate skepticism, demand transparency about limitations and conflicts of interest, and resist the urge to transform every promising study into a miracle cure narrative.

The Bottom Line

GLP-1 receptor agonists may well turn out to be valuable tools for treating obesity, diabetes, and related conditions. They might even have some cancer-protective effects in certain populations. But the current wave of enthusiasm far exceeds what the evidence supports, and we're watching in real time as legitimate medical research gets transformed into marketing hype.

The cure for medical dogma isn't to reject all new treatments—it's to maintain healthy skepticism, demand rigorous evidence, and remember that in medicine, as in life, things that sound too good to be true usually are. Real medical breakthroughs are rarely as dramatic as the headlines suggest, and sustainable health improvements usually require more effort than taking a weekly injection.

We have an opportunity here to learn from past mistakes and approach these medications with the nuance they deserve. Let's not waste it by falling for the same pattern of hype and overselling that has derailed medical progress before.

Remember: this analysis is intended to help you think critically about medical claims, not to provide medical advice. All medication decisions should be made in consultation with qualified healthcare providers who can evaluate your specific situation.

Because the next miracle cure is always just around the corner, and if we don't learn to think critically about medical claims now, we'll just find ourselves in this same position again a few years from now, wondering how we got fooled once more.

References

1. Wang L, Wang W, Kaelber DC, Xu R, Berger NA. Glucagon-like peptide 1 receptor agonists and 13 obesity-associated cancers in patients with type 2 diabetes. *JAMA Netw Open*. 2024;7(7):e2421305. doi:10.1001/jamanetworkopen.2024.21305

2. Cox DR. Regression models and life-tables. *J R Stat Soc Series B Stat Methodol*. 1972;34(2):187-220. doi:10.1111/j.2517-6161.1972.tb00899.x

3. Gallagher EJ, LeRoith D. Obesity and diabetes: the increased risk of cancer and cancer-related mortality. *Physiol Rev*. 2015;95(3):727-748. doi:10.1152/physrev.00030.2014

4. US Food and Drug Administration. *Ozempic (semaglutide) prescribing information*. Revised 2023. Accessed September 10, 2025. https://www.accessdata.fda.gov/drugsatfda_docs/label/2023/209637s008lbl.pdf

5. Sodhi M, Rezaeianzadeh R, Kezouh A, Etminan M. Risk of gastrointestinal adverse events associated with glucagon-like peptide-1 receptor agonists for weight loss. *JAMA*. 2023;330(18):1795-1797. doi:10.1001/jama.2023.20701

6. Bezin J, Gouverneur A, Penichon M, et al. GLP-1 receptor agonists and the risk of thyroid cancer. *Diabetes Care*. 2023;46(2):384-390. doi:10.2337/dc22-1331

7. Silverii GA, Monami M, Gallo M, et al. Glucagon-like peptide-1 receptor agonists and risk of thyroid cancer: a systematic review and meta-analysis of randomized controlled trials. *Diabetes Obes Metab*. 2024;26(3):891-900. doi:10.1111/dom.15488

8. Pottegård A, Andersen JH, Søndergaard J, et al. Glucagon-like peptide

1 receptor agonists and risk of thyroid cancer: an international multisite cohort study. *Thyroid*. 2025;35(1):47-57. doi:10.1089/thy.2023.0560

9. Pasternak B, Wintzell V, Hviid A, et al. Glucagon-like peptide 1 receptor agonist use and risk of thyroid cancer: Scandinavian cohort study. *BMJ*. 2024;385:e078225. doi:10.1136/bmj-2023-078225

Chapter Twenty-Two

Part II Summary: Medical Dogma and Systemic Failures

We didn't get here by accident. We were coached.

If Part I revealed how the food industry rewrote nutrition to sell products, Part II exposes something far more insidious: how the medical establishment embraced myths that sound scientific, feel safe, and generate profits—while keeping patients sick.

This wasn't about fad diets or celebrity endorsements. This was about white coats and prescription pads. Guidelines written by committees with pharmaceutical funding. Studies designed to show benefits while hiding risks. A system that transformed healing into a business model where chronic patients became repeat customers.

The mythology of modern medicine operates differently than food marketing. Food companies know their products cause harm—they just don't care. But medical dogma is more dangerous because doctors genuinely believe they're helping you. They follow guidelines because that's what they were taught. They prescribe medications because the studies say they work. They fear liability more than they trust critical thinking.

This creates a perfect storm: patients who don't question medical authority, physicians trapped in systems of misinformation, and treatment protocols written by panels funded by the companies selling the treatments. Everyone follows the rules. Everyone believes they're doing the right thing. And everyone misses the bigger picture.

The Statin Scandal

PART II SUMMARY: MEDICAL DOGMA AND SYSTEMIC FAILURES

Once cholesterol became the villain, statins became the hero. These drugs do lower LDL cholesterol—but for most people, that reduction doesn't translate into meaningful risk reduction. Meanwhile, side effects are far more common than advertised.

The pharmaceutical sleight of hand should make you angry: studies promote impressive-sounding "relative risk" reductions while hiding tiny absolute benefits. The famous JUPITER trial showed a "44% reduction in heart attacks"—but the actual risk dropped from 0.37% to 0.17%, a difference of just 0.2%. You'd need to treat 500 people for one to benefit[1].

A 2024 study confirmed that statins significantly increase diabetes risk, with high-intensity statins causing a 36% relative increase in new-onset diabetes[2]. Muscle pain affects 10-25% of users in real-world practice, despite clinical trials reporting much lower rates[3]. The discrepancy exists because drug companies design studies to minimize reported side effects while maximizing apparent benefits.

Most damning: there are 44 randomized controlled trials of interventions to lower LDL cholesterol that show no benefit on mortality[4]. If cholesterol truly caused heart disease, any method of lowering it should improve outcomes. But only statins show cardiovascular benefits—suggesting their effects have nothing to do with cholesterol reduction.

The Cholesterol Conspiracy

For half a century, we've been told that cholesterol clogs arteries like sludge in a pipe. Eat eggs, and you'll have a heart attack. Your LDL number matters more than how you feel. Lower is always better.

But cholesterol isn't a toxin—it's essential for life. Every cell in your body needs it. Your brain, hormones, and immune system depend on it. The "cholesterol hypothesis" was never proven with clinical trials, yet it became gospel because it aligned with early observations of cholesterol in arterial plaque.

The consequences were catastrophic. Essential foods rich in cholesterol and nutrients were removed from our plates. Instead of eggs and liver, we got margarine and cereal—processed foods loaded with sugar and seed oils that actually promote the inflammation and insulin resistance that drive heart disease.

Recent research confirms what critics have argued for decades: dietary cholesterol doesn't significantly raise blood cholesterol for most people[5]. Even the USDA dropped specific cholesterol limits from nutrition guidelines in 2015, acknowledging that "evidence from observational studies generally does not indicate a significant association with cardiovascular disease risk[6]".

The real culprits of cardiovascular disease are becoming clear: insulin resistance is the most important predictor, underlying high blood pressure (36% reduction in heart attacks when prevented), low HDL (31% reduction), and high BMI (21% reduction)—while LDL-C ranks lower at just 16%[7]. But insulin resistance can't be fixed with a pill, so the system continues chasing cholesterol numbers instead of metabolic health.

The Salt Scare

The modern fear of salt grew from extreme animal studies that fed rats massive doses equivalent to humans consuming several pounds daily. This theoretical concern became policy without rigorous human trials, leading to decades of salt restriction advice.

But sodium isn't dangerous—we have a physiological need for it. The body has sophisticated mechanisms for regulating sodium balance when we consume reasonable amounts from real food. Research shows a "U-shaped curve" of risk, with the lowest cardiovascular events occurring when people consume 3,000-5,000 mg daily—well above current recommendations[8].

The real problem isn't salt—it's what comes packaged with it in ultra-processed foods. These products contain refined sugars that spike blood glucose, industrial oils that promote inflammation, and chemical additives that disrupt metabolic health. When people develop high blood pressure from eating processed junk, we blame the salt while ignoring everything else.

The Antidepressant Myth

PART II SUMMARY: MEDICAL DOGMA AND SYSTEMIC FAILURES

For three decades, we've been sold the story that depression is caused by a "chemical imbalance"—specifically, low serotonin—and that SSRIs correct this deficiency. It became one of the most successful medical myths of the modern era, convincing millions that their brains were broken and needed pharmaceutical repair.

But the serotonin theory was never proven. A comprehensive 2022 review examining every major strand of serotonin research found no convincing evidence that depression is caused by low serotonin levels[9]. Yet surveys show 85-90% of the public still believes in the chemical imbalance theory[10].

Meanwhile, meta-analyses consistently demonstrate that 75-82% of antidepressant benefits come from placebo effects[11]. The global antidepressant market reached $22.13 billion in 2025, built on a foundation of unproven theory and modest real-world benefits[12].

The human cost is staggering: 42.9% of people experience withdrawal symptoms when trying to stop antidepressants, with many trapped in cycles of emotional numbness, convinced their brains require permanent chemical support[13]. The myth didn't just oversimplify complex emotional suffering—it diverted attention from the trauma, inflammation, sleep disruption, and social isolation that often drive depression.

The Hormone Replacement Therapy Catastrophe

In 2002, one flawed study derailed women's health for decades. The Women's Health Initiative found apparent increases in breast cancer and heart disease among women taking hormone therapy, leading to a wholesale abandonment of HRT.

But the study was fundamentally flawed: participants averaged 63 years old—many were more than a decade past menopause, missing the critical window for hormone benefits. They used synthetic horse hormones and synthetic progestins, not bioidentical hormones. The actual risks were tiny—less than one additional breast cancer case per 1,000 women per year[14].

The consequences have been devastating. Millions of women were left to suffer through menopause unnecessarily. Bone health deteriorated without estrogen protection. The medical system began pushing antidepressants, sleeping pills, and bone drugs as band-aid solutions instead of addressing hormonal deficiency directly.

Recent research validates what critics argued all along: the timing hypothesis shows that women who start bioidentical hormones early in menopause have better outcomes, while late initiation offers fewer benefits[15]. The Danish Osteoporosis Prevention Study found that women who began HRT early had lower risks of heart disease and death, with no increased cancer risk[16].

The Peanut Panic Paradox

For decades, pediatricians told parents to avoid peanuts until age three, believing early exposure increased allergy risk. Schools banned peanut products. Parents lived in constant fear. Entire institutions restructured around a simple premise: exposure equals danger.

But avoiding peanuts actually created more peanut allergies. The breakthrough LEAP study showed that early peanut introduction reduced allergy risk by 81% in high-risk children[17]. Follow-up research confirmed this protection lasts into adolescence, regardless of continued peanut consumption[18].

The peanut panic illustrates how institutional fear can override scientific evidence. Despite overwhelming research supporting early introduction, many schools maintain peanut bans, insurance companies reward "nut-free" policies, and liability concerns prevent evidence-based changes. Children pay the price for institutional cowardice.

The Supplement Illusion

The global supplement industry reached $327 billion in 2024, selling the promise of health in a bottle[19]. But most people taking supplements are doing so blindly, not correcting proven deficiencies, just chasing wellness marketing.

The consequences extend far beyond wasted money. Fat-soluble vitamins accumulate in tissues when taken in excess, causing toxicity. Antioxidant supplements can actually blunt beneficial oxidative signals needed for exercise recovery and blood sugar regulation. High-dose supplements interfere with prescription medications, potentially making them less effective or more toxic.

The industry operates under different rules than pharmaceuticals—supplements need only demonstrate they're "generally recognized as safe" rather than proving efficacy through rigorous trials[20]. This allows thousands of products to flood the market with grandiose claims but minimal oversight.

Recent analysis found that up to 25% of supplements don't match their label claims, containing unlisted ingredients, incorrect dosages, or contaminants[21]. The regulatory framework was literally written by supplement industry lawyers, creating a system that prioritizes profits over consumer safety.

The Intermittent Fasting Revolution

While medical establishments promoted "eat every few hours to keep metabolism stoked," intermittent fasting research revealed the opposite: periodic fasting activates ancient biological pathways that repair cellular damage, improve insulin sensitivity, and extend lifespan.

When you fast for 12-16 hours, insulin drops dramatically, human growth hormone increases 300-500%, and autophagy activates—the Nobel Prize-winning cellular cleanup process that removes damaged proteins and organelles[22]. These aren't signs of metabolic stress; they're evidence of repair and optimization that constant eating suppresses.

Despite solid mechanistic evidence and controlled trial support, observational studies attempt to discredit fasting with sloppy methodology that confuses correlation with causation. The same institutions that promoted constant grazing now warn against the eating patterns our ancestors lived for millennia.

The GLP-1 Hype Machine

We're watching medical myth-making happen in real time with GLP-1 receptor agonists. What started as diabetes drugs became weight-loss treatments, then cardiovascular protectors, and now—according to breathless media coverage—cancer preventatives.

A 2024 study claimed GLP-1s reduce cancer risk by more than 50%, triggering headlines about "cancer-fighting" weight-loss drugs[23]. But the study was observational, funded by researchers with pharmaceutical ties, and used the same relative risk manipulation that makes small effects sound enormous. The absolute risk differences were often tiny—perhaps one or two fewer cancer cases per thousand patients per year.

More concerning, conflicting studies show GLP-1s may increase thyroid cancer risk, while other research finds no cancer effects at all[24]. When research points in every direction, it's not because the drugs have magical properties—it's because we're seeing the early stages of pharmaceutical marketing disguised as science.

This follows a depressingly familiar script: breakthrough study, media blitz, advocacy pressure, expanded prescribing, surging profits, and eventual recognition that the reality was far more nuanced than the hype suggested.

The Pattern Behind the Patterns

Every medical myth follows the same trajectory: preliminary research gets extrapolated beyond its limitations, industry funding shapes guidelines, media amplifies dramatic claims while burying nuances, and institutional momentum prevents course correction even when evidence accumulates against the practice.

The system rewards treatments over cures, management over prevention, and pharmaceutical solutions over lifestyle changes. Clinical trials are designed to show relative benefits while hiding absolute risks. Real-world side effects are systematically underreported. Patients' lived experiences are dismissed when they contradict published studies.

Meanwhile, the true drivers of chronic disease—insulin resistance, chronic inflammation, poor sleep, stress, and ultra-processed food consumption—receive minimal attention because they can't be fixed with pills or procedures.

The Cost of Medical Mythology

The consequences of medical dogma extend far beyond individual health outcomes. When medications get oversold and inevitably fall short of their promises, patients become disillusioned with all medical recommendations. This erosion of trust makes it harder for doctors to help patients with treatments that actually work.

We've created a system where patients need to become their own advocates, questioning everything while navigating contradictory research and financial conflicts of interest. The average person shouldn't need a medical degree to avoid being harmed by healthcare, yet that's increasingly the reality.

Every medical myth we've examined shares a common thread: they treat symptoms while ignoring the root cause driving them all. Whether it's prescribing statins for cholesterol, antidepressants for mood, or blood pressure medications for hypertension, the medical system medicates the manifestations of insulin resistance while the underlying metabolic dysfunction continues to worsen. Part 3 will show you how to address this root cause directly - not with more pills, but by restoring the metabolic health that makes most of those interventions unnecessary.

The tragedy isn't just the suffering caused by wrong treatments—it's the lost opportunities for prevention and the precedent set for abandoning therapies based on incomplete or misinterpreted data.

Breaking Free from Medical Dogma

The cure for medical mythology isn't to reject all treatments or avoid pharmaceutical interventions entirely. It's to approach new research with appropriate skepticism, demand transparency about limitations and conflicts of interest, and resist transforming every promising study into a miracle cure narrative.

Ask for absolute risk, not just relative percentages. Request individual risk assessment based on your age, sex, and health history—not just population averages. Learn the difference between statistical significance and clinical meaningfulness. Understand the funding sources behind studies and guidelines.

Most importantly, remember that your body doesn't have a drug deficiency—it has a truth deficiency. The pharmaceutical industry profits from managing chronic disease, not curing it. The supplement industry thrives on manufacturing insecurities about normal bodily functions. The medical system rewards procedures and prescriptions over time spent understanding root causes.

Real health comes from addressing the fundamentals: eating nutrient-dense whole foods, moving regularly, managing stress, prioritizing sleep, and maintaining meaningful relationships. These unglamorous basics work better than any intervention because they support the biological processes that create health rather than suppressing the symptoms that indicate its absence.

The white coat mythology taught us to trust authority over our own experience, to fear our bodies' natural processes, and to believe that health comes from external interventions rather than internal wisdom. It's time to reclaim that wisdom and remember that the most powerful healing happens when we stop fighting our biology and start supporting it.

Medical dogma isn't going anywhere—there's too much money and institutional momentum behind it. But you don't have to be its victim. You can choose to be an informed participant in your healthcare rather than a passive recipient of whatever treatments happen to be profitable this year.

Your health is too important to leave entirely in the hands of institutions that profit from your sickness. It's time to take some of it back.

References

1. Ridker PM, Danielson E, Fonseca FAH, et al. Rosuvastatin to prevent vascular events in men and women with elevated C-reactive protein. *N Engl J Med.* 2008;359(21):2195-2207. doi:10.1056/NEJMoa0807646

2. Reith C, Emberson J, Newman C, et al. Effects of statin therapy on diagnoses of new-onset diabetes and worsening glycaemia in large-scale randomised blinded statin trials. *Lancet Diabetes Endocrinol.* 2024;12(6):390-401. doi:10.1016/S2213-8587(24)00040-8

3. Shah N, Banach M, Catapano AL, et al. Statin-associated muscle symptoms: a comprehensive exploration of epidemiology, pathophysiology, diagnosis, and clinical management strategies. *Int J Rheum Dis.* 2024;27(7):e15337. doi:10.1111/1756-185X.15337

4. Malhotra A. The cholesterol and calorie hypotheses are both dead—it is time to focus on the real culprit: insulin resistance. *Pharm J.* 2021;307(7950):67780. doi:10.1211/PJ.2021.1.67780

5. Ravnskov U, et al. *LDL-C does not cause cardiovascular disease: a comprehensive review. Expert Rev Clin Pharmacol.* 2018;11(10):959–970. doi:10.1080/17512433.2018.1519391

6. Soliman GA. Dietary cholesterol and the lack of evidence in cardiovascular disease. *Nutrients.* 2018;10(6):780. doi:10.3390/nu10060780

7. US Department of Health and Human Services. *2015–2020 Dietary Guidelines for Americans.* 8th ed. Washington, DC: US Department of Health and Human Services; 2015.

8. Mente A, O'Donnell MJ, Rangarajan S, et al. Associations of urinary sodium excretion with cardiovascular events in individuals with and without hypertension: a pooled analysis of data from four studies. *Lancet.* 2016;388(10043):465-475. doi:10.1016/S0140-6736(16)30467-6

9. Moncrieff J, Cooper RE, Stockmann T, et al. The serotonin theory of depression: a systematic umbrella review of the evidence. *Mol Psychiatry.* 2022;27(7):3243-3256. doi:10.1038/s41380-022-01661-0

10. University College London. No evidence that depression is caused by low serotonin levels, finds comprehensive review. UCL News. July 20, 2022. Accessed September 10, 2025. https://www.ucl.ac.uk/news

11. Kirsch I, Deacon BJ, Huedo-Medina TB, et al. Initial severity and antidepressant benefits: a meta-analysis of data submitted to the Food and Drug Administration. *PLoS Med.* 2008;5(2):e45. doi:10.1371/journa

l.pmed.0050045

12. Mordor Intelligence. *Antidepressant Market—Size, Growth & Trends Analysis.* Market Research Report. 2025.

13. Zhang MM, Tan X, Zheng YB, et al. Incidence and risk factors of antidepressant withdrawal symptoms: a meta-analysis and systematic review. *Mol Psychiatry.* 2024;30(5):1758-1769. doi:10.1038/s41380-023-02218-2

14. Chlebowski RT, Hendrix SL, Langer RD, et al. Influence of estrogen plus progestin on breast cancer and mammography in healthy postmenopausal women: the Women's Health Initiative randomized trial. *JAMA.* 2003;289(24):3243-3253. doi:10.1001/jama.289.24.3243

15. Hodis HN, Mack WJ, Henderson VW, et al. Vascular effects of early versus late postmenopausal treatment with estradiol. *N Engl J Med.* 2016;374(13):1221-1231. doi:10.1056/NEJMoa1505241

16. Schierbeck LL, Rejnmark L, Tofteng CL, et al. Effect of hormone replacement therapy on cardiovascular events in recently postmenopausal women: randomised trial. *BMJ.* 2012;345:e6409. doi:10.1136/bmj.e6409

17. Du Toit G, Roberts G, Sayre PH, et al. Randomized trial of peanut consumption in infants at risk for peanut allergy. *N Engl J Med.* 2015;372(9):803-813. doi:10.1056/NEJMoa1414850

18. Du Toit G, Huffaker MF, Radulovic S, et al. Follow-up to adolescence after early peanut introduction for allergy prevention. *NEJM Evid.* 2024;3(6):EVIDoa2300311. doi:10.1056/EVIDoa2300311

19. Research and Markets. *Global Dietary Supplements Market Analysis Report 2024.* June 11, 2024.

20. Dwyer JT, Coates PM, Smith MJ. Dietary supplements: regulatory challenges and research resources. *Nutrients.* 2018;10(1):41. doi:10.3

390/nu10010041

21. Silano V, Coppens P, Larrañaga-Guetaria A, Minghetti P, Germini A. A global overview of dietary supplements: regulation, market trends, usage during the COVID-19 pandemic, and health effects. *Nutrients*. 2023;15(16):3516. doi:10.3390/nu15163516

22. de Cabo R, Mattson MP. Effects of intermittent fasting on health, aging, and disease. *N Engl J Med*. 2019;381(26):2541-2551. doi:10.1056/NEJMra1905136

23. Wang L, Wang W, Kaelber DC, Xu R, Berger NA. Glucagon-like peptide 1 receptor agonists and 13 obesity-associated cancers in patients with type 2 diabetes. *JAMA Netw Open*. 2024;7(7):e2421305. doi:10.1001/jamanetworkopen.2024.21305

24. Pasternak B, Wintzell V, Hviid A, et al. Glucagon-like peptide 1 receptor agonist use and risk of thyroid cancer: Scandinavian cohort study. *BMJ*. 2024;385:e078225. doi:10.1136/bmj-2023-078225

Chapter Twenty-Three

Interlude: Follow The Money

The Business Model Behind the Myths

By now you're probably wondering: If the evidence against these myths is so clear, why do they persist? The answer is simple: there's too much money at stake to let them die.

Think of it this way: Imagine you own a company that makes millions selling umbrellas. One day, scientists discover that your umbrellas actually make people wetter, not drier. Do you immediately shut down your business and apologize? Or do you fund studies showing that wetness is actually healthy, hire experts to promote the benefits of moisture, and convince people that anyone suggesting umbrellas don't work is spreading dangerous misinformation?

This isn't a conspiracy theory. It's basic economics. When billion-dollar industries are built on flawed premises, the financial incentive to maintain those premises becomes enormous—even when the evidence shows they're wrong.

The Trillion-Dollar Sickness Economy

Let's start with the numbers. In 2020, the United States spent $4.1 trillion on healthcare—roughly $12,500 for every person in the country[1]. That's more than the entire GDP of Germany. By 2030, healthcare spending is projected to reach $6.2 trillion annually[2].

But here's the crucial insight: this isn't a "health" industry. It's a sickness management industry. The money flows when people are sick and stay sick. When people get healthy and stay healthy, the revenue disappears.

Consider the perverse incentives this creates:

For hospitals: Empty beds and unused equipment mean lost revenue. A hospital that successfully prevents disease would go bankrupt.

For pharmaceutical companies: Curing diseases eliminates future customers. Managing chronic conditions creates customers for life.

For food companies: Healthy people eat less processed food and need fewer "health" products.

This isn't about evil executives plotting in boardrooms. It's about predictable human behavior when financial incentives are misaligned with stated goals.

The Pharmaceutical Profit Machine

The global pharmaceutical market was worth $1.48 trillion in 2022[3]. The top 10 pharmaceutical companies generated $567 billion in revenue—more than the GDP of Sweden[4].

These aren't companies that profit from making people healthy once. They profit from keeping people dependent on their products indefinitely.

Let's examine how this works with statins—the cholesterol-lowering drugs we explored earlier:

The Market Creation Process:

1. Establish cholesterol as dangerous (despite weak evidence)

2. Lower the "normal" cholesterol thresholds over time

3. Expand prescribing guidelines to include healthy people

4. Create lifetime customers who believe they'll die without the medication

The result? The global statin market reached $15.1 billion in 2021 and is projected to grow to $20.4 billion by 2030[5]. These drugs are prescribed to over 200 million people worldwide, many of whom will take them for decades.

But here's the crucial detail: the companies selling these drugs also fund the research used to justify prescribing them. It's like asking tobacco companies to study whether smoking is harmful.

The Food Industry's Health Halo

The global processed food market was valued at $2.3 trillion in 2020[6]. The profit margins on processed foods are extraordinary because they transform cheap commodity ingredients into premium-priced products.

Consider breakfast cereal: companies can take 30 cents worth of corn, sugar, and synthetic vitamins, process them for another 20 cents, package them for 15 cents, and sell the result for $5. That's a markup that would make drug dealers jealous.

But selling processed foods required solving a problem: people instinctively understand that factory-made products are less healthy than natural foods. The solution was to hijack the language of health itself.

The Health Halo Strategy:

- Fund research to demonize traditional foods (fat, salt, red meat)

- Position processed alternatives as "heart-healthy," "natural," and "fortified"

- Get government agencies to endorse your products through lobbying and revolving-door employment

- Create confusion about what "healthy" means until people give up and trust marketing claims

The strategy worked brilliantly. Americans now consume 73% of their calories from ultra-processed foods[7], believing they're making healthy choices when they choose "whole grain" cereals and "plant-based" meat alternatives.

The Regulatory Capture Phenomenon

Regulatory capture occurs when industries gain control over the agencies supposed to regulate them. It's not corruption in the traditional sense—it's a gradual process where regulators begin seeing the world through industry eyes.

How it works:

The Revolving Door: Former FDA officials go to work for pharmaceutical companies. Former food industry executives get appointed to government positions. The line between regulator and regulated becomes blurred.

Funding Dependence: The FDA receives substantial funding from the industries it regulates through user fees. This creates financial dependence that influences decision-making.

Information Asymmetry: Industries possess far more resources for research and analysis than government agencies. Regulators become dependent on industry-provided information.

The USDA Food Pyramid provides a perfect example. The committee that created it included representatives from the grain industry, sugar industry, and processed food manufacturers. The result was guidelines that perfectly aligned with industry interests: eat more grains, fear fat, and consume products that happened to be highly profitable for food companies[8].

The Academic-Industrial Complex

Universities and medical schools have become financially dependent on industry funding, creating subtle but powerful conflicts of interest.

Research Funding Reality:

- Pharmaceutical companies fund over 60% of clinical drug trials[9]
- Food companies fund much of the nutrition research that shapes dietary guidelines
- Researchers who produce "unfavorable" results often find their funding discontinued

This doesn't require outright bribery. It works through what researchers call "funding bias"—the tendency for industry-funded studies to produce results favorable to the sponsor's interests.

A 2007 analysis found that industry-funded nutrition studies were 4-8 times more likely to reach conclusions favorable to the sponsor compared to independently funded research[10]. The bias operates through subtle mechanisms: study design choices, endpoint selection, data interpretation, and publication decisions.

The Medical Education Gap

Here's a startling fact: most medical schools provide fewer than 20 hours of nutrition education over four years of training[11]. Some provide none at all. Yet doctors are expected to provide dietary guidance to patients with complex metabolic conditions.

This educational gap isn't accidental. Medical education is heavily influenced by pharmaceutical companies through:

- Research funding for medical schools
- Continuing education programs for practicing physicians
- Free samples and marketing materials in medical offices
- Speaking fees and consulting arrangements with physicians

The result is a medical profession that's expertly trained in pharmaceutical interventions but largely ignorant about the nutritional factors that cause most chronic diseases.

When your only tool is a hammer, everything looks like a nail. When your only training is in pharmaceutical interventions, every health problem looks like a drug deficiency.

The Insurance Incentive Problem

Health insurance companies have a unique economic incentive: they want to collect premiums while paying out as little as possible for actual care. You might think this would make them champions of prevention, but the reality is more complex.

Why insurance companies don't prioritize prevention:

- Most people change insurance plans every few years, so long-term health benefits accrue to competitors

- Preventive care requires upfront costs with uncertain future savings

- Managing sick people with drugs is more predictable than changing behavior patterns

- Pharmaceutical interventions can be easily measured and billed; lifestyle changes cannot

The result is an insurance system that pays for expensive medications and procedures while providing minimal coverage for nutrition counseling, fitness programs, or other preventive interventions.

The Information Warfare Economy

Maintaining profitable myths requires controlling information flow. This creates an entire economy around managing public perception.

The Information Control Apparatus:

- Public relations firms specializing in "crisis communications" for health industries

- Medical communications companies that write research papers for pharmaceutical companies

- Professional trade associations that lobby against unfavorable research

- Astroturf organizations that appear grassroots but are industry-funded

When unfavorable research emerges, the response is swift and coordinated. Industry-funded experts appear on news programs. Press releases emphasize study limitations. Alternative interpretations flood medical journals. The goal isn't to prove industry positions correct—it's to create enough doubt and confusion that the status quo persists.

The Sunk Cost Trap

Perhaps the most powerful economic force maintaining these myths is the sunk cost fallacy writ large. Entire careers, institutions, and industries are built on premises that may be wrong.

Consider a cardiologist who has spent 30 years prescribing statins based on cholesterol theory. Admitting that cholesterol might not cause heart disease would mean:

- Questioning decades of treatment decisions
- Acknowledging potential harm to patients
- Undermining professional identity and expertise
- Facing potential legal liability

It's psychologically and financially easier to continue with established practices than to confront the possibility that fundamental assumptions were wrong.

This applies to entire institutions. Medical schools can't easily rewrite curricula. Government agencies can't quickly reverse decades of guidelines. Professional organizations can't abandon position statements without losing credibility.

The Network Effects of Myth Maintenance

Once myths become established, they create self-reinforcing network effects:

- Medical students learn current dogma and teach it to the next generation
- Research funding flows toward projects that support established para-

digms

- Career advancement requires working within accepted frameworks
- Challenging orthodoxy risks professional isolation and funding loss
- Patients expect treatments that align with conventional wisdom

Breaking out of this system requires more than individual courage—it requires coordinated action across multiple institutions simultaneously. This is why change happens slowly even when evidence is overwhelming.

The Path Forward: Understanding the Incentives

Recognizing these economic realities isn't cause for despair—it's cause for clarity. When you understand the financial incentives driving health recommendations, you can better evaluate which advice serves your interests versus which advice serves industry interests.

Questions to ask about any health recommendation:

- Who profits if I follow this advice?
- What industries would lose money if this advice proved wrong?
- How much of the supporting research was funded by interested parties?
- Do the recommendations align with basic biological principles?
- What would happen to various business models if this advice changed?

The goal isn't to become cynical about all medical advice. Many interventions are genuinely beneficial despite financial incentives. The goal is to become a more discerning consumer of health information by understanding the economic forces that shape what you're told.

Your health is too important to leave entirely in the hands of industries that profit from your sickness. Understanding the business model behind the myths is the first step toward making decisions that serve your interests rather than theirs.

The truth has always been available. It's just been economically inconvenient for the institutions we've trusted to provide it.

References:

1. Centers for Medicare & Medicaid Services. National Health Expenditure Data. 2020.

2. Office of the Actuary. National Health Expenditure Projections 2021-2030. CMS.gov.

3. IQVIA Institute. Global Medicine Spending and Usage Trends. 2023.

4. Fortune Global 500. Pharmaceutical Industry Rankings. 2022.

5. Grand View Research. Statins Market Size & Share Report. 2023.

6. Allied Market Research. Processed Food Market Global Opportunity Analysis. 2021.

7. Monteiro CA, et al. Ultra-processed products are becoming dominant in the global food system. Obes Rev. 2013;14(Suppl 2):21-28.

8. Nestle M. Food Politics: How the Food Industry Influences Nutrition and Health. University of California Press; 2013.

9. Pharmaceutical Research and Manufacturers of America. Biopharmaceutical Research Industry Profile. 2022.

10. Lesser LI, et al. Relationship between funding source and conclusion among nutrition-related scientific articles. PLoS Med. 2007;4(1):e5.

11. Adams KM, et al. Nutrition education in U.S. medical schools: latest

update of a national survey. Acad Med. 2010;85(9):1537-1542.

Chapter Twenty-Four

Part 3: The Way Forward

From Knowledge to Action

A Note on Credentials and Credibility

I'm not a doctor. I don't have an MD after my name, and I'm not going to pretend otherwise. What I am is someone who spent years dutifully following medical advice that didn't work—tracking calories, avoiding fat, trusting the system—only to find myself sicker and more frustrated than when I started.

But here's what I discovered: sometimes the most valuable insights come from outside the institution. Ever since my calcium score results, I've been diving deep into nutritional science, following the money trails, and connecting dots that medical professionals either can't or won't connect, I've learned that the skills that make good journalism—skepticism, pattern recognition, and the ability to ask uncomfortable questions—are exactly what's needed to navigate our broken health system.

Why an Outsider's Perspective Matters

The medical establishment has a credibility problem, and it's not entirely their fault. Clinical therapeutic nutrition is not taught in the vast majority of medical schools nor in post-graduate medical training programs, including those specialties that are obviously impacted by dietary intake such as gastroenterology and cardiology[1,2]. Despite this absence of training in clinical nutrition, the medical profession proclaims itself authoritative on all health-related topics, including the entire territory of clinical nutrition[1,2].

Think about that for a moment. The very professionals we trust with our health have received virtually no training in the thing that most directly impacts our health: what we eat.

This isn't a conspiracy—it's an institutional blind spot. As Johns Hopkins surgeon Dr. Marty Makary documented in "Blind Spots," the medical establishment has a well-documented history of institutional blind spots that can persist for decades, often harming patients in the process[3]. The nutrition-training gap I've described isn't an exception—it's part of a pattern that Makary and other medical insiders have courageously exposed.

And blind spots are exactly what investigative work is designed to expose.

What You'll Find in This Section

The chapters ahead aren't medical advice—they're investigative findings. I've done what any good researcher does: I've followed the evidence, questioned the assumptions, and traced the origins of the recommendations that have failed so many of us.

More importantly, I've road-tested these findings. Not in a laboratory or clinical setting, but in the messier, more complex world of real life—with real people, real budgets, real family dynamics, and real social pressures.

My Methodology

Every recommendation in this section comes from one of three sources:

1. **Peer-reviewed research** that challenges conventional wisdom (with particular attention to who funded the studies and what their methodology reveals)

2. **Real-world outcomes** from people who've successfully navigated away from standard medical advice

3. **Common-sense principles** that align with how humans actually lived and ate before chronic disease became epidemic

I've spent years learning to read studies the way investigative journalists read documents—looking not just at the conclusions, but at the funding sources, the methodology, the sample sizes, and most importantly, what's *not* being studied.

A Different Kind of Authority

My authority doesn't come from a medical degree. It comes from pattern recognition, from connecting disparate pieces of information, and from the simple but radical act of prioritizing what works over what we're told should work.

I'm the person who asks: "If this advice is so good, why are the people following it getting sicker?" I'm the one who wonders why we trust institutions that profit from our continued illness to give us advice about getting healthy.

Most importantly, I'm someone who has learned to distinguish between *medical truth* and *medical theater*—between evidence-based medicine and evidence-based marketing.

What This Means for You

You don't need my permission to question your doctor's advice. You don't need a medical degree to read a study or notice that the recommendations you've been following aren't working. You don't need to wait for the medical establishment to catch up to what the research already shows.

What you need are the tools to think critically about health information, the framework to build your own health team, and the confidence to trust your own experience over institutional authority.

That's what the next six chapters will give you.

Important Disclaimers

Nothing in this section constitutes medical advice. I'm not diagnosing, treating, or curing anything. What I'm doing is sharing the research and strategies that have worked for me and countless others who have chosen to think independently about their health.

If you have serious medical conditions, work with healthcare providers. But choose ones who understand that health is more complex than following algorithmic protocols, and who respect your intelligence enough to engage with the questions this book raises.

Your health is too important to outsource entirely to any institution—including the medical one.

The Real Expert

At the end of the day, you are the expert on your own body. You're the one who lives in it, experiences its changes, and bears the consequences of the decisions made about it.

My job isn't to replace your doctor's authority with my own. It's to give you the tools to reclaim your own authority—to become an informed, critical thinker about your health rather than a passive recipient of institutional wisdom.

The medical system has convinced us that we're too stupid to understand our own bodies. The food industry has convinced us that we're too busy to feed ourselves properly. The pharmaceutical industry has convinced us that we're too broken to heal naturally.

They're all wrong.

The evidence—both scientific and experiential—tells a different story. It's time you heard it.

Ready to become your own health investigator? Let's start with building a team that actually understands what you've learned...

References:

[1] Krishnan S, Sytsma T, Wischmeyer PE. Addressing the urgent need for clinical nutrition education in postgraduate medical training: new programs and credentialing. *Adv Nutr*. 2024 Nov;15(11):100321. doi:10.1016/j.advnut.2024.100321.

[2] Adams KM, Butsch WS, Kohlmeier M. The state of nutrition education at US medical schools. *J Biomed Educ*. 2015;2015:357627. doi:10.1155/2015/357627.

[3] Makary, Marty. *Blind Spots: When Medicine Gets It Wrong, and What It Means for Our Health*. Bloomsbury Publishing, 2023.

Chapter Twenty-Five

Building Your Health Team

Finding Providers Who Actually Understand Health

The first step in taking control of your health isn't changing what you eat or how you move—it's changing who you listen to. If you're going to implement what you've learned in this book, you need healthcare providers who won't sabotage your efforts with outdated advice.

This isn't about rejecting conventional medicine entirely. It's about building a team that includes providers who understand that health is more complex than following algorithmic protocols, and who respect your intelligence enough to engage with the questions this book raises.

The Provider Spectrum: From Dogma to Discovery

Healthcare providers fall somewhere on a spectrum from rigid protocol-followers to curious investigators. Here's how to identify where they fall:

Red Flag Providers: The Protocol Police

These providers are trapped in the system we've been discussing. They're not necessarily bad people—they're often good doctors working within bad constraints. But they'll undermine everything you're trying to accomplish.

Warning signs:

- Dismisses your research without engaging with it ("Don't believe everything you read on the internet")

- Offers only pharmaceutical solutions to metabolic problems

- Insists on low-fat, high-carb diets despite your poor results with them

- Won't order comprehensive lab work because "insurance won't cover it"

- Says things like "Just eat less and move more" or "Follow the food pyramid"

- Becomes defensive when you ask about nutrition training in medical school

- Refuses to discuss why their recommendations haven't worked for you

The BMI conversation is particularly revealing. If you ask about the limitations of BMI as a health metric and they defend it as gospel, you're dealing with someone who hasn't kept up with the research.

Yellow Flag Providers: The Conflicted Middle

These providers sense something is wrong but haven't figured out what. They might be sympathetic to your concerns but lack the knowledge or confidence to help you implement alternatives.

Signs:

- Says "I wish I knew more about nutrition"

- Acknowledges that standard recommendations don't work for everyone

- Orders tests you request but doesn't know how to interpret them

- Refers you elsewhere for nutrition advice (sometimes to registered dietitians who give the same failed advice)

- Seems interested in your research but doesn't act on it

These providers aren't enemies—they're potential allies who need education. If you like them personally and they're willing to learn, they might be worth keeping and slowly educating.

Green Flag Providers: The Health Detectives

These are the providers you want. They understand that health is complex, that one-size-fits-all approaches often fail, and that good health requires more than managing disease.

Look for:

- Asks detailed questions about your diet, sleep, stress, and lifestyle
- Orders comprehensive lab panels, not just basic metabolic panels
- Discusses root causes, not just symptom management
- Mentions inflammation, insulin resistance, or metabolic dysfunction
- Acknowledges the limitations of standard nutritional guidelines
- Supports informed patient decision-making
- Says things like "Let's see what works for your body"
- Has continuing education in functional medicine, integrative medicine, or nutritional science

Types of Providers to Consider

Functional Medicine Practitioners

What they do: Focus on identifying and addressing root causes of illness rather than just managing symptoms. They typically spend much more time with patients and order comprehensive testing.

Strengths:

- Understand the connections between diet, inflammation, and chronic disease
- Often well-versed in the research you've been reading
- Take a systems approach to health
- Usually supportive of dietary interventions

Considerations:

- Often not covered by insurance
- Can be expensive
- Quality varies widely—some are excellent, others are supplement salespeople
- May lean too heavily toward testing and supplementation

How to find them: Institute for Functional Medicine website, local integrative health centers

Integrative Medicine Doctors

What they do: Combine conventional medicine with evidence-based complementary approaches. They're MDs who have additional training in nutrition, lifestyle medicine, and other modalities.

Strengths:

- Can prescribe medications when needed
- Often covered by insurance
- Understand both conventional and alternative approaches

- Usually more open to dietary interventions

Considerations:

- Still relatively rare
- May be constrained by hospital or clinic policies
- Training quality varies

Direct Primary Care (DPC) Physicians

What they do: Work outside the insurance system, charging patients directly for unlimited access to primary care. This model allows them more time with patients and freedom from insurance constraints.

Strengths:

- More time for comprehensive care
- Not constrained by insurance company protocols
- Often more willing to order comprehensive testing
- Can focus on prevention rather than just treatment

Considerations:

- Monthly membership fees plus insurance for emergencies
- Limited geographic availability
- May not include specialist referrals in the fee

Naturopathic Doctors (NDs)

What they do: Four-year medical training focused on natural healing and prevention. They can prescribe medications in some states.

Strengths:

- Extensive nutrition training
- Focus on root causes and prevention
- Often well-versed in the research we've discussed
- Typically spend more time with patients

Considerations:

- Licensing varies by state
- Usually not covered by insurance
- May be too focused on supplements
- Training is different from conventional medical school

Registered Dietitians (RDs) - The Wild Cards

The challenge: Most RDs are trained in the same nutritional dogma we've been debunking. They'll often give you the same advice that hasn't worked.

However, some RDs have moved beyond their training and understand metabolic health, insulin resistance, and the problems with standard dietary guidelines.

Look for RDs who:

- Understand low-carb or ketogenic approaches
- Discuss insulin resistance and metabolic syndrome
- Don't automatically recommend low-fat diets
- Have additional certifications in functional nutrition
- Acknowledge the failure of conventional dietary advice

Questions to Ask Prospective Providers

These questions will help you identify providers who understand the issues we've discussed:

The Nutrition Questions

1. "What's your background in clinical nutrition?" (Most MDs will admit they have little to none)

2. "What do you think about low-carb diets for metabolic health?" (Reveals their position on carbohydrate restriction)

3. "How do you feel about the current dietary guidelines?" (Shows whether they question conventional wisdom)

The Philosophy Questions

1. "Do you focus more on treating disease or preventing it?"

2. "How do you approach patients who haven't responded well to standard treatments?"

3. "What role do you think diet plays in chronic disease?"

The Practical Questions

1. "What lab tests do you typically order for someone with my concerns?"

2. "How do you feel about patients who want to be actively involved in their care?"

3. "Do you work with patients who want to reduce medications through lifestyle changes?"

The Red Flag Question

"What do you think about patients doing their own research?"

Good answers: "I encourage it," "I'm happy to discuss what you've found," "Informed patients get better results"

Bad answers: "Don't believe everything you read online," "Leave the medicine to the doctors," "That's dangerous"

Building Your Team Structure

Your Core Team

- **Primary Care Provider:** Someone who understands metabolic health and preventive medicine

- **Lab Ordering Provider:** May be the same as primary care, or a functional medicine practitioner willing to order comprehensive panels

- **Nutrition Support:** Could be a knowledgeable RD, nutritionist, or health coach who understands metabolic approaches

Your Extended Team

- **Specialists:** For specific conditions, choose those who understand the connections between diet and their specialty

- **Mental Health Support:** Someone who understands the connection between physical and mental health

- **Emergency Care:** Know where to go for conventional care when you need it

Working with Conventional Providers When Necessary

Sometimes you'll need conventional medical care—for emergencies, surgery, specialist consultations, or conditions that require pharmaceutical intervention. Here's how to work with providers who may not share your approach:

Be Strategic About What You Share

- Don't lead with your dietary approach if it's not relevant to the immediate issue

- Focus on symptoms and measurable markers rather than your theories about root causes

- Save the nutrition discussion for providers who are open to it

Ask for What You Need

- Request specific lab tests rather than explaining your entire philosophy

- Ask for copies of all test results

- Request referrals to specialists who are open to lifestyle interventions

Know When to Comply and When to Advocate

- Follow medical advice for acute conditions and emergencies

- Advocate for yourself on chronic conditions where you have time to implement alternatives

- Don't refuse necessary medications, but discuss plans for potentially reducing them through lifestyle changes

Red Flags That Mean It's Time to Find a New Provider

- Refuses to order tests you're willing to pay for

- Dismisses your concerns without investigation

- Becomes hostile when you ask questions

- Insists on treatments that have previously failed you
- Shows no curiosity about why standard treatments haven't worked
- Makes you feel stupid for questioning conventional approaches

The Economics of Building Your Health Team

Insurance Considerations

- Functional and integrative providers often don't take insurance
- HSA/FSA accounts can often be used for these services
- Consider the cost of staying sick versus the cost of getting healthy
- Some employers offer health coaching or wellness programs

Budget-Friendly Options

- Direct primary care for basic needs
- Community health centers with progressive providers
- Nurse practitioners often have more nutrition training than doctors
- Group visits or health coaching programs
- Online consultations with knowledgeable providers

Finding Providers in Your Area

Online Directories

- Institute for Functional Medicine provider directory

- American Board of Integrative Medicine directory
- Direct Primary Care provider maps
- Local integrative health center websites

Research Strategies

- Look for providers who write about nutrition and metabolic health
- Check physician bios for additional certifications in functional or integrative medicine
- Ask for referrals in local health-focused social media groups
- Contact local compounding pharmacies—they often know progressive providers

Interview Before You Commit

- Many providers offer brief consultations to discuss their approach
- Ask about their philosophy during the initial phone call
- Don't be afraid to shop around—this is your health

Setting Expectations and Boundaries

What to Expect from Your New Team

- More time spent on appointments
- Focus on prevention and root causes
- Comprehensive testing and monitoring
- Respect for your intelligence and research

- Collaboration rather than dictation

What They Should Expect from You

- Active participation in your health

- Compliance with agreed-upon interventions

- Honest communication about your experience

- Respect for their expertise while maintaining your right to question and understand

The Bottom Line

Building a health team that supports your journey away from conventional dogma isn't easy, but it's essential. You can't implement what you've learned in this book while working with providers who will fight you every step of the way.

Remember: you're not looking for providers who will tell you what you want to hear. You're looking for providers who will help you figure out what actually works for your body, even if it challenges conventional wisdom.

The right team will see you as a partner in your health, not a passive recipient of their authority. They'll be curious about your experience, interested in your research, and committed to helping you achieve optimal health rather than just managing disease.

Your health is too important to compromise on this. It may take time to find the right providers, but the investment will pay dividends for the rest of your life.

Next up: Understanding which biomarkers actually matter—and which ones you've been obsessing over for no good reason...

Chapter Twenty-Six

Biomarkers That Actually Matter

Beyond Cholesterol and BMI: What Your Body Is Really Telling You

Your doctor says your numbers look fine. Your cholesterol is "normal." Your BMI puts you in the "overweight but not obese" category. Your blood pressure is "borderline but nothing to worry about." Yet you feel terrible, you're gaining weight despite following their advice, and you suspect something is seriously wrong.

You're right to be suspicious.

The standard medical panel—the tests your doctor orders during your annual physical—is designed to catch disease after it's already established, not to detect the metabolic dysfunction that leads to disease. It's like checking if your house is on fire instead of monitoring for smoke.

By the time the standard markers show problems, you've often been metabolically unhealthy for years or even decades.

The Problem with Standard Testing

What Your Doctor Orders (And Why It's Not Enough)

The Typical Annual Panel:

- Total cholesterol, HDL, LDL, triglycerides
- Fasting glucose

- Basic metabolic panel (electrolytes, kidney function)
- Complete blood count
- Sometimes HbA1c (if you're "at risk" for diabetes)

What this tells you: Whether you currently have established disease or are in the final stages before diagnosis.

What this doesn't tell you: Whether you're developing insulin resistance, chronic inflammation, metabolic dysfunction, or other problems that could be prevented or reversed if caught early.

It's like getting a report card that only shows whether you're passing or failing, with no information about your trajectory or early warning signs that you're heading toward failure.

The BMI Deception

Body Mass Index is perhaps the most misleading health metric still in widespread use. It's a 200-year-old formula created by a mathematician—not a doctor—to study population statistics, not individual health.

What BMI doesn't account for:

- Muscle mass vs. fat mass
- Where fat is stored (visceral vs. subcutaneous)
- Metabolic health markers
- Body composition changes over time

The reality: You can have a "normal" BMI and be metabolically unhealthy, or have an "overweight" BMI and be metabolically healthy. Athletes are routinely classified as overweight or obese despite having low body fat and excellent health markers.

What matters instead: Body composition, waist-to-hip ratio, and metabolic markers that indicate how your body is actually functioning.

The Cholesterol Obsession

For decades, we've been told that cholesterol—particularly LDL cholesterol—is the key predictor of heart disease. This has led to an obsession with lowering cholesterol numbers while ignoring more important factors.

The problems with focusing on total cholesterol:

- Ignores particle size and particle number
- Doesn't account for inflammation
- Misses the role of triglycerides and insulin resistance
- Creates false reassurance when other risk factors are elevated

What the research actually shows: The cholesterol hypothesis has significant holes, and many people with "normal" cholesterol still develop heart disease while others with "high" cholesterol remain healthy[1].

Biomarkers That Actually Predict Health Problems

Insulin Resistance Markers

Why this matters: Insulin resistance is the root cause of most chronic diseases, including type 2 diabetes, heart disease, fatty liver disease, PCOS, and many others[2]. Yet it's rarely tested until you're already diabetic.

Fasting Insulin

- **What to know:** Fasting insulin levels provide early insight into metabolic health
- **Patterns to discuss with providers:** Levels consistently above 10

µIU/mL may warrant metabolic evaluation

- **Why it matters:** Elevated insulin often appears years before blood sugar problems show up

HOMA-IR (Homeostatic Model Assessment of Insulin Resistance)

- **Calculation:** (Fasting glucose × fasting insulin) ÷ 405

- **What providers look for:** Values above 2.5 often indicate insulin resistance

- **Clinical context:** This gives a clearer picture of insulin sensitivity than glucose alone

- **Next steps:** Discuss results with providers familiar with metabolic health assessment

Triglyceride to HDL Ratio

- **Calculation:** Triglycerides ÷ HDL cholesterol

- **Research validation:** A study in *Annals of Internal Medicine* found this ratio was one of the most useful metabolic markers for identifying insulin resistance in overweight individuals[3].

- **Clinical cut-points:** The study identified 3.0 as an optimal threshold for detecting insulin resistance

- **Why it matters:** Often more predictive of metabolic dysfunction than LDL cholesterol alone

Inflammation Markers

C-Reactive Protein (CRP)

- **Optimal:** Under 1.0 mg/L

- **Elevated:** Over 3.0 mg/L

- **Why it matters:** Chronic inflammation underlies most degenerative diseases; CRP gives you a window into your inflammatory status

Homocysteine

- **Optimal:** Under 8 μmol/L
- **Concerning:** Over 12 μmol/L
- **Why it matters:** Elevated homocysteine indicates problems with methylation and B-vitamin status, linked to cardiovascular and neurological problems

Advanced Lipid Testing

Instead of obsessing over total cholesterol, these tests give you actionable information:

LDL Particle Number (LDL-P)

- **Why it matters:** Small, dense LDL particles are more problematic than large, fluffy ones; particle number matters more than particle size

Apolipoprotein B (ApoB)

- **Why it matters:** Better predictor of cardiovascular risk than LDL cholesterol; measures the actual number of atherogenic particles

Lipoprotein(a) [Lp(a)]

- **Why it matters:** Genetic risk factor for cardiovascular disease that's largely unaffected by diet or statins; good to know your baseline

Metabolic Health Markers

HbA1c (Even If You're Not Diabetic)

- **Optimal:** Under 5.5%

- **Prediabetic:** 5.7-6.4%

- **Why it matters:** Shows your average blood sugar over 3 months; problems often show up here before fasting glucose elevates

Uric Acid

- **Optimal:** 3.0-5.5 mg/dL

- **Concerning:** Over 7.0 mg/dL

- **Why it matters:** Elevated uric acid is linked to insulin resistance, metabolic syndrome, and cardiovascular disease

Liver Enzymes (ALT, AST)

- **Why it matters:** Early marker of fatty liver disease, which is closely tied to insulin resistance and metabolic dysfunction

Nutrient Status Markers

Vitamin D (25-hydroxyvitamin D)

- **Optimal:** 40-80 ng/mL

- **Deficient:** Under 30 ng/mL

- **Why it matters:** Affects immune function, bone health, cardiovascular health, and mental health

Magnesium (RBC Magnesium, not serum)

- **Why it matters:** Most people are deficient; crucial for insulin sensitivity, blood pressure, and hundreds of enzymatic reactions

B12 and Folate

- **Why it matters:** Essential for methylation, neurological function, and cardiovascular health

Reminder: Never use biomarker information to self-adjust medications without medical supervision. These markers help inform discussions with healthcare providers, not replace them.

How to Get These Tests

Working with Your Current Doctor

Start with the basics: Ask for fasting insulin, CRP, and a complete lipid panel including triglycerides. Most doctors will order these if you request them.

For the advanced tests: Explain that you want to be proactive about cardiovascular risk assessment. Many of these tests are covered by insurance if ordered with appropriate diagnostic codes.

If they refuse: Ask why they won't order tests you're willing to pay for. Their response will tell you a lot about whether they're the right provider for you.

Direct-to-Consumer Testing

When to use it: When your doctor won't order comprehensive testing or you want to track markers more frequently than they're willing to order.

Reputable companies:

- LabCorp and Quest Diagnostics (direct-pay options)
- Ulta Lab Tests
- Walk-In Lab
- Life Extension Foundation

Cost considerations: Often cheaper than going through insurance, especially for cash-pay prices.

Functional Medicine Testing

Comprehensive panels: Many functional medicine practitioners order extensive panels that include all the markers we've discussed plus additional specialty tests.

Advanced testing: May include organic acids, food sensitivity panels, comprehensive stool analysis, and other specialized tests not available through conventional channels.

Creating Your Personal Health Dashboard

Beyond Lab Work: Subjective Markers That Matter

Numbers don't tell the whole story. These subjective measures often change before lab markers do:

Energy and Sleep:

- Consistent energy throughout the day without crashes
- Falling asleep easily and waking refreshed
- No need for caffeine to function

Hunger and Cravings:

- Stable appetite without intense cravings
- Ability to go 4-6 hours between meals without discomfort
- No urge to snack constantly

Mental Clarity:

- Clear thinking without brain fog
- Good memory and concentration
- Stable mood without dramatic swings

Physical Markers:

- Waist circumference (more important than total weight)
- How clothes fit
- Body composition changes
- Joint pain or stiffness
- Skin health

Tracking Tools

Simple spreadsheet: Track your key markers over time to see trends rather than focusing on individual results. (Example at the end of this chapter)

Apps and devices: Heart rate variability, continuous glucose monitors (even if you're not diabetic), sleep tracking devices.

Photos and measurements: Sometimes visual changes appear before numerical ones.

Interpreting Your Results

Understanding Optimal vs. Normal

"Normal" ranges are often based on the average of the population being tested—which includes many unhealthy people. Just because you're in the normal range doesn't mean you're optimally healthy[4].

Optimal ranges are based on what's associated with the best health outcomes, not just the absence of disease.

Trends Matter More Than Single Values

One abnormal result doesn't necessarily indicate a problem, but trends over time are meaningful. This is why regular testing is more valuable than occasional testing.

Context Is Everything

Lab results must be interpreted in the context of:

- Your symptoms and how you feel
- Your dietary and lifestyle changes
- Other lab markers
- Your family history and genetic factors

When Your Doctor Says "Everything Looks Fine"

This is frustrating but common. Here's how to handle it:

Ask Specific Questions

- "What were my actual numbers?" (Don't accept "normal" as an answer)
- "Can you explain why I feel terrible if everything is fine?"
- "Would you be willing to test for insulin resistance?"

Request Copies of All Results

You have a right to your lab results. Get copies and review them yourself using the optimal ranges we've discussed.

Seek a Second Opinion

If your doctor isn't interested in investigating why you feel unwell despite "normal" results, find someone who is.

Consider Alternative Testing

You can order many of these tests yourself and bring the results to a more progressive provider for interpretation.

Red Flags in Lab Results

Metabolic dysfunction warning signs:

- Fasting insulin over 8 µIU/mL
- Triglycerides over 150 mg/dL
- HDL under 40 mg/dL (men) or 50 mg/dL (women)
- Waist circumference over 35 inches (women) or 40 inches (men)
- Blood pressure consistently over 130/85
- Fasting glucose over 95 mg/dL

Don't wait for diabetes diagnosis: If you have several of these markers, you're likely developing insulin resistance and should take action immediately.

The Testing Schedule

Initial Baseline

Get comprehensive testing before making any major dietary or lifestyle changes so you have a true baseline to compare against.

Follow-up Testing

- **Basic markers:** Every 3-6 months while making changes
- **Advanced markers:** Every 6-12 months
- **Yearly comprehensive:** Full panel annually to track long-term trends

Adjust Based on Changes

If you're making significant dietary changes, more frequent testing can help you see what's working and what isn't.

What to Do with This Information

Don't Panic

Abnormal results are information, not a death sentence. Most metabolic dysfunction can be improved significantly with dietary and lifestyle changes.

Prioritize the Big Three

Focus on insulin resistance, inflammation, and nutrient deficiencies first. These underlying issues often improve multiple markers simultaneously.

Work with Knowledgeable Providers

Use this information to find providers who understand functional testing and can help you interpret results in context.

Track Your Progress

Regular testing allows you to see the impact of your changes and adjust your approach based on results.

The Bottom Line

The biomarkers your doctor routinely checks are designed to diagnose disease, not prevent it. By the time they show problems, you've often been developing metabolic dysfunction for years.

The markers we've discussed in this chapter can catch problems early when they're still reversible. They can also help you track your progress as you implement the changes outlined in this book.

Remember: optimal health isn't just the absence of disease—it's having energy, mental clarity, stable mood, and a body that functions well. The right biomarkers can help you achieve and maintain that level of health.

Don't wait for your doctor to order these tests. Take charge of your own health monitoring and use the information to make informed decisions about your wellness strategy.

Your body is constantly communicating with you. These biomarkers help you understand what it's trying to say—before it has to start shouting through symptoms and disease.

Next: How to transition to real food without losing your mind (or your social life)...

References:

1. Ravnskov U, Diamond DM, Hama R, et al. Lack of an association or an inverse association between low-density-lipoprotein cholesterol and mortality in the elderly: a systematic review. **BMJ Open.** 2016;6(6):e010401. doi:10.1136/bmjopen-2015-010401

2. Reaven GM. Insulin resistance: the link between obesity and cardiovascular disease. **Med Clin North Am.** 2011;95(5):875-892. doi:10.1016/j.mcna.2011.06.002

3. McLaughlin T, Reaven G, Abbasi F, et al. Use of metabolic markers to identify overweight individuals who are insulin resistant. **Ann Intern Med.** 2003;139(10):802-809. doi:10.7326/0003-4819-139-10-200311

180-00007

4. Goodman E. Interpreting Functional Lab Results. **Elissa Goodman** website. Published March 23, 2022. Accessed September 10, 2025. https://elissagoodman.com

Chapter Twenty-Seven

Transitioning to Real Food

Practical Implementation Strategies Without Losing Your Mind

You understand the problems with processed food. You know the research about metabolic health. You've found healthcare providers who won't sabotage your efforts. Now comes the hard part: actually changing what you eat in a world designed to make that as difficult as possible.

This isn't another "just eat real food" lecture. You already know you should eat real food. The challenge is figuring out how to do it consistently in a culture that profits from your poor health, with a food system that's deliberately confusing, while managing work, family, social obligations, and a lifetime of ingrained habits.

The Implementation Challenge

Why "Just Eat Real Food" Doesn't Work

Most nutrition advice treats food choices as if they happen in a vacuum. It assumes you have unlimited time, money, cooking skills, and willpower. It ignores the fact that you're fighting against:

- **Food industry manipulation** - Products designed to be irresistible and addictive
- **Social pressures** - Family, friends, and colleagues who think you're being extreme
- **Economic incentives** - Processed food is often cheaper and more con-

venient

- **Institutional obstacles** - Workplace cafeterias, school lunches, hospital food

- **Psychological factors** - Emotional eating, stress responses, ingrained habits

- **Information overload** - Conflicting advice from endless "experts"

Telling someone to "just eat real food" is like telling someone to "just be happy" or "just stop worrying." It's not actionable advice—it's a goal without a strategy.

The Transition Strategy: Phases, Not Perfection

Your 90-Day Health Transformation Roadmap

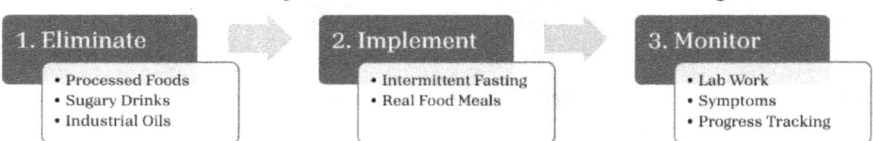

Phase 1: Elimination (Weeks 1-4)

Goal: Remove the worst offenders without trying to replace everything perfectly.

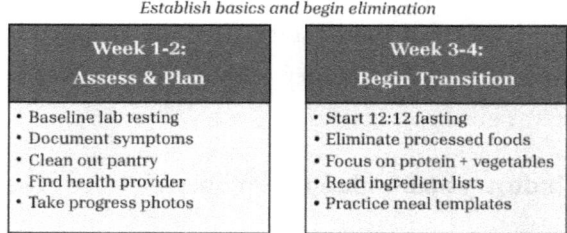

Priority removals:

1. **Sugary drinks** - Soda, fruit juice, sports drinks, flavored coffee drinks

2. **Industrial seed oils** - Anything with vegetable oil, canola oil, soybean

oil

3. **High-fructose corn syrup** - Read labels; it's in everything from bread to salad dressing

4. **Trans fats** - Anything with "partially hydrogenated" oils

5. **Artificial sweeteners** - Diet sodas, sugar-free products with aspartame, sucralose

Why these first: These are the most metabolically damaging and often the easiest to identify and eliminate.

Implementation strategy:

- Don't try to replace everything immediately
- Focus on removal, not substitution
- Read ingredient lists, not nutrition facts panels
- When in doubt, choose the option with fewer ingredients

Phase 2: Substitution (Weeks 5-8)

Goal: Replace processed foods with whole food alternatives.

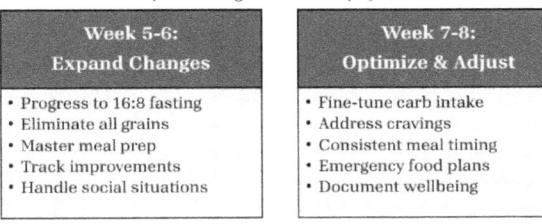

Key substitutions:

- **Grains and starches:** Replace with vegetables. Period. If you must keep some starches, white rice is less inflammatory than brown rice, but vegetables should be your default carbohydrate source.

- *Why:* All grains spike insulin and contribute to metabolic dysfunction. Your body doesn't need dietary carbohydrates to function optimally.

- **Snack foods:** Replace chips and crackers with nuts, seeds, cheese, or vegetables with fat

  - *Why:* Processed snacks are designed to be addictive and spike blood sugar. Protein and fat provide stable energy without metabolic disruption.

- **Breakfast foods:** Replace cereals and pastries with eggs, meat, or vegetables cooked in fat

  - *Why:* Starting your day with carbohydrates sets you up for blood sugar swings and cravings all day. Protein and fat provide sustained energy.

- **Cooking fats:** Replace industrial oils with butter, ghee, olive oil, avocado oil, or coconut oil

  - *Why:* Industrial seed oils are inflammatory and metabolically damaging. Traditional fats have sustained human health for millennia.

- **Sweeteners:** Eliminate all sweeteners if possible. If absolutely necessary, monk fruit is the least problematic option.

  - *Why:* Any sweet taste can trigger insulin responses and maintain sugar cravings. The goal is to retrain your palate away from sweetness.

Implementation strategy:

- Focus on one meal at a time

- Master breakfast first (it's usually the most routine)

- Prep ingredients in advance

- Don't aim for perfect meals, aim for better meals

Phase 3: Optimization (Weeks 9-12)

Goal: Fine-tune your approach based on how you feel and respond.

MONTH 3: Integration & Sustainability
Solidify systems and plan long-term

Week 9-10: System Refinement	Week 11-12: Long-term Planning
• Repeat lab testing • Adjust based on results • Solidify provider relationships • Master restaurant eating • Help interested family	• Create sustainable systems • Plan for challenges • Monitoring protocols • Document lessons learned • Set optimization goals

What to evaluate:

- Energy levels throughout the day
- Sleep quality and mood
- Hunger and satiety patterns
- Weight and body composition changes
- Digestive health
- Lab marker improvements

Potential adjustments:

- Carbohydrate timing and quantity
- Meal frequency and intermittent fasting
- Specific food sensitivities
- Supplement needs

The Shopping Revolution

Grocery Store Navigation

Rule #1: Shop the perimeter The healthiest foods are usually around the edges: produce, meat, dairy, eggs.

Rule #2: Read ingredient lists, not marketing claims

- "Natural," "healthy," and "organic" are marketing terms
- If you can't pronounce it, don't eat it
- More than 5 ingredients is usually a red flag

Rule #3: Price per nutrient, not price per calorie

- Grass-fed beef is expensive per pound but cheap per unit of nutrition
- Organic vegetables cost more but provide better nutrient density
- Processed foods seem cheap but are nutritionally bankrupt

Your Weekly Shopping Foundation

Proteins	Vegetables	Healthy Fats
• Grass-Fed Ground Beef	• Broccoli & Cauliflower	• Grass-Fed Butter
• Chicken Thighs/Breasts	• Spinach & Kale	• Extra Virgin Olive Oil
• Wild-Caught Fish	• Bell Peppers	• Avocados
• Pasture-Raised Eggs	• Zucchini & Squash	• Nuts & Seeds
• Organic Bacon/Sausage	• Brussels Sprouts	• Coconut Oil

The 80/20 Shopping List

80% of your cart should come from these categories:

Proteins:

- Grass-fed beef, lamb, bison
- Pasture-raised chicken, turkey, eggs

- Wild-caught fish and seafood
- Organ meats (if you're adventurous)

Fats:

- Avocados and avocado oil
- Olive oil (extra virgin, cold-pressed)
- Coconut oil and coconut products
- Nuts and seeds (almonds, walnuts, macadamias)
- Grass-fed butter or ghee

Vegetables:

- Leafy greens (spinach, kale, arugula)
- Cruciferous vegetables (broccoli, cauliflower, Brussels sprouts)
- Low-starch vegetables (zucchini, peppers, asparagus)
- Alliums (onions, garlic, leeks)

Optional carbohydrates (only if metabolically healthy and active):

- Sweet potatoes and squash (in small amounts)
- Berries (lowest sugar fruits)
- White rice (if you must have grains - less inflammatory than brown)

Important note: Most people with metabolic dysfunction should minimize or eliminate these entirely until their health markers improve significantly.

20% flexibility for:

- Social situations

- Family preferences
- Convenience items during busy periods
- Foods you're testing for tolerance

Meal Timing and Intermittent Fasting

Why When You Eat Matters

Constant eating is metabolically damaging:

- Keeps insulin elevated throughout the day
- Prevents fat burning and cellular repair processes
- Contributes to insulin resistance
- Disrupts natural hunger and satiety signals

Intermittent fasting is not optional for metabolic health - it's how humans naturally ate before food became available 24/7.

Starting with 12:12

Minimum recommendation: 12 hours without eating, 12-hour eating window

- Example: Stop eating at 7 PM, don't eat again until 7 AM
- *Why this works:* Allows insulin to drop and fat burning to begin

Benefits you'll notice:

- Better sleep (no late-night digestion)
- Clearer morning mental state
- Natural appetite regulation

- Improved energy stability

Progressing to 16:8

Once 12:12 feels easy, extend to 16:8:

- Example: Stop eating at 6 PM, first meal at 10 AM (or whatever schedule fits your life)

- *Why it's better:* Deeper metabolic benefits, enhanced fat burning, cellular cleanup (autophagy)[1]

A Natural Side Effect: Fewer Meals When you eat protein and fat instead of carbohydrates, you'll naturally feel satisfied longer. Many people find they naturally drop to two meals a day without effort or hunger.

Three meals a day is a modern invention, not a biological necessity. When you're eating foods that provide stable blood sugar, your body won't demand constant feeding.

Important: Don't use your eating window as an excuse to eat more carbohydrates. Quality still matters more than quantity. Additionally, people taking blood pressure medications, diabetes medications, or antidepressants should consult healthcare providers before making significant dietary changes or attempting intermittent fasting, as these interventions can affect medication requirements.

The Metabolically Optimal Approach

What Dr. Robert Lufkin and other metabolic health experts recommend:[2]

1. **Eggs** - Perfect protein with all essential amino acids

2. **Animal proteins** - Grilled, roasted, or slow-cooked (beef, fish, poultry)

3. **Low-carb vegetables** - Leafy greens, cruciferous vegetables, above-ground vegetables

4. **High-quality fats** - From animals and plants (butter, olive oil, avocados)

5. **Full-fat dairy** - If tolerated (cheese, heavy cream)

Why this order matters:

- **Protein stabilizes blood sugar** and provides building blocks for repair

- **Fat provides sustained energy** without insulin spikes

- **Vegetables provide nutrients** with minimal metabolic impact

- **This combination eliminates** the foods that drive insulin resistance and inflammation

Is this "extreme"? Not compared to the extreme processed food diet that's making everyone sick. This is how humans ate for thousands of years before chronic disease became epidemic.

The Template Approach

Instead of rigid meal plans, use flexible templates based on metabolic health principles:

Breakfast Template:

- Protein + vegetables + healthy fat (no carbohydrates)

- Examples: Eggs with spinach cooked in butter; leftover steak with sautéed mushrooms

- *Why:* Starting with protein and fat stabilizes blood sugar and prevents mid-morning crashes

Lunch Template:

- Protein + large salad + fat-based dressing

- Examples: Salmon salad with olive oil; chicken with avocado and greens
- *Why:* Maintains stable energy without the afternoon slump from carbohydrate crashes

Dinner Template:

- Protein + cooked vegetables + fat
- Examples: Grass-fed beef with roasted broccoli in butter; fish with asparagus
- *Why:* Provides satiety without disrupting sleep with blood sugar swings

Batch Cooking Strategies

Sunday prep that actually works:

- Cook large batches of protein (whole chickens, roasts, ground meat)
- Wash and chop vegetables for the week
- Make large batches of bone broth or soup
- Prepare grab-and-go snacks (hard-boiled eggs, cut vegetables)

Don't try to prep complete meals - prep components that can be combined differently throughout the week.

Dealing with Cravings and Withdrawal

What to Expect

Week 1-2: The withdrawal phase

- Intense cravings for sugar and processed foods
- Possible headaches, irritability, fatigue

- Sleep disruption
- Digestive changes

Week 3-4: The adaptation phase

- Cravings begin to diminish
- Energy starts to stabilize
- Sleep improves
- Digestive system adjusts

Week 5+: The optimization phase

- Stable energy without crashes
- Reduced cravings
- Improved mental clarity
- Better sleep and mood

Managing Cravings

Understand the difference:

- **Physical hunger:** Gradual onset, satisfied by any food, can wait
- **Cravings:** Sudden onset, specific food desires, urgent feeling

Strategies that work:

- Eat more protein and fat to increase satiety
- Stay hydrated (often we mistake thirst for hunger)
- Get adequate sleep (sleep deprivation increases cravings)

- Manage stress (cortisol drives food-seeking behavior)
- Have healthy alternatives readily available

Emergency protocols:

- Keep nuts, hard-boiled eggs, or other protein-rich snacks available
- When craving something sweet, try berries with full-fat cream
- When craving something crunchy, try vegetables with guacamole or hummus
- Remember: cravings are temporary and will pass

Social Situations and Family Dynamics

Navigating Social Pressure

Common responses and how to handle them:

"You're being too extreme"

- Response: "I'm just trying to feel better. This approach works for me."

"Everything in moderation"

- Response: "I've tried moderation and it didn't work for my body."

"You're no fun anymore"

- Response: "I'm actually having more fun now that I feel better."

"One bite won't hurt"

- Response: "Thanks, but I'm really satisfied with what I have."

Family Strategies

When you're cooking for others:

- Make the protein and vegetables the star; offer starches on the side
- Use cooking methods everyone enjoys (roasting, grilling)
- Focus on foods that are naturally appealing (who doesn't like bacon and eggs?)

When others are cooking:

- Offer to bring a dish you can eat
- Eat beforehand if necessary
- Focus on the social aspect, not the food

With children:

- Model good eating without making it a battle
- Involve them in shopping and cooking
- Don't turn food into reward/punishment systems
- Remember that children often need multiple exposures to accept new foods

Restaurant and Travel Strategies

Restaurant Navigation

Questions to ask:

- What oil do you cook with?
- Can you prepare this without the sauce/dressing on the side?
- Do you have any dishes that are just meat and vegetables?

Safe bets at most restaurants:

- Grilled or roasted meats and fish
- Salads with oil and vinegar dressing
- Vegetables prepared simply
- Eggs (for breakfast places)

Red flags:

- Anything fried (probably in industrial oils)
- Complicated sauces (often contain sugar and poor-quality oils)
- "Healthy" menu items (often highly processed)

Travel Planning

Pack portable foods:

- Nuts and seeds
- Beef jerky (check ingredients)
- Hard-boiled eggs
- Avocados

Research ahead:

- Find grocery stores near your destination
- Look up restaurants with real food options
- Consider booking accommodations with kitchen access

Don't let perfect be the enemy of good:

- Do your best with available options
- One meal or even one day won't derail your progress
- Get back to your normal routine as soon as possible

Budget-Friendly Real Food

Cost-Saving Strategies

Buy in bulk:

- Whole animals or large cuts of meat (often cheaper per pound)
- Frozen vegetables (just as nutritious as fresh, longer-lasting)
- Eggs (still one of the cheapest proteins available)

Use less expensive cuts:

- Ground meat instead of steaks
- Chicken thighs instead of breasts
- Tough cuts that become tender with slow cooking

Preserve and store properly:

- Freeze meat in meal-sized portions
- Use bone broth to add nutrients and flavor to simple meals
- Grow your own herbs and simple vegetables

Compare real costs:

- Factor in healthcare costs of staying sick
- Consider cost per nutrient, not just cost per calorie

- Remember that real food is more satisfying, so you may eat less overall

Troubleshooting Common Problems

"I Don't Have Time to Cook"

Solutions:

- Use a slow cooker or instant pot for hands-off cooking
- Cook large batches on weekends
- Keep meals simple—protein + vegetables + fat doesn't require complex recipes
- Redefine cooking—assembling salads and heating pre-cooked proteins counts

"My Family Won't Eat This Way"

Strategies:

- Start with foods everyone already likes
- Make gradual changes rather than dramatic overhauls
- Cook the same basic ingredients, but let others add grains or sauces
- Lead by example rather than trying to convert everyone

"I Feel Worse, Not Better"

Possible causes:

- Not eating enough overall calories
- Not eating enough salt (especially if cutting processed foods)

- Eating too much of foods you're sensitive to
- Not getting enough sleep or managing stress
- Underlying health issues that need professional attention

When to seek help:

- Symptoms persist beyond 4-6 weeks
- Severe digestive distress
- Significant mood changes
- Any concerning physical symptoms

Kitchen Setup for Success

Essential Equipment

You don't need a lot of fancy gadgets:

- Good knives and cutting board
- Cast iron or stainless steel pans (avoid non-stick coatings)
- Sheet pans for roasting
- Slow cooker or instant pot for convenience

Pantry Staples

Keep these on hand:

- Good quality salt (sea salt or pink salt)
- Herbs and spices for flavor variety

- Good cooking fats (coconut oil, avocado oil, butter)
- Canned fish (wild salmon, sardines)
- Nuts and seeds for quick proteins and snacks

Monitoring Your Progress

What to Track

Subjective measures (often change first):

- Energy levels and mood
- Sleep quality
- Hunger and satiety patterns
- Digestive comfort
- Mental clarity

Objective measures:

- Body composition (not just weight)
- Lab markers (as discussed in previous chapter)
- Blood pressure and resting heart rate
- Progress photos

Adjustments Based on Results

If you're not seeing improvements:

- Consider food sensitivities or intolerances

- Evaluate portion sizes and meal timing
- Look at stress management and sleep quality
- Consider working with a knowledgeable practitioner

If you're seeing good results:

- Don't fix what isn't broken
- Consider gradually increasing the strictness if you want further improvements
- Focus on making these changes sustainable long-term

The Long Game

Making It Sustainable

This isn't a diet—it's a way of eating for life:

- Build flexibility into your approach
- Don't aim for perfection, aim for consistency
- Develop cooking skills gradually
- Create systems that work with your lifestyle

Plan for setbacks:

- Holidays and celebrations
- Work travel and stress
- Family illnesses or emergencies
- Economic pressures

Remember why you started:

- Keep track of improvements in energy, mood, and health

- Remember how you felt when following conventional advice

- Focus on the positive changes, not just the restrictions

The Bottom Line

Transitioning to real food isn't just about changing what you eat—it's about changing how you think about food. Instead of seeing food as entertainment, comfort, or convenience, you start seeing it as fuel, medicine, and nourishment.

This transition takes time, patience, and often significant effort up front. But the payoff—stable energy, better mood, improved health markers, and freedom from food cravings—is worth the initial investment.

Start where you are, use what you have, do what you can. You don't need to transform everything overnight. Small, consistent changes compound over time into dramatic improvements in how you feel and function.

The food industry spent decades training you to eat processed foods. Give yourself at least a few months to retrain your palate, habits, and systems. Your body will thank you for the patience and persistence.

Next: How to handle the inevitable resistance from family, friends, and society when you start taking control of your health...

Chapter Twenty-Eight

Navigating Resistance

When Everyone Thinks You've Lost Your Mind

You've started eating real food, dropped the constant snacking, and maybe even skipped breakfast a few times. You're feeling better than you have in years. Your energy is stable, your mood is improving, and you're finally making progress on health goals that seemed impossible before.

Then it starts.

"You're being extreme." "That's not sustainable." "You need to eat breakfast—it's the most important meal of the day!" "Everything in moderation." "You're going to hurt yourself." "What about your cholesterol?"

Welcome to the resistance. It's coming from everywhere: family, friends, coworkers, and even healthcare providers who should know better. The better you feel, the more intense the pushback becomes.

This isn't accidental. You're threatening something much bigger than food choices—you're challenging the entire system that profits from keeping people sick and dependent.

Why the Resistance Is So Intense

You're Disrupting More Than Your Diet

When you change how you eat, you're inadvertently exposing several uncomfortable truths:

For your family and friends:

- Their food choices might be harming them
- The advice they've been following might be wrong
- Change is possible, which means their current situation isn't inevitable
- They might need to examine their own habits

For the medical system:

- Prevention might be more powerful than prescription drugs
- Lifestyle changes can reverse conditions they said were permanent
- Their expensive treatments might be unnecessary
- Their nutritional education might be inadequate

For the food industry:

- People can thrive without processed foods
- Addictive food design can be overcome
- Marketing claims about "healthy" foods might be false
- Profit margins on real food are lower than processed alternatives

For society generally:

- The obesity and diabetes epidemics might be preventable[1]
- Government dietary guidelines might be harmful[2]
- Individual responsibility might matter more than external interventions
- The healthcare crisis might have simple solutions

The Mirror Effect

Your success forces others to confront their own choices. When you're thriving on an approach they've been told is "dangerous" or "extreme," it creates cognitive dissonance. It's easier to convince you that you're wrong than to question everything they believe about health.

Types of Resistance You'll Encounter

The Concern Trolls

What they say: "I'm just worried about your health."

What they mean: Your success makes them uncomfortable about their own choices.

How to respond: "I appreciate your concern. I'm actually feeling the best I have in years, and my biomarkers are improving."

Don't engage with: Detailed explanations of why you're doing what you're doing. They're not genuinely interested in learning.

The False Experts

What they say: "My trainer/nutritionist/doctor says you need carbs for energy."

What they mean: I found an authority figure who validates my current beliefs.

How to respond: "Different approaches work for different people. This one is working well for me."

Don't engage with: Debates about whose expert is more credible. You can't logic someone out of a position they didn't logic themselves into.

The Moderation Police

What they say: "Everything in moderation" or "Life is too short not to enjoy food."

What they mean: Your discipline makes them feel bad about their lack of discipline.

How to respond: "I am enjoying food—probably more than I ever have. And I'm also enjoying having energy and feeling healthy."

Don't engage with: Philosophical debates about what constitutes "enjoyment" or "moderation."

The Saboteurs

What they do: Bring donuts to your office, push food on you at gatherings, make comments about your eating in front of others.

What they mean: If I can get you to break your commitment, I won't have to examine my own choices.

How to respond: Firm boundaries without explanations. "No thank you" is a complete sentence.

Don't engage with: Justifying your choices or trying to convince them you're right.

The Medical Gaslighters

What they say: "This is dangerous" or "You need to eat more carbohydrates" or "Your cholesterol will go up."

What they mean: This approach challenges everything I learned in medical school, and I'm not equipped to evaluate new information.

How to respond: "I'd like to monitor my biomarkers closely. Can we schedule follow-up testing in three months?"

Don't engage with: Trying to educate them about insulin resistance or metabolic health during an appointment. Find a different provider.

Strategic Responses for Common Situations

Family Dinners

The challenge: Family members who take your food choices as personal rejection.

Strategy:

- Focus on what you *can* eat rather than what you can't
- Bring dishes you can eat to share with everyone
- Emphasize that this isn't about them or their cooking
- Make it about your health, not their food choices

Sample response: "This looks wonderful. I'm just focusing on foods that make me feel my best right now. Can I have some of that chicken and salad?"

Work Situations

The challenge: Office food culture, team lunches, pressure to participate in food-based socializing.

Strategy:

- Be matter-of-fact, not defensive
- Focus on work performance improvements
- Don't make it about your coworkers' choices
- Have alternatives ready for social eating situations

Sample response: "I've been eating differently lately and it's really helping my energy levels. I'm going to stick with what works for me."

Social Gatherings

The challenge: Friends who think you're being antisocial or difficult.

Strategy:

- Eat before you go if necessary
- Focus on the social aspect, not the food
- Bring something you can eat to share
- Don't make your eating the center of attention

Sample response: "I'm here to spend time with you, not for the food. How have you been?"

Healthcare Appointments

The challenge: Providers who are hostile to dietary approaches that contradict their training.

Strategy:

- Lead with results, not methodology
- Request specific tests to monitor progress
- Don't try to convert them during your appointment
- Find new providers if they're unsupportive

Sample response: "I've been making some dietary changes and feeling much better. I'd like to monitor my blood work to make sure everything is moving in the right direction."

The Psychology of Resistance

Understanding the Real Issue

It's not about the food. The resistance you're facing is about:

- Fear of change
- Cognitive dissonance
- Social conformity pressure
- Economic interests
- Identity threats
- Control issues

Why Logic Doesn't Work

You can't logic someone out of an emotional position. When people resist your choices, they're not making rational arguments—they're expressing emotional discomfort with what your success implies about their situation.

Don't try to convince anyone. Your job is to take care of your health, not to convert others to your approach.

Boundary Setting Strategies

The Broken Record Technique

Pick a simple response and repeat it verbatim:

- "This approach works for me."
- "I'm feeling great with these changes."

- "My doctor and I are monitoring my progress."

Don't elaborate. Don't justify. Don't explain. Just repeat your chosen phrase.

The Information Diet

Stop sharing details about your eating approach unless someone specifically asks for help. Your eating choices don't need to be a topic of conversation.

Share results, not methods. If people comment on how you look or your energy, thank them. You don't need to explain how you achieved it.

The Subject Change

Master the art of redirection:

- "Thanks for your concern. How are things with you?"
- "I appreciate you thinking of me. Did you see that game last night?"
- "That's sweet of you to worry. How's your project going?"

When to Engage vs. When to Disengage

Signs Someone Is Genuinely Interested

- They ask specific questions about your experience
- They want to know about resources or books you've found helpful
- They're dealing with health issues they can't solve
- They ask for your advice rather than giving you theirs
- They're willing to consider that conventional advice might be wrong

Signs Someone Is Just Resisting

- They immediately list reasons why your approach won't work
- They cite authorities or studies without actually reading them
- They make it about their concern for your health rather than their own curiosity
- They argue with your personal experience
- They become emotional or defensive when you share your results

The "Don't Engage" List

Never try to convince:

- People who are emotionally invested in being right
- Family members who take your choices as personal criticism
- Healthcare providers during appointments (find better ones instead)
- Anyone who starts their response with "But..."
- People who ask questions just to argue with your answers

Handling Specific Accusations

"You're Being Extreme"

Response: "Eating the way humans ate for thousands of years isn't extreme. What's extreme is the processed food diet that's making everyone sick."[3]

Or simply: "This works for my body."

"That's Not Sustainable"

Response: "I'm not trying to sustain anything except my health. This approach is working well for me."

Internal reality: It's actually much more sustainable than the constant hunger and cravings from processed foods.

"You Need Balance"

Response: "I am balanced. I have more energy and feel better than I have in years."

Internal reality: There's nothing "balanced" about eating foods that make you sick.

"What About Your Social Life?"

Response: "My social life is better than ever. Turns out people like spending time with me when I have energy and feel good."

Internal reality: Real friends care about your wellbeing, not whether you eat their food.

"You're Going to Develop an Eating Disorder"

Response: "I'm actually developing a healthy relationship with food for the first time in my life."

Internal reality: Eating disorders involve obsession, guilt, and loss of control. This approach typically reduces all three.

Building Your Support Network

Finding Your Tribe

Look for:

- Online communities focused on metabolic health

- Local groups interested in real food
- Healthcare providers who understand functional medicine
- Friends and family members who support your health goals
- People who are results-oriented rather than dogma-oriented

Avoid:

- Groups that focus on food restriction rather than health optimization
- People who make dietary choices into moral issues
- Communities that demonize anyone who thinks differently
- Support groups that focus on problems rather than solutions

Creating Supportive Relationships

With family:

- Lead by example rather than trying to convert them
- Focus on how you feel rather than what you eat
- Cook foods that everyone can enjoy
- Don't make food choices a source of family conflict

With friends:

- Suggest activities that don't revolve around food
- Be flexible about social eating when it matters
- Find friends who care about your wellbeing
- Don't let food become a barrier to relationships that matter

With coworkers:

- Keep your eating approach private unless asked
- Focus on work performance improvements
- Don't become the "food police" in your office
- Pack your own food and don't comment on others' choices

The Long-Term Perspective

Consistency Speaks Louder Than Arguments

Your results will do the talking. After months or years of sustained energy, better health markers, and improved quality of life, the resistance will start to fade. Some people will even start asking for advice.

Becoming a Quiet Example

Don't evangelize. Just live well. When people see you thriving over time, they'll start to question their own assumptions. Your consistent wellbeing is more persuasive than any argument.

Handling Success

As you get healthier, the resistance may actually intensify before it diminishes. Success threatens people's beliefs more than failure does. Be prepared for this and don't let it derail your progress.

Emergency Protocols

When You're Tempted to Give In

Remember why you started:

- How you felt when following conventional advice
- The energy and mental clarity you've gained
- The health improvements you've seen
- The freedom from constant hunger and cravings

Have a support system ready:

- People you can text when you're struggling
- Online communities where you can vent safely
- Healthcare providers who understand your approach
- Books or resources that reinforce your knowledge

When Family Events Become Battlegrounds

Strategies for high-stakes situations:

- Eat beforehand so you're not hungry
- Bring food you can eat to share
- Have an exit strategy if things get heated
- Remember that one meal won't destroy your progress
- Focus on relationships, not food choices

When Healthcare Providers Undermine You

Protect your progress:

- Don't let them shame you back into failed approaches
- Request specific tests rather than accepting general advice

- Find providers who understand metabolic health

- Remember that you're the expert on how you feel

- Don't let medical degrees override your personal experience

The Bottom Line

The resistance you face when changing your diet isn't really about food—it's about challenging systems, beliefs, and identities that people have invested in heavily. Your success threatens those investments.

You don't need anyone's permission to take care of your health. You don't need to convince anyone that your approach is right. You don't need to defend your choices to people who aren't genuinely interested in understanding them.

Your job is simple: Take care of your health, monitor your progress, and let your results speak for themselves. The people who matter will support your efforts to feel better. The people who don't support your health improvements probably shouldn't have much influence over your life decisions anyway.

Remember: The same voices telling you to "be reasonable" and "eat in moderation" are often the same voices that got you into health trouble in the first place. Trust your experience over their opinions.

The resistance is temporary. Your health improvements are lasting.

Next: Emergency protocols—when conventional medicine is actually necessary and how to navigate it without derailing your progress...

References

1. Ludwig DS, Ebbeling CB. The carbohydrate-insulin model of obesity: beyond "calories in, calories out." *JAMA Intern Med.*

2018;178(8):1098-1103. doi:10.1001/jamainternmed.2018.2933

2. Teicholz N. *The Big Fat Surprise: Why Butter, Meat and Cheese Belong in a Healthy Diet.* New York, NY: Simon & Schuster; 2014.

3. Cordain L, Eaton SB, Sebastian A, et al. Origins and evolution of the Western diet: health implications for the 21st century. *Am J Clin Nutr.* 2005;81(2):341-354. doi:10.1093/ajcn/81.2.341

Chapter Twenty-Nine

Emergency Protocols

When Conventional Medicine Is Actually Necessary

Let's be clear: this book is not anti-medicine. It's pro-appropriate medicine. There are times when conventional medical intervention is not just helpful—it's lifesaving. The key is knowing when you need it, how to navigate it, and how to maintain your health improvements while dealing with medical emergencies or acute conditions.

The goal isn't to avoid doctors forever. It's to use the medical system strategically while maintaining the metabolic health improvements you've worked so hard to achieve.

When You Absolutely Need Conventional Medicine

True Medical Emergencies

Don't hesitate to seek immediate medical care for:

- Chest pain or heart attack symptoms
- Stroke symptoms (sudden weakness, speech changes, vision changes)
- Severe injuries requiring surgery
- Acute infections that aren't responding to rest and supportive care
- Diabetic ketoacidosis or other metabolic emergencies

- Severe allergic reactions
- Any condition where delay could result in permanent damage or death

Your dietary approach is irrelevant in these situations. Get the care you need immediately.

Acute Conditions Requiring Medical Management

Situations where medical intervention is appropriate:

- Bacterial infections requiring antibiotics
- Broken bones requiring setting or surgery
- Acute appendicitis or other surgical emergencies
- Severe pneumonia or other respiratory infections
- Blood clots requiring anticoagulation
- Mental health crises requiring immediate intervention

The principle: When your body's normal healing mechanisms are overwhelmed or when structural repair is needed, conventional medicine excels.

Chronic Conditions Requiring Careful Monitoring

Some conditions require ongoing medical supervision even while optimizing lifestyle:

- Type 1 diabetes (though dietary approaches can reduce insulin needs)
- Severe heart disease (lifestyle can improve outcomes but may need medication management)
- Advanced kidney disease
- Autoimmune conditions requiring immunosuppressive medications

- Cancer treatment
- Certain hormonal disorders

The approach: Work with knowledgeable providers to optimize lifestyle factors while maintaining necessary medical treatments.

Preparing for Medical Interactions

Documentation Strategy

Keep detailed records of:

- Your current medication list (including supplements)
- Recent lab results and trends
- Your dietary approach and how long you've been following it
- Any health improvements you've experienced
- Contact information for your regular healthcare providers

Why this matters: Emergency providers need accurate information quickly, and your regular approach to health may affect treatment decisions.

Medical Information Summary

Create a one-page summary that includes:

- Current health status and improvements
- Medications and supplements you're taking
- Any drug allergies or sensitivities
- Your primary care provider's contact information

- Any specific concerns about standard treatments

Keep copies: In your wallet, on your phone, and with emergency contacts.

Communication Strategy

Be strategic about what you share:

- Focus on medical facts, not dietary philosophy
- Emphasize your commitment to monitoring and follow-up
- Avoid arguing about approaches during emergency situations
- Save dietary discussions for non-urgent appointments

Navigating Hospital Stays

Food Challenges

Hospital food is notoriously problematic - high in processed carbohydrates, industrial oils, and sugar. Here's how to handle it:

If you're able to eat:

- Request the "diabetic" or "cardiac" diet (often slightly better options)
- Ask family to bring allowed foods from outside
- Focus on any protein and vegetables available
- Avoid the bread, desserts, and processed items

If you're NPO (nothing by mouth):

- This is temporary - don't stress about breaking your routine
- Focus on healing rather than perfect nutrition

- Resume your normal eating as soon as medically cleared

IV nutrition concerns:

- Most IV fluids contain dextrose (sugar)
- This is medically necessary in many situations
- Don't fight this during acute illness
- Your body can handle short-term glucose administration

Medication Interactions

Common concerns with metabolic health approaches:

Blood sugar medications:

- Your dietary approach may lower blood sugar
- Monitor glucose carefully if you're on diabetes medications
- Work with providers to adjust medications as needed
- Don't stop medications without medical supervision

Blood pressure medications:

- Dietary changes often improve blood pressure
- Monitor readings regularly
- May need medication adjustments as health improves
- Discuss changes with your provider, don't adjust on your own

Cholesterol medications:

- Providers may be concerned about dietary fat intake

- Focus on your actual lab results, not theoretical concerns
- Request comprehensive lipid panels, not just basic cholesterol
- Be prepared to find providers who understand advanced testing

Surgery and Recovery

Pre-surgery preparation:

- Continue your normal eating until instructed to fast
- Your metabolic health may improve surgical outcomes[1]
- Discuss any supplements with your surgical team
- Don't make dramatic dietary changes right before surgery

Post-surgery recovery:

- Protein is crucial for healing
- Don't worry about perfect macronutrient ratios during acute recovery
- Resume your normal approach as soon as medically appropriate
- Focus on nutrient-dense foods to support healing

Working with Hospital Staff

Nursing Staff Communication

Nurses often have more time for discussion than doctors:

- Explain your normal eating pattern briefly
- Ask for help identifying the best available food options

- Request to speak with a dietitian if concerned about meal plans

- Be polite but firm about your dietary needs

What to emphasize:

- Your commitment to following medical advice

- Your desire to support healing through good nutrition

- Your willingness to work within hospital constraints

- Your understanding that some compromises may be necessary

Physician Communication

During hospital rounds:

- Keep discussions brief and focused

- Lead with your commitment to recovery

- Ask specific questions about medication interactions

- Save dietary philosophy discussions for later

Sample approach: "I've been following a low-carbohydrate diet that's improved my metabolic health. Are there any concerns with my current medications, and how should I adjust as I recover?"

Discharge Planning

Before leaving the hospital:

- Get clear instructions about medication changes

- Ask about activity restrictions

- Understand follow-up appointment schedules

- Get contact information for questions

Medication reconciliation:

- Review all medications with discharge staff
- Understand which are new, which are temporary, and which are ongoing
- Ask about interactions with supplements you normally take
- Get written instructions for any dosage changes

Medication Management

Working with Necessary Medications

Don't view medications as failure:

- Some conditions require pharmaceutical intervention
- Lifestyle optimization can often reduce medication needs over time
- Work with providers to find the minimum effective doses
- Monitor for side effects and discuss alternatives when appropriate

Reducing Medications Safely

As your health improves, you may need fewer medications:

Blood pressure medications:

- Monitor readings regularly at home
- Work with providers to reduce doses gradually
- Never stop suddenly (can cause rebound hypertension)

- Track improvements in a log to share with providers

Diabetes medications:

- Monitor blood sugar carefully with dietary changes
- Work with providers familiar with low-carb approaches
- May need rapid adjustments to prevent hypoglycemia
- Consider continuous glucose monitoring during transitions

Other medications:

- Discuss reduction plans with prescribing providers
- Make changes gradually under medical supervision
- Antidepressant discontinuation requires gradual tapering to prevent withdrawal syndrome.
- Monitor for return of symptoms
- Have a plan for increasing doses if needed

Supplement Interactions

Common interactions to be aware of:

Blood thinning effects:

- Fish oil, vitamin E, and some herbs can increase bleeding risk
- Important before surgery or if taking anticoagulants
- Discuss with providers before procedures

Blood pressure effects:

- Magnesium and potassium can lower blood pressure

- May enhance effects of blood pressure medications
- Monitor readings carefully

Blood sugar effects:

- Chromium, alpha-lipoic acid, and berberine can lower blood sugar
- Important if taking diabetes medications
- May need medication adjustments

Specialist Consultations

Preparing for Specialist Visits

Cardiologists:

- Bring comprehensive lipid panels, not just basic cholesterol
- Focus on inflammatory markers and metabolic health
- Be prepared to discuss particle size and particle number
- Emphasize improvements in blood pressure and other risk factors

Endocrinologists:

- Document blood sugar improvements if diabetic
- Track insulin sensitivity changes
- Monitor thyroid function if relevant
- Discuss hormone optimization approaches

Gastroenterologists:

- Track digestive improvements with dietary changes

- Document any food sensitivities or intolerances
- Discuss microbiome health and inflammation
- Be prepared to explain elimination diets if relevant

Finding Specialists Who Understand

Look for providers who:

- Understand metabolic health and nutrition
- Are open to lifestyle interventions
- Monitor comprehensive biomarkers
- Support patient empowerment and education

Red flags in specialists:

- Dismiss dietary approaches without consideration
- Focus only on medications without lifestyle discussion
- Refuse to monitor comprehensive labs
- Become defensive when questioned about standard treatments

Mental Health Considerations

Stress and Anxiety During Medical Issues

Health crises can trigger anxiety about:

- Losing progress you've made
- Being forced back into unhealthy patterns

- Medical providers undermining your approach

- Family pressure to "just follow doctor's orders"

Coping strategies:

- Remember that temporary medical interventions don't erase long-term progress

- Focus on what you can control in the current situation

- Maintain perspective about short-term vs. long-term health

- Seek support from people who understand your approach

Depression and Mood Changes

Medical issues can affect mood through:

- Disrupted sleep and routine

- Inflammatory effects of illness or surgery

- Medication side effects

- Stress about health and recovery

Protective factors:

- Maintain good nutrition as much as possible within medical constraints

- Prioritize sleep and stress management

- Stay connected with supportive people

- Consider counseling if struggling with adjustment

Recovery and Returning to Normal

Post-Illness Recovery

Gradually resume your normal approach:

- Start with gentle foods that are easy to digest
- Gradually increase back to your normal eating pattern
- Don't rush back to intensive fasting or exercise
- Listen to your body's recovery needs

Monitor your progress:

- Track energy levels and how you're feeling
- Resume regular lab monitoring
- Note any changes in your response to foods
- Adjust your approach based on how you're recovering

Learning from Medical Experiences

Use medical interactions to improve your approach:

- What providers were most helpful and knowledgeable?
- What gaps in your preparation became apparent?
- How can you better communicate your approach in the future?
- What backup plans do you need for future medical situations?

Building a Medical Emergency Plan

Create Your Medical Team

Primary care provider: Someone who understands and supports your metabolic health approach

Emergency contacts: Include providers who know your history and approach

Specialist backup: Know which specialists in your area are open to lifestyle approaches

Pharmacy relationship: Find pharmacists who understand supplement interactions

Emergency Information Kit

Keep readily accessible:

- Current medication and supplement list
- Recent lab results
- Medical history summary
- Emergency contact information
- Insurance information
- Advance directives if applicable

Family Education

Make sure family members understand:

- Your normal approach to health and why you follow it
- When to seek emergency care vs. when to support home recovery
- How to communicate your approach to medical providers
- Your preferences for medical decision-making

The Bottom Line

Conventional medicine excels at acute care, emergency interventions, and managing severe disease. Your metabolic health approach excels at preventing disease and optimizing long-term health. They're not mutually exclusive—they're complementary when used appropriately.

The key principles:

- Use conventional medicine for acute care and emergencies
- Maintain your metabolic health approach for prevention and optimization
- Work with providers who understand both approaches
- Don't let perfect be the enemy of good during medical crises
- Resume your normal approach as soon as medically appropriate

Remember: Taking antibiotics for a bacterial infection doesn't negate months of metabolic health improvements. Having surgery doesn't erase the benefits of insulin sensitivity. Temporary compromises during medical treatment don't require permanent abandonment of your health optimization approach.

Your job is to be a smart consumer of medical care—using it when you need it, avoiding it when you don't, and maintaining your health improvements through both scenarios.

The goal isn't to avoid all medical intervention. The goal is to need less of it over time while being prepared to use it effectively when necessary.

Finally: How to raise healthy children and break generational cycles of poor health...

Reference

1. Cassie S, Menezes C, Birch DW, Xinzhe Shi, Shahzeer Karmali. Effect of preoperative weight loss in bariatric surgical patients: a systematic review. *Surg Obes Relat Dis.* 2011 Nov-Dec;7(6):760-767. doi:10.1016/j.soard.2011.08.011

Chapter Thirty

Raising Healthy Children

Breaking Generational Cycles of Poor Health

You've taken control of your own health. You understand the problems with processed food, you've found healthcare providers who support your approach, and you're seeing real improvements in how you feel and function. Now comes perhaps the most important question: How do you give your children the metabolic health advantages you wish you'd had?

This isn't about putting children on restrictive diets or creating food anxiety. It's about normalizing real food, establishing healthy patterns early, and protecting children from the metabolic damage that leads to a lifetime of chronic disease.

The stakes couldn't be higher. For the first time in modern history, children are expected to have shorter lifespans than their parents[1]. Childhood obesity, type 2 diabetes, and fatty liver disease—once extremely rare in children—are now common. The metabolic dysfunction that took decades to develop in previous generations is now appearing in elementary school children.

But you have the power to change this trajectory for your family.

The Childhood Metabolic Health Crisis

What's Different Now

Children today face metabolic challenges that previous generations never experienced:

- Ultra-processed foods designed to be irresistible to developing brains

- Constant access to high-sugar, high-carbohydrate foods

- Marketing specifically targeting children with addictive food products

- School meal programs built around processed foods and food industry donations

- Reduced physical activity and increased screen time

- Sleep disruption from overstimulation and blue light exposure

Early Warning Signs

Metabolic dysfunction in children often appears as:

- Difficulty concentrating or ADHD-like symptoms

- Mood swings and behavioral problems

- Frequent illnesses or slow recovery from illness

- Sleep problems or difficulty waking up

- Skin issues like acne or eczema

- Early puberty or delayed development

- Weight gain or difficulty maintaining healthy weight

- Constant hunger or food cravings

- Dental problems despite good hygiene

These aren't just "normal childhood issues"—they're often signs of metabolic dysfunction that can be addressed with dietary changes.

Age-Appropriate Strategies

Infants and Toddlers (0-3 years)

This is the most critical period for establishing metabolic health patterns.

Breastfeeding advantages:

- Provides optimal nutrition for brain development
- Establishes healthy gut microbiome
- Reduces risk of obesity and metabolic dysfunction later in life[2]
- Creates natural eating patterns based on hunger and satiety

First foods strategy:

- Skip baby cereals and processed baby foods
- Start with nutrient-dense whole foods (avocado, egg yolk, soft-cooked vegetables)
- Avoid fruit juices and sweetened foods entirely
- Let children explore textures and flavors without forcing consumption
- Don't use food as entertainment or comfort

What to avoid:

- Baby cereals and processed baby foods
- Fruit juices (even "natural" ones)
- Crackers, puffs, and processed snack foods
- Using food to stop crying or as rewards
- Forcing children to "clean their plate"

Preschoolers (3-6 years)

Goals at this age:

- Establish real food as normal and desirable
- Develop natural hunger and satiety cues
- Create positive associations with family meals
- Begin simple food preparation involvement

Practical strategies:

- Serve family meals with slight modifications for children (less spice, softer textures)
- Include children in grocery shopping and food preparation
- Make vegetables and proteins the stars of meals
- Offer choices between healthy options ("Would you like broccoli or asparagus?")
- Don't become a short-order cook making separate meals

Handling resistance:

- Children may need 10+ exposures to a food before accepting it
- Don't force eating, but don't offer alternatives
- Keep offering refused foods without pressure
- Model enjoyment of healthy foods yourself
- Stay calm about food battles—they're temporary

School-Age Children (6-12 years)

New challenges emerge:

- Peer pressure and social eating situations
- School meal programs with poor food options
- Marketing and advertising targeting children
- Birthday parties and social events centered around processed foods
- Increased independence and food choices

Education strategies:

- Teach children about how food affects their energy and mood
- Explain why their family eats differently without demonizing other families
- Help them understand marketing tricks used by food companies
- Involve them in meal planning and preparation
- Give them language to use in social situations

School navigation:

- Pack lunches with foods your child enjoys and that travel well
- Communicate with teachers about classroom food policies
- Volunteer for school events to influence food choices when possible
- Teach children how to make the best choices from available options
- Don't make school food battles more important than your child's social relationships

Teenagers (13+ years)

The ultimate test of the foundation you've built. Teenagers will make their own food choices, often in opposition to parental preferences.

Strategies for success:

- Focus on how food affects performance (sports, academics, appearance)
- Respect their growing autonomy while maintaining family meal traditions
- Stock the house with healthy options they actually like
- Avoid food battles that damage your relationship
- Trust the foundation you've built during earlier years

Common teenage challenges:

- Peer pressure to eat like friends
- Desire to rebel against family food rules
- Busy schedules that promote convenience eating
- Body image concerns that may lead to restriction or overconsumption
- Limited cooking skills and independence

Creating a Healthy Food Environment

Kitchen and Pantry Setup

Make healthy choices the easy choices:

- Keep processed foods out of the house (you can't eat what isn't there)
- Stock plenty of real food options that children enjoy
- Prepare healthy snacks in advance (cut vegetables, hard-boiled eggs, nuts)
- Make water the default beverage

- Keep fruit available but don't make it the primary snack

Age-appropriate food access:

- Toddlers: Healthy foods at their eye level and reach
- School-age: Pre-portioned healthy snacks they can grab independently
- Teenagers: Ingredients and skills to prepare their own healthy meals

Family Meal Strategies

Make family meals a priority:

- Aim for at least one family meal per day
- Turn off screens during meals
- Focus on conversation and connection, not food policing
- Include children in meal planning and preparation
- Model enjoyment of healthy foods

Meal composition for families:

- Protein as the centerpiece (meat, fish, eggs)
- Vegetables prepared in appealing ways (roasted with butter, grilled, etc.)
- Healthy fats (avocado, olive oil, nuts)
- Optional starches served on the side for family members who want them

Handling Social Situations

Birthday Parties and Social Events

Teaching balance without compromise:

- Discuss strategies beforehand ("eat the protein from the pizza, skip the cake")
- Focus on the social aspect rather than the food
- Don't make your child feel different or deprived
- Have them eat something nutritious before going to events where food options are poor
- Teach them that occasional poor food choices won't ruin their health

Sample language for children:

- "I'm not hungry right now, thanks"
- "My stomach feels better when I eat different foods"
- "I brought my own snack that I really like"
- "This looks great, but I'm saving room for dinner"

School Challenges

Working within the system:

- Pack lunches when possible
- Teach children to identify better options in school cafeterias
- Communicate with teachers about classroom food rewards and celebrations
- Volunteer for school events to influence food choices
- Focus on long-term patterns, not daily perfection

Lunch packing strategies:

- Include foods your child will actually eat
- Make lunches appealing and easy to eat
- Include some foods that don't require heating or refrigeration
- Ask your child for input on lunch preferences
- Don't pack foods that will embarrass your child socially

Extended Family and Caregivers

Managing different food philosophies:

- Communicate your family's approach clearly but respectfully
- Focus on health rather than rules ("These foods help our family feel our best")
- Pick your battles—don't let food become a relationship destroyer
- Provide healthy alternatives when your children are in others' care
- Trust that occasional exposure to processed foods won't undo your foundation

Addressing Common Parental Concerns

"My Child Is Too Thin/Too Heavy"

Focus on health, not weight:

- Children's weight naturally fluctuates during growth
- Metabolically healthy children will find their natural weight
- Restricting food can create unhealthy relationships with eating

- Adding processed foods to increase weight often causes metabolic problems

- Work with healthcare providers who understand childhood nutrition

Signs of healthy development:

- Consistent energy levels throughout the day

- Good sleep patterns

- Normal growth velocity (not necessarily size)

- Stable mood and behavior

- Good immune function

"My Child Won't Eat Vegetables"

Practical solutions:

- Start with vegetables they can tolerate and gradually expand

- Include them in vegetable preparation and gardening

- Serve vegetables with fats and flavors they enjoy (butter, cheese, salt)

- Don't make vegetables a battle—keep offering without pressure

- Remember that some children are naturally more sensitive to certain tastes

Alternative approaches:

- Hide vegetables in foods they already like (cauliflower in mac and cheese)

- Start with sweeter vegetables (carrots, sweet potatoes)

- Try different preparation methods (roasted vs. steamed vs. raw)

- Make vegetables part of dishes rather than separate sides
- Consider that some children do fine with fewer vegetables if they're eating nutrient-dense animal foods

"My Child Has ADHD/Behavioral Issues"

Dietary factors that can affect behavior:

- Blood sugar swings from processed carbohydrates
- Food additives and artificial colors
- Food sensitivities or intolerances
- Nutrient deficiencies (especially B vitamins, magnesium, omega-3s)
- Poor sleep quality affected by diet

Working with healthcare providers:

- Find providers who understand nutrition's role in behavior
- Consider elimination diets to identify trigger foods
- Monitor the relationship between food intake and behavioral symptoms
- Don't abandon necessary medical treatments, but optimize nutrition alongside them

"My Child Is Constantly Hungry"

This often indicates blood sugar instability:

- Increase protein and fat in meals and snacks
- Eliminate or reduce processed carbohydrates that spike blood sugar
- Ensure adequate calorie intake from nutrient-dense foods

- Consider meal timing and frequency adjustments
- Address any underlying health issues with appropriate providers

Building Food Skills and Knowledge

Age-Appropriate Cooking Involvement

Toddlers (2-4 years):

- Washing vegetables and fruits
- Stirring ingredients in bowls
- Tearing lettuce for salads
- Simple measuring with supervision

School-age (5-12 years):

- Basic knife skills with appropriate supervision
- Following simple recipes
- Understanding basic cooking methods
- Planning meals and making grocery lists

Teenagers (13+ years):

- Independent meal preparation
- Understanding nutrition and how food affects the body
- Budget-conscious shopping and meal planning
- Cooking for the family occasionally

Teaching Food Literacy

Help children understand:

- How to read ingredient lists
- The difference between real food and processed food products
- How different foods affect energy, mood, and performance
- Basic nutrition principles without obsessive detail
- How to make good choices in various situations

Avoid:

- Labeling foods as "good" or "bad" in moralistic terms
- Creating guilt or shame around food choices
- Obsessive calorie counting or macro tracking
- Using food as reward or punishment
- Making children responsible for family members' food choices

Special Considerations

Children with Medical Conditions

Type 1 Diabetes:

- Low-carb approaches can significantly reduce insulin needs[3]
- Work with endocrinologists who understand nutritional management
- Monitor blood sugars carefully during dietary transitions
- Teach children to manage their condition with food choices

ADHD and Behavioral Issues:

- Eliminate artificial additives and colors
- Consider elimination diets to identify trigger foods
- Ensure stable blood sugar through protein and fat intake
- Work with providers who understand nutrition's role in brain function

Digestive Issues:

- Consider food sensitivities and intolerances
- Focus on gut-healing foods (bone broth, fermented foods)
- Avoid inflammatory foods (processed grains, industrial oils)
- Work with practitioners who understand functional gut health

Eating Disorders Prevention

Creating a healthy relationship with food:

- Focus on health and how food makes you feel, not appearance or weight
- Avoid diet mentality or restriction language
- Don't use food as emotional regulation tool
- Model balanced attitudes toward food and body image
- Teach children to trust their hunger and satiety cues

Warning signs to watch for:

- Obsessive food restrictions beyond family health guidelines
- Excessive exercise or compensatory behaviors

- Preoccupation with body size or weight
- Social withdrawal around food situations
- Mood changes related to eating or food choices

Working with Schools and Other Institutions

Advocating for Better School Food

Strategies that work:

- Volunteer for school wellness committees
- Bring nutrition expertise to parent-teacher organizations
- Advocate for policies that reduce classroom food rewards
- Support farm-to-school programs when possible
- Focus on student performance and health outcomes

What doesn't work:

- Attacking school staff or administrators
- Making demands without offering solutions
- Ignoring budget and practical constraints
- Creating division among parents over food philosophy

Sports and Activities

Optimizing performance through nutrition:

- Focus on real food for sustained energy rather than sports drinks and energy bars

- Teach children that good nutrition enhances athletic performance
- Work with coaches who understand performance nutrition
- Avoid the sports culture of junk food rewards and team celebrations

The Long-Term Perspective

Building Independence

The goal is raising adults who:

- Understand how food affects their health and performance
- Can prepare nutritious meals for themselves and their families
- Make good food choices independently
- Have a healthy relationship with food without obsession or restriction
- Can navigate social food situations confidently

Measuring Success

Success looks like:

- Children who choose healthy foods when given options
- Family meals that everyone enjoys
- Children who understand the connection between food and how they feel
- Reduced illness and stable energy in your children
- Positive relationships with food that don't involve guilt or shame

Success doesn't require:

- Perfect compliance with family food guidelines
- Children who never eat processed foods
- Conflict-free food relationships at all times
- Other families adopting your approach
- Children who proselytize about nutrition to their friends

Practical Implementation

Starting Where You Are

If your children are already used to processed foods:

- Make gradual changes rather than dramatic overhauls
- Start with foods they already like in healthier versions
- Involve them in the process of improving family nutrition
- Focus on addition before subtraction (add vegetables before removing desserts)
- Be patient—taste preferences can change over time

Weekly Planning

Make healthy eating easier:

- Plan meals that work for the whole family
- Prep vegetables and proteins in advance
- Keep healthy snacks readily available
- Involve children in meal planning and preparation

- Have backup plans for busy days

Budget Considerations

Healthy food on a budget:

- Buy whole chickens and use every part
- Focus on eggs as an affordable protein source
- Buy frozen vegetables when fresh is too expensive
- Use less expensive cuts of meat in slow-cooker meals
- Grow simple vegetables if you have space

The Generational Impact

Breaking Family Patterns

Many parents are breaking cycles of:

- Poor food relationships modeled by their own parents
- Using food for emotional regulation
- Diet mentality and weight obsession
- Accepting poor health as inevitable
- Lacking knowledge about nutrition and cooking

Creating New Family Traditions

Establish traditions that support health:

- Family cooking and meal preparation

- Gardening and food sourcing
- Active family recreation rather than food-centered entertainment
- Teaching children about their food choices and their effects
- Celebrating with experiences rather than just food

The Ripple Effect

Children who grow up with metabolic health advantages will:

- Have better academic and athletic performance
- Experience fewer chronic health issues
- Develop better decision-making skills around food
- Pass healthy patterns on to their own children
- Require less medical intervention throughout their lives

The Bottom Line

Raising metabolically healthy children isn't about perfect compliance with dietary rules. It's about creating an environment where healthy choices are normal, teaching children the skills they need to take care of themselves, and building positive relationships with real food.

The most important factors:

- Model the behavior you want to see
- Make healthy foods available and appealing
- Teach without preaching
- Focus on health and performance rather than weight or appearance

- Trust the foundation you're building, even when children make choices you wouldn't make

Remember: You're not just feeding your children—you're teaching them how to feed themselves and their future families. The patterns you establish now will influence generations.

The investment in your children's metabolic health pays dividends not just in their childhood, but throughout their entire lives. You're giving them advantages that most of their peers won't have: stable energy, better mood regulation, stronger immune systems, and the knowledge and skills to maintain their health independently.

This is perhaps the greatest gift you can give them—not just better health for today, but the foundation for a lifetime of vitality and the knowledge to pass it on to their own children.

The cycle of metabolic dysfunction can end with your family. The cycle of metabolic health can begin with your choices today.

Congratulations. You now have the tools to take control of your health, build an effective healthcare team, and create lasting change for yourself and your family. The knowledge is yours. The choice is yours. Your health is yours to reclaim.

Citations for Chapter 29

1. Olshansky SJ, Passaro DJ, Hershow RC, et al. A potential decline in life expectancy in the United States in the 21st century. *N Engl J Med.* 2005;352(11):1138-1145. doi:10.1056/NEJMsr043743

2. Horta BL, Loret de Mola C, Victora CG. Long-term consequences of breastfeeding on cholesterol, obesity, systolic blood pressure and type 2 diabetes: a systematic review and meta-analysis. *Acta Paediatr.* 2015;104(S467):30-37. doi:10.1111/apa.13133

3. Lennerz BS, Barton A, Bernstein RK, et al. Management of type 1 diabetes with a very low-carbohydrate diet. *Pediatrics.* 2018;141(6):e20173349. doi:10.1542/peds.2017-3349

Chapter Thirty-One

Part 3 Summary: Your Implementation Roadmap

Putting It All Together for Lasting Change

You now have the complete toolkit for taking control of your health. Six chapters of practical strategies, proven approaches, and real-world solutions. But having the tools isn't the same as using them effectively. This summary will help you turn knowledge into action with a clear, prioritized implementation plan.

The Big Picture: What You've Learned

Chapter 1: Building Your Health Team

- How to identify providers who understand metabolic health
- Questions to ask and red flags to avoid
- Working with conventional medicine when necessary

Chapter 2: Biomarkers That Actually Matter

- Which tests reveal real health status vs. misleading metrics
- How to get comprehensive testing and interpret results
- Creating your personal health dashboard

Chapter 3: Transitioning to Real Food

- Phase-by-phase approach to changing what you eat

- Practical strategies for shopping, cooking, and meal planning
- The critical importance of intermittent fasting

Chapter 4: Navigating Resistance

- Understanding why others resist your health changes
- Scripts and strategies for handling social pressure
- Protecting your progress from external influences

Chapter 5: Emergency Protocols

- When conventional medicine is necessary and helpful
- How to maintain your health improvements during medical treatment
- Working strategically with the medical system

Chapter 6: Raising Healthy Children

- Age-appropriate strategies for building metabolic health in children
- Breaking generational cycles of poor health
- Creating family food environments that support long-term success

Your 90-Day Implementation Plan

Month 1: Foundation Building

Week 1-2: Assess and Plan

- Complete baseline biomarker testing (fasting insulin, CRP, comprehensive lipid panel)
- Document current symptoms, energy levels, and health concerns

- Take progress photos and measurements
- Clean out pantry and kitchen of processed foods
- Find one healthcare provider who understands metabolic health

Week 3-4: Begin Food Transition

- Eliminate sugary drinks, industrial oils, and high-fructose corn syrup
- Start 12:12 intermittent fasting
- Focus on protein and vegetables for each meal
- Begin reading ingredient lists instead of nutrition facts panels
- Practice basic meal templates (protein + vegetables + fat)

Month 2: Building Momentum

Week 5-6: Expand Changes

- Progress to 16:8 intermittent fasting if 12:12 feels comfortable
- Eliminate remaining processed foods and grains
- Master batch cooking and meal prep strategies
- Begin tracking subjective improvements (energy, sleep, mood)
- Handle first major social food situation using chapter 4 strategies

Week 7-8: Optimize and Adjust

- Fine-tune carbohydrate intake based on your response
- Address any persistent cravings or adjustment challenges
- Establish consistent meal timing and eating windows

- Create emergency food plans for travel and busy periods
- Document improvements in energy, sleep, and overall wellbeing

Month 3: Integration and Sustainability

Week 9-10: System Refinement

- Repeat biomarker testing to track objective improvements
- Adjust approach based on lab results and how you feel
- Solidify relationships with supportive healthcare providers
- Master restaurant and social eating strategies
- Begin helping family members who express interest

Week 11-12: Long-term Planning

- Create sustainable systems for maintaining changes
- Plan for upcoming challenges (holidays, travel, life changes)
- Establish ongoing monitoring and adjustment protocols
- Document lessons learned and what works best for your body
- Set goals for continued optimization

Priority Order: What to Tackle First

Highest Priority (Do These First)

1. **Eliminate processed foods** - Biggest metabolic impact
2. **Start intermittent fasting** - Immediate benefits for insulin sensitivity

3. **Find one supportive healthcare provider** - Essential for monitoring progress

   4. **Get baseline lab testing** - Establishes your starting point

Medium Priority (Do These Second)

   1. **Optimize meal composition** - Focus on protein, vegetables, healthy fats

   2. **Establish consistent meal timing** - Supports metabolic regulation

   3. **Create supportive food environment** - Makes healthy choices easier

   4. **Develop social situation strategies** - Protects your progress

Lower Priority (Do These Once Basics Are Solid)

   1. **Advanced biomarker testing** - Fine-tune based on initial results

   2. **Supplement optimization** - Address specific deficiencies identified

   3. **Exercise integration** - Support metabolic health improvements

   4. **Advanced fasting protocols** - Only after basics are mastered

Troubleshooting Common Challenges

"I'm Not Seeing Results"

Check these factors:

- Are you truly eliminating processed foods, or making exceptions?
- Is your intermittent fasting window consistent?
- Are you eating enough protein and fat to maintain satiety?

- Are hidden carbohydrates or sweeteners stalling progress?
- Do you need to address stress management or sleep quality?

Timeline expectations:

- Energy improvements: 1-2 weeks
- Mood and mental clarity: 2-4 weeks
- Weight changes: 4-8 weeks
- Lab marker improvements: 8-12 weeks[1]

"The Social Pressure Is Overwhelming"

Remember:

- You don't need anyone's permission to take care of your health
- Results speak louder than arguments
- Consistent behavior over time reduces resistance
- Find your tribe of supportive people
- Focus on how you feel, not others' opinions

"I Keep Having Setbacks"

This is normal. Strategies:

- View setbacks as learning opportunities, not failures
- Get back to your routine immediately, don't wait for Monday
- Identify triggers and create better plans for next time
- Remember that consistency over time matters more than perfection

- Focus on progress, not perfection

Measuring Success: What to Track

Objective Measures

- **Lab markers:** Fasting insulin, triglycerides, HDL, CRP, HbA1c
- **Body composition:** Waist circumference, body fat percentage
- **Vital signs:** Blood pressure, resting heart rate
- **Performance metrics:** Sleep quality, exercise capacity

Subjective Measures (Often Change First)

- **Energy levels:** Stable throughout the day without crashes
- **Mental clarity:** Improved focus and cognitive function
- **Mood stability:** Less anxiety, depression, or emotional volatility
- **Sleep quality:** Falling asleep easily, waking refreshed
- **Appetite regulation:** Natural hunger/satiety cues, reduced cravings
- **Physical comfort:** Less joint pain, digestive issues, skin problems

Success Milestones

3 Months

- Stable energy without afternoon crashes
- Improved sleep quality and morning alertness

- Reduced cravings for processed foods
- Initial improvements in biomarkers
- Established sustainable eating patterns
- Confidence in handling social food situations

6 Months

- Significant improvements in lab markers
- Stable mood and mental clarity
- Body composition improvements
- Mastery of meal planning and preparation
- Strong support network and healthcare team
- Ability to help others interested in similar changes

1 Year

- Reversal or significant improvement in metabolic dysfunction
- Optimal energy and mental performance
- Sustainable lifestyle that doesn't feel restrictive
- Positive influence on family and close friends
- Deep understanding of how food affects your body
- Confidence in long-term health optimization

Building Your Support System

Essential Team Members

- **Healthcare provider** who understands metabolic health
- **Accountability partner** following similar approach
- **Online community** for questions and support
- **Family members** who support your health goals

Resources to Keep Handy

- **Emergency meal plans** for busy or stressful periods
- **Restaurant guides** for your area
- **Travel strategies** for maintaining routine away from home
- **Biomarker tracking sheets** to monitor progress
- **Response scripts** for handling social pressure

The Long Game

This Isn't a Diet—It's a Life Upgrade

Remember why you started:

- The conventional approach wasn't working
- You deserve to feel energetic and healthy
- Small changes compound into dramatic improvements
- You're breaking cycles for future generations

Keep the bigger picture in mind:

- Health improvements continue for years, not just months
- You're developing skills and knowledge for life
- Your success influences others to improve their health
- You're creating a legacy of health for your family

Continuous Improvement

As you master the basics:

- Fine-tune based on your body's responses
- Stay curious about new research and approaches
- Help others who are ready for change
- Continue learning about optimizing health
- Adapt strategies as your life circumstances change

Your Action Plan Starts Now

Today:

1. Choose one action from the Week 1-2 list
2. Schedule baseline lab testing
3. Clean one area of your kitchen
4. Plan tomorrow's meals using the protein + vegetables + fat template

This Week:

1. Complete the Week 1-2 checklist
2. Find one healthcare provider to research

3. Begin elimination of processed foods

   4. Start 12:12 intermittent fasting

This Month:

   1. Complete Month 1 objectives

   2. Document improvements in energy and wellbeing

   3. Handle your first challenging social food situation

   4. Begin planning Month 2 strategies

Final Reminders

You have everything you need to transform your health. The knowledge is proven, the strategies are practical, and the benefits are life-changing.

Progress isn't linear. Expect good days and challenging days. What matters is the overall trajectory over weeks and months, not daily perfection.

Your health is worth the effort. The investment you're making now pays dividends for decades. Better energy, clearer thinking, improved mood, and reduced disease risk are all achievable when you apply these principles consistently.

You're not alone. Millions of people have successfully made these changes. You have access to the same information and strategies that have worked for them.

Start where you are, use what you have, do what you can. You don't need to be perfect to make progress. You just need to begin.

The time for excuses is over. The time for action is now.

Your health transformation starts today.

Reference

1. Volek JS, et al. "Metabolic characteristics of keto-adapted ultra-endurance runners." *Metabolism.* 2012;61(10):1456-1464. doi:10.1016/j.metabol.2012.03.007.

Chapter Thirty-Two

Appendix

How to Read Studies Like an Investigative Journalist

You don't need a medical degree to evaluate research—you need the skills of an investigative journalist. After years of following advice based on flawed studies, I learned to read research the way I read any other document that might be trying to sell me something: with healthy skepticism and attention to what's not being said. Also, never forget, bias can cut both ways - advocates for alternative approaches can also cherry-pick favorable evidence. Apply the same critical thinking to all health claims, regardless of source.

The Journalist's Approach to Medical Research

Step 1: Follow the Money First

Before you read a single word of the study, investigate the funding.

Look for:

- Who funded the study? (Check the "Funding" or "Disclosures" section)

- Do any authors have financial relationships with companies that would benefit from certain results?

- Was it funded by industry groups, government agencies, or independent foundations?

Red flags:

- Studies on statins funded by statin manufacturers
- Nutrition research funded by food companies
- Studies where authors have consulting relationships with companies whose products are being studied

Example: The famous sugar industry studies from the 1960s that blamed fat for heart disease were directly funded by sugar companies, but this wasn't disclosed for decades.

How to check: Look at the end of any study for "Conflicts of Interest," "Funding Sources," or "Author Disclosures." If this information is missing or vague, be suspicious.

Step 2: Understand Study Types and Their Limitations

Not all studies are created equal. Here's the hierarchy:

Observational Studies (Weakest Evidence)

- **What they are:** Researchers observe people and track what happens over time
- **Example:** Following people who eat red meat and seeing if they get cancer
- **Why they're weak:** Correlation ≠ causation. People who eat lots of red meat might also smoke, drink, avoid exercise, and eat processed foods
- **Red flag phrases:** "Associated with," "linked to," "correlated with"

Randomized Controlled Trials (RCTs) (Stronger Evidence)

- **What they are:** Researchers randomly assign people to different treatments and measure outcomes
- **Example:** Giving half the participants a drug and half a placebo, then

measuring results

- **Why they're better:** Randomization helps control for confounding variables
- **Limitations:** Often short-term, may not reflect real-world conditions

Meta-analyses (Potentially Strongest)

- **What they are:** Studies that combine results from multiple other studies
- **Why they can be good:** Larger sample sizes, more statistical power
- **Why they can be misleading:** "Garbage in, garbage out"—combining flawed studies doesn't make the conclusions valid

Step 3: Read the Study Like a Detective

Start with these questions:

Who was studied?

- Young, healthy college students or older adults with multiple health conditions?
- Men only, women only, or both?
- What was their baseline health status?
- How many people dropped out of the study?

What exactly was tested?

- Was it the specific intervention you're interested in?
- What doses were used? (Often much higher or lower than real-world use)

- How long did the study last? (Many studies are too short to show meaningful results)

How were outcomes measured?

- Objective measures (blood tests, imaging) or subjective reports (surveys, questionnaires)?

- Were the measures clinically meaningful or just statistically significant?

- Did they measure what actually matters to patients?

Step 4: Decode Statistical Manipulation

The most common tricks used to make small effects look dramatic:

Relative Risk vs. Absolute Risk

- **Relative risk:** "50% increase in heart attacks!"

- **Absolute risk:** Heart attacks increased from 2 per 1000 people to 3 per 1000 people

- **Reality check:** Ask "50% of what?" and "How many actual people does this affect?"

Statistical Significance vs. Clinical Significance

- **Statistical significance:** The result probably didn't happen by chance

- **Clinical significance:** The result actually matters for real people

- **Red flag:** Results that are "statistically significant" but have tiny effect sizes

Surrogate Endpoints vs. Clinical Outcomes

- **Surrogate endpoints:** Cholesterol levels, blood pressure numbers, biomarkers

- **Clinical outcomes:** Heart attacks, strokes, death, quality of life
- **Problem:** Changes in biomarkers don't always translate to improvements in actual health

Example: A drug might lower cholesterol by 30% (impressive surrogate endpoint) but only prevent 1 heart attack per 1000 people treated (modest clinical outcome).

Step 5: Look for What's Missing

Investigative journalists always ask: "What aren't they telling me?"

Common omissions:

- **Negative results:** Studies that didn't show benefits often don't get published
- **Side effects:** May be minimized or buried in supplementary data
- **Long-term follow-up:** Many studies are too short to show real-world effects
- **Dropout rates:** If lots of people quit the study, the results may not be meaningful
- **Subgroup analyses:** Sometimes only certain groups benefited, but this gets lost in overall results

Step 6: Check the Conclusions Against the Data

Read the actual results section, not just the abstract or conclusions.

Warning signs:

- Conclusions that seem stronger than the data supports
- Abstract emphasizes benefits but downplays risks

- Authors claim "proof" when they only showed correlation
- Recommendations that go beyond what the study actually tested

Example: A study might show a drug reduced relative risk by 20%, but the conclusion claims it "significantly reduces heart disease risk" without mentioning that absolute risk reduction was 0.2%.

How to Find and Evaluate Conflicting Research

The Reality of Medical Research

Here's what no one tells you: For almost every health topic, you can find studies supporting opposite conclusions. This isn't a bug in the system—it's a feature that you need to understand and navigate.

Why Studies Conflict

1. Different Populations

- Study A: Healthy 25-year-olds
- Study B: Sick 65-year-olds
- Result: Completely different outcomes for the same intervention

2. Different Methodologies

- Study A: Observational study over 20 years
- Study B: Randomized trial over 6 months
- Result: Different conclusions about the same treatment

3. Different Definitions

- Study A: Defines "low-carb" as under 40% of calories from carbs

- Study B: Defines "low-carb" as under 10% of calories from carbs
- Result: Appears to be studying the same thing, but isn't

4. Different Funding Sources

- Study A: Funded by pharmaceutical company
- Study B: Funded by independent foundation
- Result: Different conclusions about the same drug

Your Conflicting Research Strategy

Step 1: Expect Conflicts Don't assume that conflicting studies mean we "don't know anything." Instead, ask why they conflict and what that tells you.

Step 2: Look for Patterns in the Conflicts

- Do industry-funded studies consistently show benefits while independent studies show problems?
- Do short-term studies show benefits while long-term studies show harm?
- Do studies in healthy people show different results than studies in sick people?

Step 3: Weight the Evidence Give more credibility to:

- Longer-term studies over short-term ones
- Studies with hard endpoints (death, heart attacks) over surrogate markers (cholesterol levels)
- Studies with fewer conflicts of interest
- Studies that match the population you're interested in (yourself)

- Randomized controlled trials over observational studies

Step 4: Consider the Biological Plausibility Ask yourself: "Does this make sense based on what we know about human biology?"

Examples:

- Does it make sense that humans suddenly need to avoid foods we've eaten for millennia?

- Does it make sense that industrial chemicals are healthier than traditional foods?

- Does it make sense that the body can't function without constant feeding?

Red Flags in Conflicting Research

When you see studies with opposite conclusions, look for these warning signs:

1. Industry Influence Patterns

- Studies funded by sugar companies consistently exonerate sugar

- Studies funded by pharmaceutical companies consistently support pharmaceutical solutions

- Studies funded by food companies consistently support processed food consumption

2. Methodology Shopping

- Researchers changing study designs until they get the results they want

- Post-hoc analyses that weren't planned from the beginning

- Switching primary endpoints mid-study when the original endpoint doesn't show benefits

3. Publication Bias

- Only positive results get published while negative results get buried
- Industry-sponsored studies are more likely to be published if they show benefits
- Journals may be reluctant to publish studies that contradict established medical dogma

Practical Research Evaluation Tools

Questions to Ask About Any Study:

1. **Who paid for this research?**
2. **How long did it last?** (Longer is usually better)
3. **Who was studied?** (Does it match you?)
4. **What exactly was tested?** (Dose, duration, specific intervention)
5. **What was actually measured?** (Biomarkers or real health outcomes?)
6. **How big was the effect in absolute terms?** (Not just percentages)
7. **How many people dropped out?** (High dropout rates = questionable results)
8. **Do the conclusions match the data?** (Read beyond the abstract)
9. **Are there obvious confounding factors?** (What else might explain the results?)
10. **Does this make biological sense?** (Trust your common sense)

Building Your Research Literacy

Start Simple

- Begin with one health topic you care about (like the ones covered in this book)
- Find 3-5 studies on that topic and practice reading them using this framework
- Don't worry about understanding every statistical term—focus on the big picture

Use Quality Sources

- PubMed (pubmed.ncbi.nlm.nih.gov) for peer-reviewed research
- Cochrane Reviews for systematic reviews and meta-analyses
- Be skeptical of press releases and news articles about studies

Learn to Love Uncertainty

- Good science often gives you ranges and probabilities, not definitive answers
- Be suspicious of anyone who claims "the science is settled" on complex health topics
- Comfortable uncertainty is better than false certainty

The Power of Pattern Recognition

After reading dozens of studies on health topics, you'll start to notice patterns:

- Industry-funded studies almost always favor industry interests
- Short-term studies often show different results than long-term studies
- Studies that measure biomarkers often show different results than stud-

ies that measure actual health outcomes

- The same statistical tricks appear across different health topics

This pattern recognition is your most powerful tool. It allows you to quickly identify likely biases and limitations without needing to understand every technical detail.

When Experts Disagree

What to do when credible experts reach opposite conclusions:

1. Look at their funding sources and potential conflicts2. Examine what type of evidence they're relying on3. Consider their track record on previous recommendations4. Ask whether their recommendations make biological sense5. Consider trying the intervention yourself (if safe) and monitoring your own response

Your Personal Research Protocol

For any health claim you encounter:

1. **Check the source:** Who's making the claim and why?

2. **Find the original study:** Don't rely on news articles or summaries

3. **Apply the evaluation framework:** Use the questions listed above

4. **Look for conflicting evidence:** Search for studies with opposite conclusions

5. **Consider your context:** Does this apply to someone like you?

6. **Monitor your own response:** How does your body react to interventions?

The Bottom Line on Research Evaluation

You don't need to become a statistician to be an informed consumer of medical research. You need to think like an investigative journalist: follow the money, question the methodology, look for what's missing, and trust patterns over individual studies.

Remember:

- No single study proves anything definitively

- Industry-funded research should be viewed with extreme skepticism

- Your personal response to interventions is data too

- Common sense and biological plausibility matter

- It's okay to act on incomplete information if the intervention is safe and you monitor your response

The goal isn't to become a research expert—it's to avoid being manipulated by research that's designed to sell you something rather than help you optimize your health.

Most importantly, don't let the complexity of medical research paralyze you into inaction. The current medical establishment is built on studies that often wouldn't pass the evaluation framework outlined here. You can make better decisions by applying these principles than by blindly following conventional medical advice that may be based on flawed or biased research.

Your health is too important to outsource entirely to experts who may have conflicts of interest or who may be operating from outdated information. Use these tools to become an informed participant in your own healthcare rather than a passive recipient of whatever treatment happens to be profitable this year.

About the author

David L. Etheridge is an entrepreneur, writer, and pricing consultant who turned his analytical skills toward questioning mainstream health advice. With an MBA and a career built on analytical problem-solving, he applies these skills to examining the evidence behind widely accepted medical guidance.

His wake-up call came with a coronary calcium score of 450—despite following conventional guidance and taking statins for two decades. That shock drove him to ask hard questions about the disconnect between his health outcomes and the treatments he was prescribed. His investigation led him to trace funding sources, evaluate study methodologies, and expose patterns of influence across food, pharmaceutical, and medical institutions—uncovering how nutritional myths became accepted wisdom despite contradictory evidence.

This book brings together the results of that research and his personal journey back to metabolic health, so readers can make better-informed choices and take back control of their health.

Action Guide

Use QR Code to Receive Bonus Material

Point Your Camera At QR Code for Action Guide

www.ingramcontent.com/pod-product-compliance
Lightning Source LLC
Chambersburg PA
CBHW020530030426
42337CB00013B/794